RADIOLOGY

CASE REVIEW SERIES | **Pediatric Imaging**

RADIOLOGY

CASE REVIEW SERIES | Pediatric Imaging

Arie Franco, MD, PhD

Associate Professor of Radiology
Department of Radiology
Medical College of Georgia at Georgia Regents University
Augusta, Georgia

Jacques F. Schneider, MD

Head of Pediatric Radiology
Department of Pediatric Radiology
University Children's Hospital Basel (UKBB)
Basel, Switzerland

SERIES EDITOR

Roland Talanow, MD, PhD

President
Department of Radiology Education
Radiolopolis, a subdivision of InnoMed, LLC
Stateline, Nevada

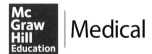

New York   Chicago   San Francisco   Athens   London
Madrid   Mexico City   Milan   New Delhi   Singapore
Sydney   Toronto

Radiology Case Review Series: Pediatric Imaging

1 2 3 4 5 6 7 8 9 0   CTP/CTP   18 17 16 15 14

ISBN 978-0-07-177548-9
MHID 0-07-177548-X

This book was set in Times LT Std. by Thomson Digital.
The editors were Michael Weitz and Brian Kearns.
The production supervisor was Catherine H. Saggese.
Project management was provided by Ritu Joon, Thomson Digital.
The designer was Elise Lansdon; the cover designer was Thomas DePierro.
China Translation & Printing Services, Ltd., was printer and binder.

This book is printed on acid-free paper.

Library of Congress Cataloging-in-Publication Data

Franco, Arie, author.
  Pediatric imaging / Arie Franco, Jacques F. Schneider ; editor, Roland Talanow.
    p. ; cm. — (Radiology case review series)
  Includes bibliographical references and index.
  ISBN 978-0-07-177548-9 (pbk. : alk. paper) — ISBN 0-07-177548-X
  I. Schneider, Jacques F., author. II. Talanow, Roland, editor. III. Title. IV. Series: Radiology case review series.
  [DNLM: 1. Diagnostic Imaging—methods—Case Reports. 2. Diagnostic Imaging—methods—Problems and Exercises. 3. Child. 4. Infant. 5. Pediatrics—methods—Case Reports. 6. Pediatrics—methods—Problems and Exercises. WN 18.2]
  RJ51.R33
  618.92'007575—dc23
                                                                    2014006470

This book is dedicated to my wife Emma, my daughter Liran and my son-in-law Paul, my daughter Eynat, and my lovely grandson Ethan. My family has been very supportive and helpful in allowing and giving me the opportunity to spend many hours in the organization and preparation of this book.

—Arie Franco, MD, PhD

To my parents Nicole and Fernand, and to my partner Hans, who gave me their love, time, and continuous support.

—Jacques F. Schneider, MD

Contents

Contributors

Neil M. Borden, MD
Associate Professor of Radiology
Department of Radiology
Medical College of Georgia at Georgia
   Regents University
Augusta, Georgia

Ramon E. Figueroa, MD
Professor of Radiology
Department of Radiology
Medical College of Georgia at Georgia
   Regents University
Augusta, Georgia

Chetan Shah, MD, MBA
Assistant Professor of Radiology, Mayo Clinic
Courtesy Faculty at University of Florida
Nemours, Jacksonville, Florida
Jacksonville, Florida

Series Preface

Maybe I have an obsession for cases, but when I was a radiology resident I loved to learn especially from cases, not only because they are short, exciting, and fun—similar to a detective story in which the aim is to get to "the bottom" of the case—but also because, in the end, that's what radiologists are faced with during their daily work. Since medical school, I have been fascinated with learning, not only for my own benefit but also for the sake of teaching others, and I have enjoyed combining my IT skills with my growing knowledge to develop programs that help others in their learning process. Later, during my radiology residency, my passion for case-based learning grew to a level where the idea was born to create a case-based journal: integrating new concepts and technologies that aid in the traditional learning process. Only a few years later, the *Journal of Radiology Case Reports* became an internationally popular and PubMed indexed radiology journal—popular not only because of the interactive features but also because of the case-based approach. This led me to the next step: why not tackle something that I especially admired during my residency but that could be improved—creating a new interactive case-based review series. I imagined a book series that would take into account new developments in teaching and technology and changes in the examination process.

As did most other radiology residents, I loved the traditional case review books, especially for preparation for the boards. These books are quick and fun to read and focus in a condensed way on material that will be examined in the final boards. However, nothing is perfect and these traditional case review books had their own intrinsic flaws. The authors and I have tried to learn from our experience by putting the good things into this new book series but omitting the bad parts and exchanging them with innovative features.

What are the features that distinguish this series from traditional series of review books?

To save space, traditional review books provide two cases on one page. This requires the reader to turn the page to read the answer for the first case but could lead to unintentional "cheating" by seeing also the answer of the second case. Doesn't this defeat the purpose of a review book? From my own authoring experience on the *USMLE Help* book series, it was well appreciated that we avoided such accidental cheating by separating one case from the other. Taking the positive experience from that book series, we decided that each case in this series should consist of two pages: page 1

with images and questions and page 2 with the answers and explanations. This approach avoids unintentional peeking at the answers before deciding on the correct answers yourself. We keep it strict: one case per page! This way it remains up to your own knowledge to figure out the right answer.

Another example that residents (including me) did miss in traditional case review books is that these books did not highlight the pertinent findings on the images: sometimes, even looking at the images as a group of residents, we could not find the abnormality. This is not only frustrating but also time consuming. When you prepare for the boards, you want to use your time as efficiently as possible. Why not show annotated images? We tackled that challenge by providing, on the second page of each case, the same images with annotations or additional images that highlight the findings.

When you are preparing for the boards and managing your clinical duties, time is a luxury that becomes even more precious. Does the resident preparing for the boards truly need lengthy discussions as in a typical textbook? Or does the resident rather want a "rapid fire" mode in which he or she can "fly" through as many cases as possible in the shortest possible time? This is the reality when you start your work after the boards! Part of our concept with the new series is providing short "pearls" instead of lengthy discussions. The reader can easily read and memorize these "pearls."

Another challenge in traditional books is that questions are asked on the first page and no direct answer is provided, only a lengthy block of discussion. Again, this might become time consuming to find the right spot where the answer is located if you have doubts about one of several answer choices. Remember: time is money—and life! Therefore, we decided to provide explanations to *each* individual question, so that the reader knows exactly where to find the right answer to the right question. Questions are phrased in an intuitive way so that they fit not only the print version but also the multiple-choice questions for that particular case in our online version. This system enables you to move back and forth between the print version and the online version.

In addition, we have provided up to 3 references for each case. This case review is not intended to replace traditional textbooks. Instead, it is intended to reiterate and strengthen your already existing knowledge (from your training) and to fill potential gaps in your knowledge.

However, in a collaborative effort with the *Journal of Radiology Case Reports* and the international radiology community Radiolopolis, we have developed an online repository with more comprehensive information for each case, such as demographics, discussions, more image examples, interactive image stacks with scroll, a window/level feature, and other interactive features that almost resemble a workstation. In addition, we are planning ahead toward the new Radiology Boards format and are providing rapid fire online sessions and mock examinations that use the cases in the print version. Each case in the print version is crosslinked to the online version using a case ID. The case ID number appears to the right of the diagnosis heading at the top of the second page of each case. Each case can be accessed using the case ID number at the following web site: www.radiologycasereviews.com/case/ID, in which "ID" represents the case ID number. If you have any questions regarding this web site, please e-mail the series editor directly at roland@talanow.info.

I am particularly proud of such a symbiotic endeavor of print and interactive online education and I am grateful to McGraw-Hill for giving me and the authors the opportunity to provide such a unique and innovative method of radiology education, which, in my opinion, may be a trendsetter.

The primary audience of this book series is the radiology resident, particularly the resident in the final year who is preparing for the radiology boards. However, each book in

this series is structured on difficulty levels so that the series also becomes useful to an audience with limited experience in radiology (nonradiologist physicians or medical students) up to subspecialty-trained radiologists who are preparing for their CAQs or who just want to refresh their knowledge and use this series as a reference.

I am delighted to have such an excellent team of US and international educators as authors on this innovative book series. These authors have been thoroughly evaluated and selected based on their excellent contributions to the *Journal of Radiology Case Reports*, the Radiolopolis community, and other academic and scientific accomplishments.

It brings especially personal satisfaction to me that this project has enabled each author to be involved in the overall decision-making process and improvements regarding the print and online content. This makes each participant not only an author but also part of a great radiology product that will appeal to many readers.

Finally, I hope you will experience this case review book as it is intended to be: a quick, pertinent, "get to the point" radiology case review that provides essential information for the radiology boards in the shortest time available, which, in the end, is crucial for preparation for the boards.

Roland Talanow, MD, PhD

Preface

This case review book is part of a series and contains more than 200 cases in the different subspecialties of the pediatric radiology. Each case is summarized in two pages. The first page of each case contains a short history, images, and five questions. The verso of the first page contains the diagnosis, the same images with annotations and legends, answers to the questions, and pearls that are pertinent to the case. For maximal learning benefit, it is suggested that the reader tries initially to figure out the diagnosis and the answers to the questions before turning the page.

Due to space constraints, only very essential information is provided in the second page of each case. The online version of the book contains a detailed discussion.

The book is intended for use by radiology and pediatric residents and fellows, medical students, radiologists, and physicians who want to learn and increase their knowledge in the field of pediatric radiology. Radiology residents may find this book helpful in preparation for their board certification examination.

Arie Franco, MD, PhD
Jacques F. Schneider, MD

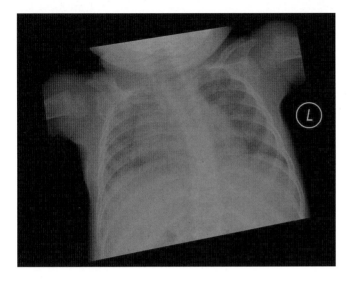 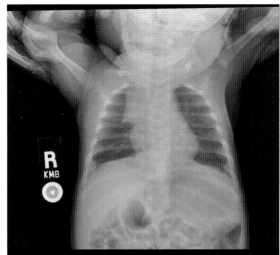

1. Describe the findings.

2. Where is the thymus anatomically located?

3. What is the thymic sail sign?

4. What is the thymic wave sign?

5. How and when is the spinnaker sign formed?

Case ranking/difficulty:

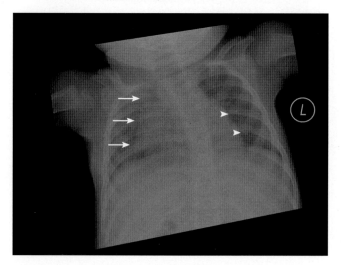

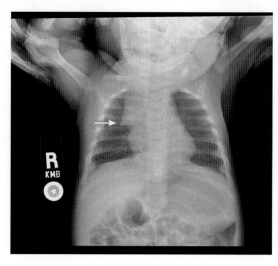

Frontal radiograph of the chest demonstrates the sail sign of normal thymus appearance (*arrows*). The thymus has a wavy appearance that is noted between the ribs (*arrowheads*).

Frontal view of the chest of another 2-month-old male represents the sail sign (*arrow*).

Answers

1. The sail sign and the wave sign are seen consistent with normal thymus in an infant.

2. The thymus occupies the anterior and superior mediastinum, located behind the sternum in the midline. In infancy, the upper border of the thymus extends almost to the thyroid gland in the neck and the lower margin overlaps the upper part of the heart, occasionally extending as far as the diaphragm.

3. The sail sign seen in 8.8% of children describes a triangular soft tissue density forming either the right, left, or both mediastinal borders.

4. The wave sign is normal indentation of the thymus laterally by the adjacent anterior ribs. The thymic notch is an indentation seen at the junction of the thymic and the cardiac outlines.

5. The spinnaker or angels wing sign describes the elevation of the thymus in the presence of pneumomediastinum.

Pearls

- The thymus is an organ located in the superior and anterior mediastinum.
- It consists of two asymmetric lobes, usually large during infancy and can occupy most of the anterior mediastinum.
- The thymus normally decreases in size after infancy and childhood.

Suggested Readings

Correia-Pinto J, Henriques-Coelho T. Images in clinical medicine. Neonatal pneumomediastinum and the spinnaker-sail sign. *N Engl J Med.* 2010;363(22):2145.

Han DH. Thymic sail sign: unique to paediatric chest radiographs? *Pediatr Radiol.* 2010;40(3):375-376.

1-day-old male who underwent abdominal sonographic study

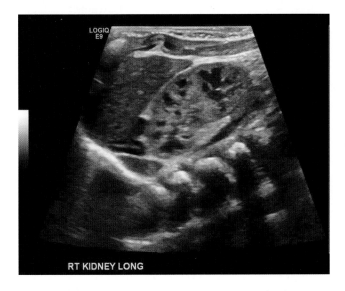

RT KIDNEY LONG

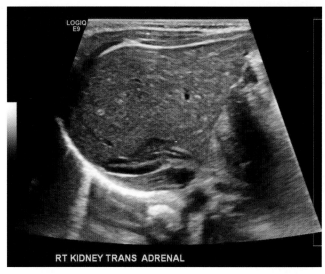

RT KIDNEY TRANS ADRENAL

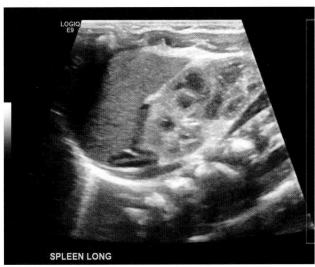

SPLEEN LONG

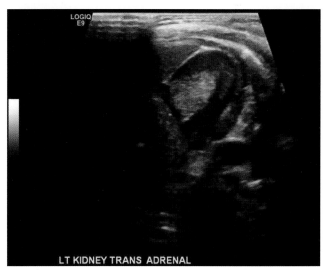

LT KIDNEY TRANS ADRENAL

1. What are the principal landmarks for visualization of the right adrenal gland in neonatal ultrasound?

2. What are the principal landmarks for visualization of the left adrenal gland in neonatal ultrasound?

3. Where is the upper pole of the left kidney normally located in relation to the left adrenal gland?

4. How does the cortex of the normal adrenal glands appear in neonatal ultrasound?

5. How does the central medulla of the normal adrenal glands appear in neonatal ultrasound?

Case ranking/difficulty:

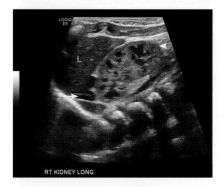

Longitudinal sonogram of the right upper quadrant of the abdomen demonstrates normal appearance of the right adrenal gland (*arrow*), normal right kidney (*arrowhead*), and liver (L).

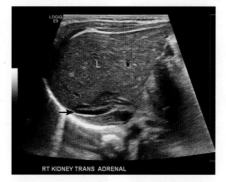

Transverse sonogram of the right upper quadrant of the abdomen demonstrates normal appearance of the right adrenal gland (*arrow*) and normal liver (L).

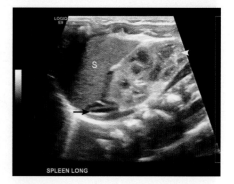

Longitudinal sonogram of the left upper quadrant of the abdomen demonstrates normal appearance of the left adrenal gland (*arrow*), normal left kidney (*arrowhead*), and spleen (S).

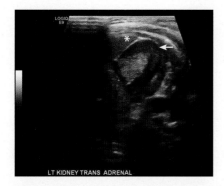

Transverse sonogram of the left upper quadrant of the abdomen demonstrates normal appearance of the left adrenal gland (*arrow*) and normal appearance of the edge of the spleen (*asterisk*).

Pearls

- The adrenal glands are located within the retroperitoneum.
- The normal adrenals are seen well in ultrasound images in a neonate.
- They have a typical Y-shape and the central medulla is hyperechoic with a hypoechoic cortex.
- The right adrenal gland is located superomedial to the upper pole of the right kidney and posterolateral to the inferior vena cava.
- The left adrenal gland is situated more anteromedial than superior to the upper pole of the left kidney.

Answers

1. The right adrenal gland is supramedial to the right kidney. The right kidney is posterolateral to the inferior vena cava.

2. The key landmarks are the aorta medially, the left inferior crus of the diaphragm, and the lower pole of the spleen or upper renal pole laterally.

3. The upper pole of the left kidney is normally located laterally and inferiorly in relation to the left adrenal gland.

4. The cortex of the normal adrenal glands is hypoechoic in neonatal ultrasound.

5. The central medulla of the normal adrenal glands is hyperechoic in neonatal ultrasound.

Suggested Readings

Oppenheimer DA, Carroll BA, S Yousem S. Sonography of the normal neonatal adrenal gland. *Radiology*. 1983;146:157-160.

Prokop M, Galanski M, Schaefer-Prokop C. Spiral and multislice computed tomography of the body. *George Thieme Verlag*. 2003. ISBN:0865778701.

Yeh HC. Sonography of the adrenal glands: normal glands and small masses. *AJR Am J Roentgenol*. 1980;135(6):1167-1177.

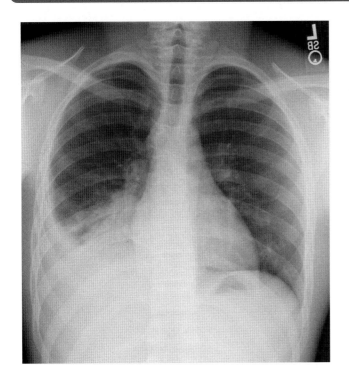 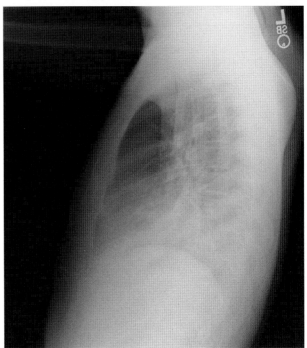

1. What are the findings in the frontal view of the chest?

2. What are the findings in the lateral view of the chest?

3. In which lobe is the opacity seen in the images located?

4. What is the most likely underlying diagnosis?

5. What is the etiology of the disease?

Case ranking/difficulty: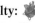

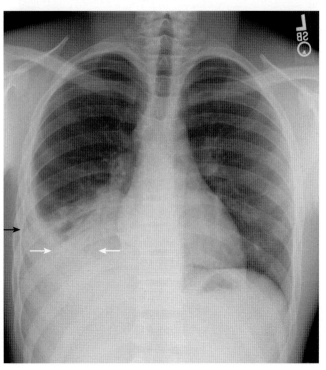

Frontal radiograph of the chest reveals opacity of the right lower lobe. There is silhouetting of the right hemidiaphragm (*white arrows*). There is obscuration of the right costophrenic sulcus (*black arrow*) representing right-sided pleural effusion.

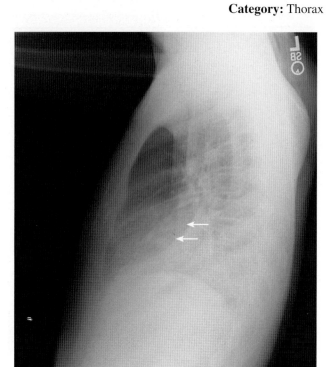

Lateral radiograph of the chest reveals opacity of the posterior lower lung zone, posterior to the major fissure (*white arrows*). In comparison to the frontal view, it represents right lower lobe air-space disease.

Answers

1. Findings are silhouetting of the right hemidiaphragm and obscuration of the right costophrenic sulcus.

2. Findings are opacity in the lower lung zone posterior to the major fissure and silhouetting of the posterior aspect of the diaphragm.

3. The opacity seen in the images is located in the right lower lobe.

4. The most likely diagnosis is community-acquired pneumonia.

5. The etiology is infectious.

Pearls

- In a healthy adolescent presenting with cough and fever, community-acquired pneumonia is most common.
- Community-acquired pneumonia may affect people of all ages.

- Immunosuppression, airway obstruction, and chronic lung disease are risk factors.
- Clinical picture includes respiratory distress, fever, cough, malaise, and fatigue.
- Plain radiograph is the first and a simple imaging modality for diagnosis.
- CT is the second imaging modality of choice if complications may be present such as empyema.

Suggested Readings

Arnold FW, Ramirez JA, McDonald LC, Xia EL. Hospitalization for community-acquired pneumonia: the pneumonia severity index vs clinical judgment. *Chest*. 2003;124(1):121-124.

Claudius I, Baraff LJ. Pediatric emergencies associated with fever. *Emerg Med Clin North Am*. 2010;28(1):67-84, vii-viii.

3-year-old female with fever and cough

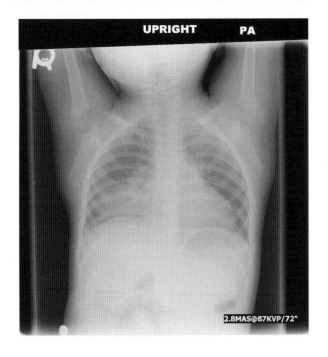 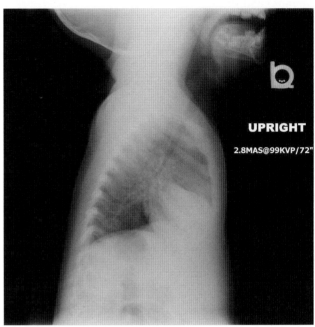

1. How are patients with this entity present clinically?

2. What are the borders of the opacity in the lateral view of the chest?

3. Why is the right heart border in the frontal view of the chest obscured?

4. What is the most common organism causing this entity?

5. What is the treatment option?

Case ranking/difficulty:

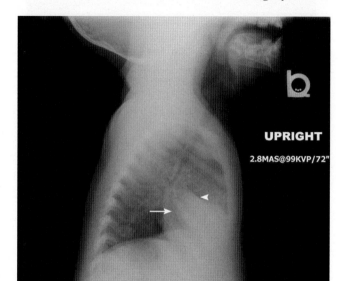

Frontal radiograph of the chest shows opacity in the medial aspect of the right lower lung zone with the silhouette sign involving the right heart border (*arrow*) that indicates a process in the right middle lobe. The entire right hemi-diaphragm is seen, meaning that the right lower lobe is not involved.

Lateral radiograph of the chest shows consolidation that appears as a wedge-shaped density overlying the heart, bordered superiorly by the minor fissure (*arrowhead*) and inferiorly by the major fissure (*arrow*).

Answers

1. Clinical presentation includes fever, cough, wheezing, and tachypnea.

2. The opacity is bordered by the minor fissure superiorly and major fissure inferiorly.

3. In the frontal view, the right heart border is obscured by the right middle lobe opacity.

4. Most likely etiology is gram-positive bacteria such as *Streptococcus pneumoniae*.

5. Treatment is antibiotics.

- Right middle lobe pneumonia can occur at any age.
- Among the differential diagnoses are foreign body aspiration, endotracheal tumors, and mucus plugging.
- In frontal plain radiograph, there is silhouetting of the right heart border.
- In lateral radiograph, there is a wedge-shaped opacity overlying the heart bordered superiorly by the minor fissure and inferiorly by the major fissure.

Suggested Readings

Dees SC, Spock A. Right middle lobe syndrome in children. *JAMA*. 1966;197(1):8-14.

Lutfiyya MN, Henley E, Chang LF. Diagnosis and treatment of community-acquired pneumonia. *Am Fam Physician*. 2006;73:442-450.

Pearls

- In children, more than 50% of right middle lobe collapse is due to bacterial infection.
- Differential diagnosis includes right middle lobe collapse, which is widely under-diagnosed, frequently unrecognized, and usually occurs in children aged 1 to 2 years.

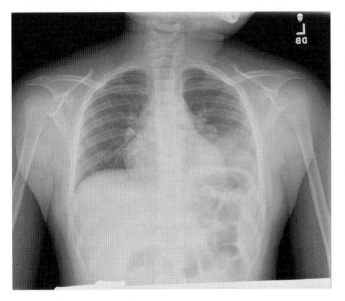 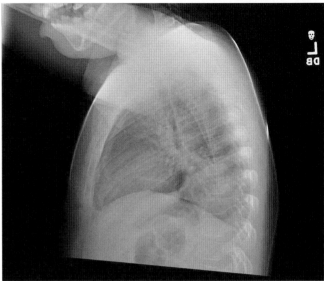

1. Describe the findings.

2. What may be the complications of such entity?

3. What constituents can be found in exudate of this entity?

4. What are the most common organisms causing community-acquired pneumonia?

5. What are the most common organisms causing pneumonia in the neonatal period?

Case ranking/difficulty: 🐢

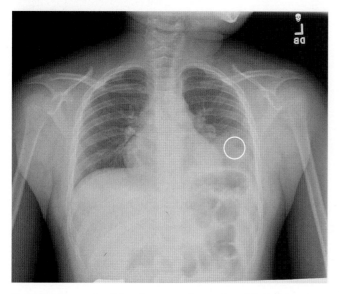

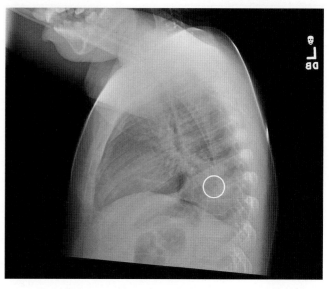

Frontal radiograph of the chest reveals opacity of the left lower lobe (*circle*). Compared to the upper-left lung zone there is density in the lateral aspect of the lower lung zone. The left heart border is preserved. There is obscuration of the left hemidiaphragm.

Lateral radiograph of the chest reveals a retrocardiac density in the posterior lower lung zone (*circle*). Normally posteriorly as we look caudally, the lung should become more lucent. In this image, the lung becomes more dense posteriorly.

Answers

1. There is retrocardiac opacity. In lateral view, there is density in the lower posterior lung zone. There is loss of the left hemidiaphragm ("silhouette sign") and preservation of the left heart border, indicating involvement of the left lower lobe and sparing of the lingula of the left upper lobe.

2. Complication of pneumonia may include pulmonary failure, pleural effusion, pneumatocele, and necrotizing pneumonitis.

3. In the exudate due to pneumonia, there are proteins such as fibrin, and pus is found with white blood cells.

4. The most common organisms causing community-acquired pneumonias are *Chlamydia pneumoniae*, *Haemophilus influenzae*, *Mycoplasma pneumoniae*, *Streptococcus pneumoniae*, and a variety of respiratory viruses.

5. The most common organisms causing pneumonia in the neonatal period are Group B Streptococcus, *Listeria monocytogenes*, *Klebsiella pneumoniae*, and *Escherichia coli*.

Pearls

- In chest radiograph, left lower lobe pneumonia demonstrates retrocardiac opacity, silhouetting of the left hemidiaphragm, and preservation of the left heart borders.
- Complications may include pleural effusion, pneumothorax, pneumatoceles, respiratory failure, and more.
- Most are community-acquired.
- The exudate that fills the alveoli has increased proteins, fibrin, and white blood cells.
- Treatment is antibiotics.

Suggested Reading

Thompson BH, Berbaum KS, George MJ, Ely JW. Identifying left lower lobe pneumonia at chest radiography: performance of family practice residents before and after a didactic session. *Acad Radiol.* 1998;5(5):324-328.

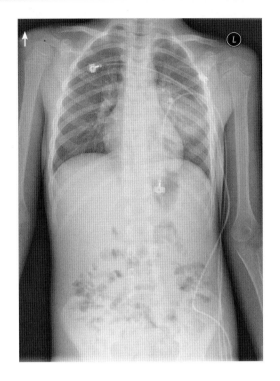 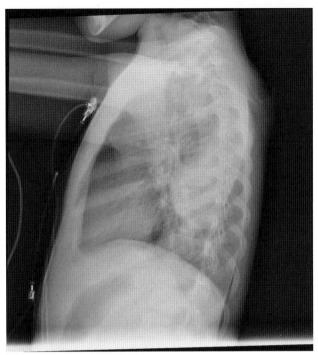

1. What are the findings?

2. What is the differential diagnosis?

3. What is the underlying pathophysiology of this entity?

4. What is the most causative agent of this entity?

5. What should be the appropriate management?

Case ranking/difficulty:

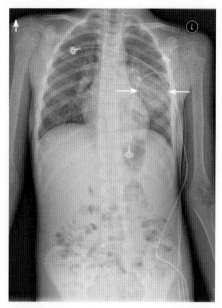

Frontal view of chest radiograph reveals round opacity in the superior segment of the left lower lobe (*arrows*).

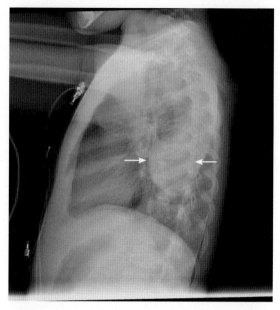

Lateral view of chest radiograph reveals round opacity in the superior segment of the left lower lobe (*arrows*).

Answers

1. There is a rounded opacity in the superior segment of the left lower lobe.

2. Posterior mediastinal mass, round pneumonia, and loculated pleural fluid.

3. The pathophysiology of round pneumonia is the absence of collateral air communicating pathways in children (ie, pores of Kohn, canals of Lambert), which limit spread of infection.

4. Round pneumonia is caused by bacterial infection, with *Streptococcus pneumoniae* being the most common causative organism.

5. Ultrasound can help confirm the diagnosis of round pneumonia by demonstration of sonographic air bronchogram as linear branching echogenic structures within the lesion. Repeat radiograph in 1 to 2 weeks after antibiotics treatment would show improvement in lung opacity. CT scan has much higher radiation and should be avoided.

Pearls

- Round pneumonia is more common in children under 8 years of age. However, 15% cases occur between 8 and 12 years of age.
- Most round pneumonias are located posteriorly within the lower lobes.
- Sonographic air bronchogram demonstrates linear branching echogenic structures within the lesion.
- Repeat radiograph in 1 to 2 weeks after antibiotics treatment would show an improvement in lung opacity.

Suggested Readings

Kim YW, Donnelly LF. Round pneumonia: imaging findings in a large series of children. *Pediatr Radiol.* 2007;37(12):1235-1240.

Restrepo R, Palani R, Matapathi UM, Wu YY. Imaging of round pneumonia and mimics in children. *Pediatr Radiol.* 2010;40(12):1931-1940.

Shah CC, Greenberg SB. Pediatric chest. In: Rumack CM, Wilson SR, eds. *Diagnostic Ultrasound.* 4th ed. Philadelphia, PA: Elsevier; 2011:1768-1799.

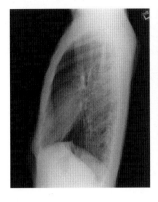 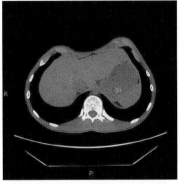 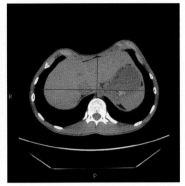 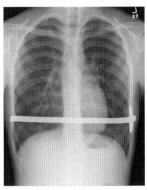

1. Describe the findings of the first three figures.

2. Describe the findings of the last figure.

3. What is the Haller index?

4. What are the complications of this entity?

5. What are the treatment options?

Case ranking/difficulty: 🦂

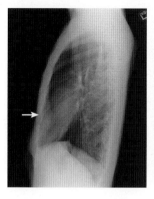

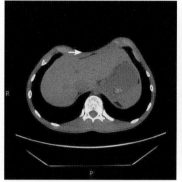

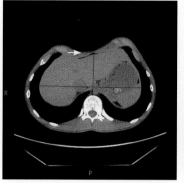

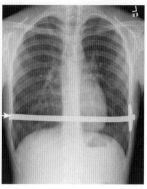

Lateral radiograph of the chest demonstrates concave appearance of the lower anterior chest wall (*arrow*).

Non-contrast CT of the chest demonstrates concave appearance of the lower anterior chest wall (*arrow*). The level of the CT is the narrowest antero-posterior diameter.

Non-contrast CT of the chest demonstrates concave appearance of the lower anterior chest wall (*arrow*). The level of the CT is the narrowest antero-posterior diameter. The blue line is a line drawn to measure the narrowest frontal diameter of the inner chest. The red line was drawn to measure the inner transverse diameter of the chest at the level of the narrowest antero-posterior diameter. These measurements were performed for calculation of Haller index.

Frontal view of the chest following surgical correction demonstrates the pectus bar (*arrow*).

Answers

1. There is concave appearance of the lower anterior chest wall due to a decrease in the antero-posterior diameter of the lower chest.

2. The bar seen in the lower chest was placed during the surgical correction of pectus excavatum. This is the Lorenz pectus bar, which is a convex transverse bar placed under the anterior chest wall.

3. Haller index is derived by dividing the transverse chest diameter by the antero-posterior diameter. This is done at the narrowest antero-posterior diameter of the chest. An index of more than 3.2 has been correlated with a severe deformity that requires surgery.

4. Depending on the severity, pectus excavatum can impair cardiac and respiratory function and cause pain in the chest and back.

5. Treatment is performed with the Nuss procedure and with the placement of a Lorenz pectus bar.

Pearls

- Pectus excavatum is a deformity of the anterior chest wall.
- The sternum and the ribs are abnormal and this creates an abnormal caved-in appearance of the anterior chest wall.
- This abnormality may create deformities in the heart and in the lungs and may impair the cardiovascular function.

- Plain radiograph and CT of the chest demonstrate a decrease in the lower antero-posterior diameter of the chest.
- Radiologists need to be aware and know how to determine the Haller index, which is derived by dividing the transverse chest diameter by the antero-posterior diameter.
- An index of more than 3.2 has been correlated with a severe deformity that requires surgery.

Suggested Readings

Donnelly LF, Frush DP. Abnormalities of the chest wall in pediatric patients. *AJR Am J Roentgenol.* 1999;173(6):1595-1601.

Mortellaro VE, Iqbal CW, Fike FB, et al. The predictive value of Haller index in patients undergoing pectus bar repair for pectus excavatum. *J Surg Res.* 2011;170(1): 104-106.

Redlinger RE Jr, Kelly RE Jr, Nuss D, Kuhn MA, Obermeyer RJ, Goretsky MJ. One hundred patients with recurrent pectus excavatum repaired via the minimally invasive Nuss technique-effective in most regardless of initial operative approach. *J Pediatr Surg.* 2011;46(6):1177-1181.

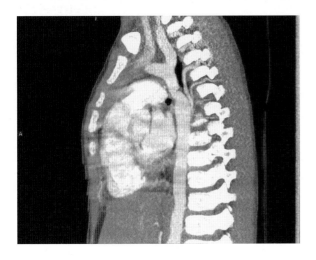 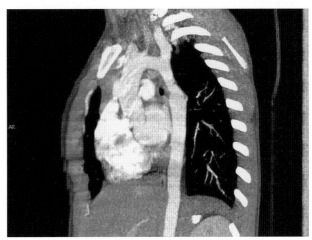

1. What are the findings?

2. What is the clinical presentation?

3. What are the possible complications?

4. What is the sign of the shown entity in frontal chest radiograph?

5. What is the most common location of the shown entity?

Case ranking/difficulty: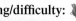

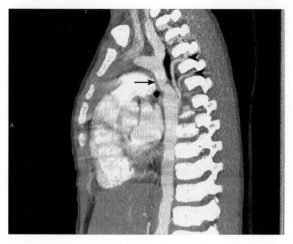

Sagittal CT of the chest reveals narrowing of the aorta distal to the branching point of the left subclavian vein (*arrow*). Collateral vessels are seen (*arrowheads*).

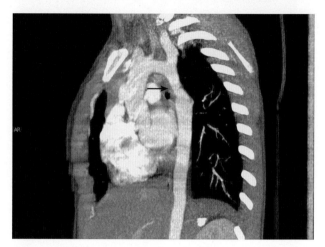

Sagittal CT of the chest reveals narrowing of the aorta distal to the branching point of the left subclavian vein (*arrow*).

Answers

1. There is stricture of the aorta distal to the branching point of the left subclavian artery.

2. Clinical presentation usually varies. Patients may be asymptomatic or present with various clinical signs such as hypertension, chest pain, dizziness, or cold feet and legs.

3. Possible complications of coarctation of aorta include heart failure, severe hypertension, aortic rupture, and endocarditis.

4. Poststenotic dilation of the aorta results in a classic "figure 3 sign" on x-ray. When the esophagus is filled with barium, a reverse three or E sign is often seen and represents a mirror image of the areas of prestenotic and poststenotic dilatation.

5. The most common location of coarctation of the aorta is distal to the branching point of the left subclavian artery.

Pearls

- There are three types of aortic coarctation: preductal, ductal, and postductal.
- Narrowing of a segment of the aorta is seen.
- Treatment consists of segmental resection of the narrowed portion of the aorta and reanastomosis. Symptomatic treatment of complication is necessary.

Suggested Readings

de Roos A, Roest AA. Evaluation of congenital heart disease by magnetic resonance imaging. *Eur Radiol.* 2000;10(1):2-6.

Ferguson EC, Krishnamurthy R, Oldham SA. Classic imaging signs of congenital cardiovascular abnormalities. *Radiographics.* 2008;27(5):1323-1334.

Kimura-Hayama ET, Meléndez G, Mendizábal AL, Meave-González A, Zambrana GF, Corona-Villalobos CP. Uncommon congenital and acquired aortic diseases: role of multidetector CT angiography. *Radiographics.* 2010;30(1):79-98.

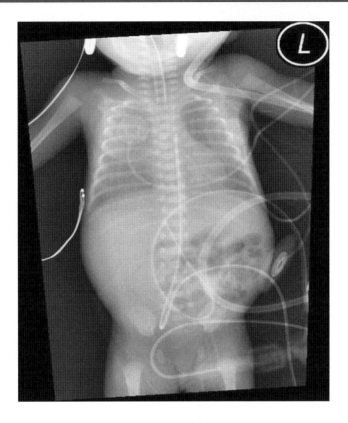

1. What is the most likely diagnosis?

2. What are the radiographic findings of this entity?

3. The disease is caused by lack of:

4. Risk factors for the disease include:

5. Treatment includes:

Case ranking/difficulty: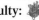

Category: Thorax

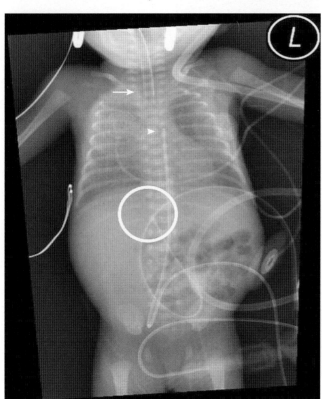

Frontal radiograph of the chest reveals hazy granularity of the lungs consistent with surfactant deficiency syndrome in a premature newborn. The *arrow* points to the distal tip of the endotracheal tube. The *arrowhead* points to the distal tip of the umbilical arterial line. The distal tip of the umbilical venous line, in the *circle*, is low in position, probably intrahepatic.

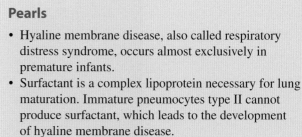

Pearls

- Hyaline membrane disease, also called respiratory distress syndrome, occurs almost exclusively in premature infants.
- Surfactant is a complex lipoprotein necessary for lung maturation. Immature pneumocytes type II cannot produce surfactant, which leads to the development of hyaline membrane disease.
- Hyaline membrane disease manifests as respiratory distress with grunting, nasal flaring, intercostals retractions, and hypoxia.
- Chest radiograph findings are ground glass appearance of the lungs with reticulogranular pattern and air bronchogram. In severe cases, whiteout of the lungs is seen.
- The risk can be reduced by antenatal steroids and early surfactant replacement therapy after birth.
- Often positive mechanical ventilation is necessary until lung maturation.

Suggested Readings

Kössel H, Versmold H. 25 years of respiratory support of newborn infants. *J Perinat Med.* 1997;25(5):421-432.

Kuhn JP, Slovis TL, Haller JO, eds. In: *Caffey's Pediatric Diagnostic Imaging.* 10th ed. Vol I. Philadelphia: Mosby; 2004:78-88.

Newman B. Imaging of medical disease of the newborn lung. *Radiol Clin North Am.* 1999;37(6):1049-1065.

Answers

1. The most likely diagnosis is hyaline membrane disease or the new name surfactant deficiency syndrome.

2. The radiographic findings of surfactant deficiency syndrome include low lung volume, ground glass appearance of the lungs, haziness and reticulogranularity of the lungs, and air-bronchogram.

3. Lack of surfactant. The disease is caused by immature type II pneumocytes that cannot produce surfactant.

4. Risk factors include prematurity, infant of diabetic mother, neonatal asphyxia, and cesarean delivery.

5. Treatment includes antenatal steroids, surfactant replacement therapy, oxygenation, continued positive airway pressure (CPAP), and assisted ventilation.

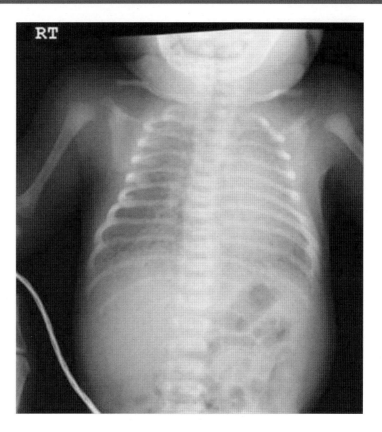

1. What is the differential diagnosis?

2. What are the radiographic findings of the case?

3. What is the pathophysiology of the case?

4. What are the risk factors?

5. What are the treatment options?

Case ranking/difficulty: 🏵

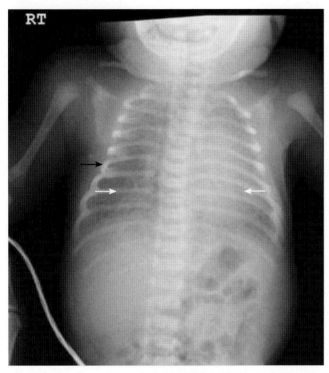

Frontal view of the chest demonstrates hyperinflation. Lungs are hazy with prominent pulmonary vascular markings (*white arrows*). Minor fissure visualized (*black arrow*) due to retained fluid.

Pearls

- Transient tachypnea of the newborn is a breathing difficulty that can be seen in the newborn shortly after delivery.
- It is being seen in full-term newborns delivered by cesarean section or in low-birth-weight babies.
- In these babies, there is lack of the vaginal squeeze of the chest that expels the fetal lung fluid from the lungs during delivery.
- Usually, this condition resolves over 24 to 48 hours.
- The chest x-ray shows hyperinflation of the lungs including prominent pulmonary vascular markings, flattening of the diaphragm, and fluid in the horizontal fissure of the right lung.

Suggested Readings

Jain L, Eaton DC. Physiology of fetal lung fluid clearance and the effect of labor. *Semin Perinatol.* 2006;30(1):34-43.

Ramachandrappa A, Jain L. Elective cesarean section: its impact on neonatal respiratory outcome. *Clin Perinatol.* 2008;35(2):373-393, vii.

Answers

1. Differential diagnosis includes hyaline membrane disease, meconium aspiration syndrome, neonatal pneumonia, and pulmonary congestion.

2. The chest x-ray shows hyperinflation of the lungs including prominent pulmonary vascular markings, hyperinflation, and fluid in the horizontal fissure of the right lung.

3. Transient tachypnea of the newborn is the result of a delay in clearance of fetal lung fluid. Infants with this syndrome are born by cesarean section or are low birth weight. There is lack of the normal vaginal squeeze that expels the lung fluid.

4. Newborns with this entity are born by cesarean section or are small for the gestational age.

5. The disease is self-limited and resolves within 24 to 48 hours after birth. No treatment is necessary. At times only oxygen supply may be given.

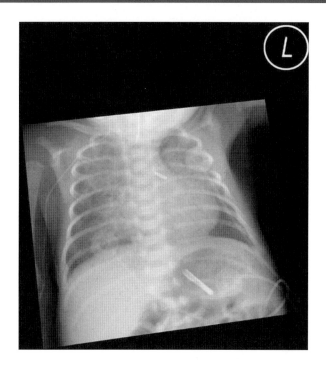

1. What is the differential diagnosis?

2. What are the risk factors?

3. What is the pathophysiology of the case?

4. What is the time frame following birth that the disease develops?

5. Chest radiograph findings are not specific. What findings may be seen?

Case ranking/difficulty: **Category:** Thorax

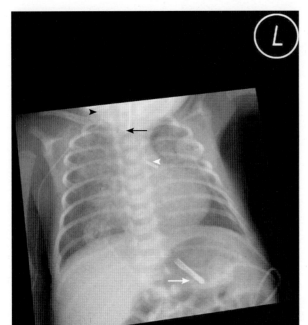

Frontal view of the chest demonstrates patchy lung opacities. Bubbly lung appearance is noted in the right upper lung zone. Subsegmental atelectatic changes are noted. The findings are nonspecific for bronchopulmonary dysplasia and the diagnosis is made by the history. *White arrow* points to the distal tip of the enteric tube. *Black arrow* points to the distal tip of the endotracheal tube. *White arrowhead* points to the PDA clip, and the *black arrowhead* points to the PICC line. The PICC line is malpositioned as it extends cranially to the right internal jugular vein.

Answers

1. Chest radiograph is very nonspecific for bronchopulmonary dysplasia. Differential diagnosis includes pulmonary congestion, atelectasis, and pneumonia.

2. Risk factors include prematurity or severe low birth weight and being on a ventilator for few weeks.

3. There is damage to alveoli due to positive airway pressure (baro-trauma) and breathing high oxygen concentration while on ventilatory support. There is pulmonary microvasculature injury and there is reduction in the overall surface area for gas exchange.

4. Newborns that get the disease are placed on ventilatory support immediately after birth to support lung function. Damage to the lungs occurs slowly. Usually the disease is formed at approximately 3 to 4 weeks after birth.

5. Chest radiograph findings are not specific. The findings seen are cyst-like changes (bubbly appearance), interstitial changes, and patchy opacities due to subsegmental atelectatic changes. Shifting atelectasis is seen in follow-up radiographs.

Pearls

- Bronchopulmonary dysplasia (BPD) is a form of chronic lung disease that develops in preterm neonates treated with oxygen and positive-pressure ventilation.
- The disease appears after being on ventilator for approximately 3 weeks.
- The disease results from toxic effect of oxygen and baro-trauma that damage the alveoli.
- Chest radiograph findings are nonspecific and represent shifting atelectatic changes, increased reticular markings, cyst-like changes (bubbly appearance), and patchy opacities.
- Diagnostic is made with chest radiographs in conjunction with clinical findings and past history.

Suggested Readings

Bancalari E, Abdenour GE, Feller R, Gannon J. Bronchopulmonary dysplasia: clinical presentation. *J Pediatr*. 1979;95(5 Pt 2):819-823.

Northway WH Jr, Rosan RC, Porter DY. Pulmonary disease following respirator therapy of hyaline-membrane disease. Bronchopulmonary dysplasia. *N Engl J Med*. 1967;276(7):357-368.

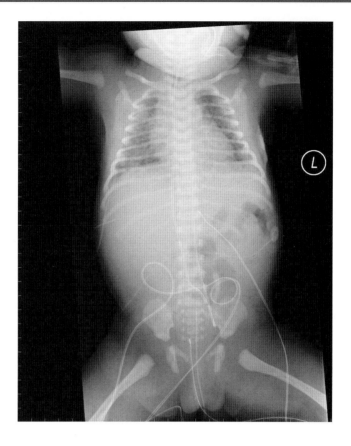

1. What are the findings?

2. What are the causes of this entity in a newborn?

3. How does the amniotic fluid looks like in this case?

4. How does the bowel respond to intrauterine distress?

5. What are the treatment options?

Case ranking/difficulty:

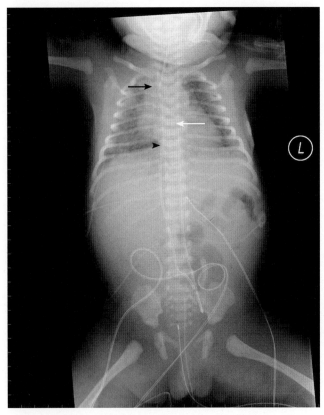

Frontal view of the chest demonstrates bilateral diffuse patchy opacities and coarse reticular findings. The *white arrow* points to the distal tip of the umbilical arterial catheter. The *arrowhead* points to the distal tip of the umbilical venous catheter. The *black arrow* points to the distal tip of the endotracheal tube.

Pearls

- Meconium aspiration syndrome is a medical condition affecting newborn infants.
- It occurs when meconium is present in the lungs during or before delivery.
- During fetal stress, meconium passes from bowel into the amniotic fluid in the uterus prior to labor and delivery. The newborn is at risk of aspirating this meconium.
- If the baby inhales the meconium-stained amniotic fluid, respiratory problems may occur. There is risk for bacterial infection and airway obstruction.
- Plain radiograph of the chest demonstrates hyperinflated lungs, areas of patchy opacities, and atelectatic changes. Coarse lung markings are noted.

Suggested Readings

Dargaville PA, Copnell B. The epidemiology of meconium aspiration syndrome: incidence, risk factors, therapies, and outcome. *Pediatrics*. 2006;117(5):1712-1721.

Wiswell TE, Tuggle JM, Turner BS. Meconium aspiration syndrome: have we made a difference? *Pediatrics*. 1990;85(5):715-721.

Answers

1. The findings include hyperinflated lungs, coarse lung markings, and bilateral patchy lung opacities representing multiple subsegmental atelectatic changes.

2. The leading three causes of meconium aspiration syndrome are due to a physiologic maturational event, a response to acute hypoxic events, and a response to chronic intrauterine hypoxia.

3. The amniotic fluid is meconium-stained.

4. Fetal distress during labor causes intestinal contractions, as well as relaxation of the anal sphincter, which allows meconium to pass into the amniotic fluid and contaminate the amniotic fluid.

5. Treatment includes intubation and ventilatory support, intrapartum suctioning of the patient's oro-pharynx, surfactant administration, and extracorporeal membranous oxygenation (ECMO) in severe cases.

Newborn with abdominal distension

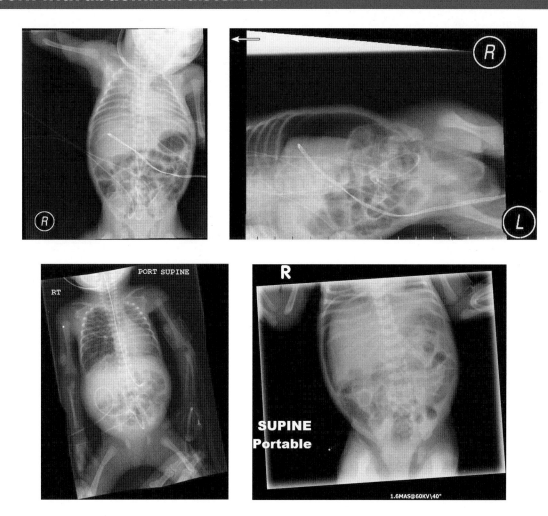

1. What are the findings?

2. What may be the etiology of the case?

3. What are the signs seen in supine radiograph of the shown case?

4. Which view is the best for confirmation of the shown case?

5. What is the treatment?

Case ranking/difficulty: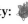

Category: Abdomen

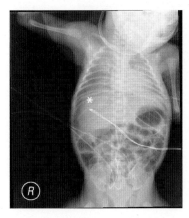

Frontal radiograph of the chest and abdomen demonstrates lucency below the diaphragm (*asterisk*) suggestive of intraperitoneal free air.

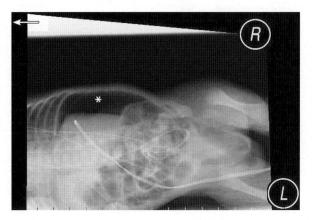

Left lateral decubitus radiograph demonstrates air above the liver (*asterisk*). This confirms the presence of intraperitoneal free air.

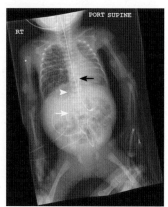

Frontal radiograph of the chest and abdomen demonstrates lucency below the diaphragm suggestive of intraperitoneal free air. Lucent intraabdominal air is a background that permits visualization of the falciform ligament (*white arrow*). The *arrowhead* points to the distal tip of the umbilical venous catheter. The *black arrow* points to the distal tip of the umbilical artery catheter.

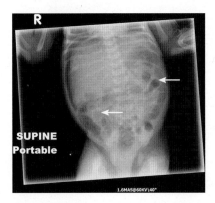

Frontal radiograph of the chest and abdomen demonstrates lucency below the diaphragm suggestive of intraperitoneal free air. The double-wall sign (Rigler sign) is shown (*arrows*) in which the inner and the outer sides of the bowel wall are visualized.

Answers

1. Frontal view of the chest and abdomen demonstrates lucency below the diaphragm suggestive of intraperitoneal free air. Left lateral decubitus view confirms this finding. In addition, the lucent air is a background that permits visualization of the falciform ligament.

2. The etiology may include necrotizing enterocolitis, surfactant deficiency syndrome, and gastric perforation. The etiology is sometimes unknown (idiopathic).

3. Football sign, Riggler sign, the double-wall sign, and the inverted V sign are seen in supine radiograph of pneumoperitoneum.

4. Left lateral decubitus is the best view to confirm pneumoperitoneum in the newborn. The air rises in this view between the liver and the right abdominal wall.

5. Exploratory laparotomy should be performed immediately upon diagnosis.

Pearls

- Intraperitoneal free air in the newborn period may be due to bowel perforation. Idiopathic cases are rare. Barotrauma in cases of respiratory distress may trigger pneumoperitoneum.
- The most frequent signs of abdominal intraperitoneal free air in a supine radiograph are lucency in the subdiaphragmatic right upper quadrant and the Rigler sign.
- Less common signs of intraperitoneal free air in the supine radiograph are air outlining the falciform ligament and the football sign.
- Confirmation of pneumoperitoneum in the newborn can be achieved by left lateral decubitus view in which the air rises between the liver and the right abdominal wall.

Suggested Readings

Brill PW, Olson SR, Winchester P. Neonatal necrotizing enterocolitis: air in Morrison pouch. *Radiology.* 1990;174:469-471.

Levine MS, Scheiner JD, Rubesin SE, Laufer I, Herlinger H. Diagnosis of pneumoperitoneum on supine abdominal radiographs. *AJR Am J Roentgenol.* 1991;156:731-735.

Ly JQ. The Rigler sign. *Radiology.* 2003;228 (3):706-707.

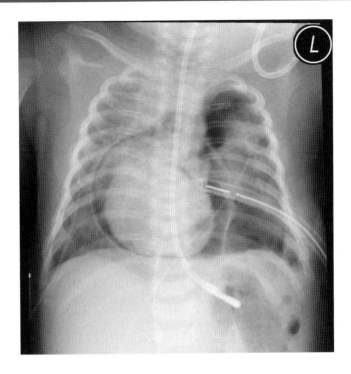

1. What are the findings?

2. What is included in the etiology of this entity?

3. What is the major differential diagnosis of this entity?

4. What is the halo sign of this entity?

5. Which two radiographic views may help in differentiating between pneumopericardium and pneumomediastinum?

Case ranking/difficulty: 🦫

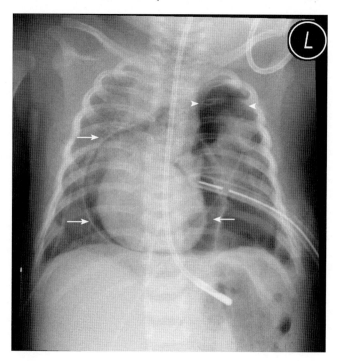

Frontal radiograph of the chest reveals lucency encircling cardiac silhouette (*arrows*) representing pneumopericardium. There is a lucency in the left apex (*arrowheads*) representing pneumothorax. The left lung is collapsed due to the pneumothorax. There is left-sided chest tube and enteric tube.

Pearls

- Pneumopericardium is collection of air or gas in the pericardial cavity.
- Etiology varies. In newborns, the most common is barotrauma.
- Spontaneous pneumopericardium can occur.
- Major differential diagnosis is pneumomediastinum.
- Posteroanterior radiograph and then taking left-side-decubitus view may help distinguish between pneumopericardium and pneumomediastinum.
- The transverse band of air sign (air in the transverse sinus of the pericardium) and the triangle sign (a hyperlucency behind the sternum, anterior to the cardiac base and the aortic root) are useful in distinguishing pneumopericardium from pneumomediastinum.

Suggested Readings

Capizzi PJ, Martin M, Bannon MP. Tension pneumopericardium following blunt injury. *J Trauma.* 1995;39:775-780.

Costa IV, Soto B, Diethelm L, Zarco P. Air pericardial tamponade. *Am J Cardiol.* 1987;60:1421-1422.

Van Gelderen WF. Stab wounds of the heart: two new signs of pneumopericardium. *Br J Radiol.* 1993;66:794-796.

Answers

1. Pneumopericardium and left-sided pneumothorax are seen. Left-sided chest tube is seen. Left lung is opacified due to compressive atelectasis from the pneumothorax.

2. The etiology of pneumopericardium varies and may include barotrauma, blunt trauma, bronchopericardial fistula, gastropericardial fistula, and thoracocentesis.

3. The major differential diagnosis is pneumomediastinum.

4. The halo sign is a radiolucent band of air partially or completely surrounding the heart in pneumopericardium.

5. A posteroanterior radiograph and then taking left-side-down decubitus radiograph will show a rapid shift of air in the pericardial sac, while air in the mediastinum will not move in the short interval between the two films.

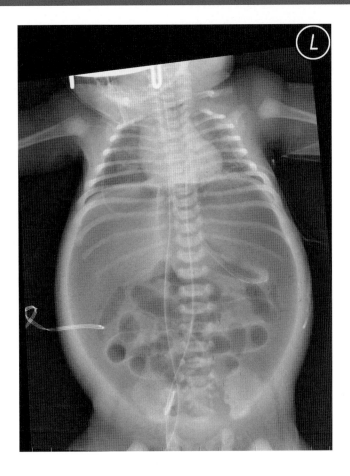

1. What are the findings?

2. Lateral to the umbilical venous catheter there is a dense line from the level of T7 to T12. What does it represent?

3. What can be an etiology of the case?

4. How is the Rigler sign being produced?

5. How is the football sign being created?

Case ranking/difficulty: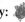

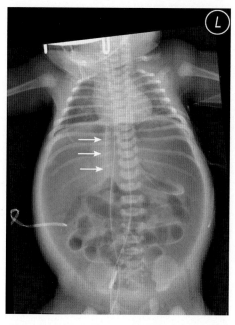

Frontal radiograph of the abdomen reveals lucency in the abdomen consistent with intraperitoneal free air. The *arrows* point to the falciform ligament.

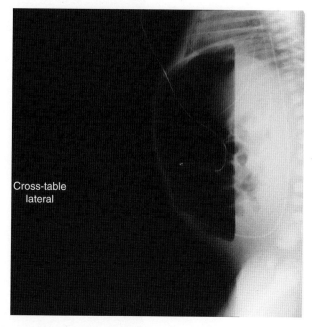

Cross-table lateral view of the abdomen confirms the presence of intraperitoneal free air.

Answers

1. There is intraperitoneal free air.

2. The falciform ligament is seen, due to the lucent background of the abdomen.

3. Cardiopulmonary resuscitation, thoracic trauma, pulmonary sepsis, and barotrauma are all causes for pneumoperitoneum.

4. Rigler sign, also known as the double wall sign, is seen on a supine radiograph of the abdomen when air is present on both sides of the bowel wall.

5. The football sign, which is seen on supine abdominal radiographs, refers to a large oval radiolucency in the shape of an American football. In the supine position, free air collects anterior to the abdominal viscera, producing a sharp interface with the parietal peritoneum and thereby creating the football outline.

Pearls

- Intraperitoneal free gas indicates a perforated abdominal viscus that requires surgical intervention.
- Rarely pneumoperitoneum can be spontaneous and not related to a perforated viscus.
- There are specific signs in the supine radiographic view that help in diagnosing pneumoperitoneum: the Rigler sign, the football sign, and the visualization of the ligamentum falciform.
- A radiograph in left lateral decubitus view is the best view to confirm intraperitoneal free air in the newborn. Air interposes between the abdominal wall and the liver and can be clearly visualized.

Suggested Readings

Cho KC, Baker SR. Extraluminal air. Diagnosis and significance. *Radiol Clin North Am*. 1994;32(5):829-844.

Levine MS, Scheiner JD, Rubesin SE, Laufer I, Herlinger H. Diagnosis of pneumoperitoneum on supine abdominal radiographs. *AJR Am J Roentgenol*. 1991;156(4):731-735.

Rampton JW. The football sign. *Radiology*. 2004;231(1):81-82.

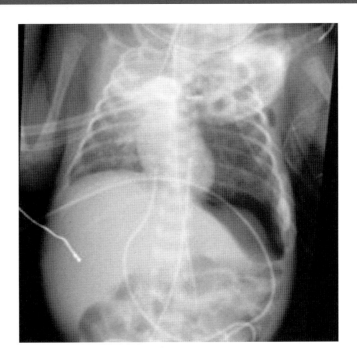

1. What are the findings?

2. What was the position of the patient when the image was taken?

3. What is the name of the sign that is demonstrated in the lower left chest?

4. In which portions of the lungs does air accumulate in the upright position?

5. How is this entity being treated?

Case ranking/difficulty: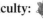

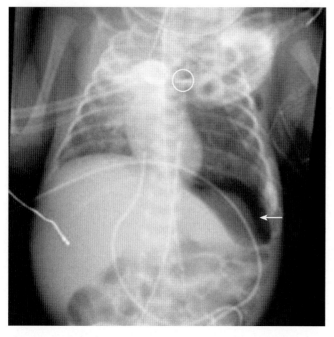

Single frontal radiograph of the chest, supine, demonstrates lucency in the left costophrenic sulcus representing the pneumothorax (*arrow*). The *circle* represents the surgical clip following the repair of the ductus arteriosus. Note is made of right upper lobe atelectasis. Patient has endotracheal tube, umbilical arterial and venous line, and enteric tube.

Pearls

- The deep sulcus sign represents pneumothorax in the supine position.
- Air tends to rise to the highest nondependent space it can get.
- The highest space of the chest in the supine position is the base of the lungs, anteriorly at the costophrenic sulcus.
- It is a lucency of the costophrenic sulcus that deepens due to collection of air.

Suggested Readings

Gordon R. The deep sulcus sign. *Radiology*. 1980;136:25-27.
Kong A. The deep sulcus sign. *Radiology*. 2003;228:415-416.

Answers

1. There is left-sided pneumothorax and right upper lobe atelectasis. The umbilical arterial and venous catheters are in good position. Small left chest wall subcutaneous emphysema is noted.

2. The patient was supine. In the supine position, the highest space of the chest is the lung base, anteriorly. Air tends to rise to the highest level. Pneumothorax in the supine position is seen in the lower chest and deepens the costophrenic sulcus.

3. The deep sulcus sign means that a pneumothorax is seen in the anterior and basal aspects of the lung, in the costophrenic sulcus. This is seen in the supine view as the air rises to the upper level it can get.

4. In the upright position, air (pneumothorax) accumulates in the apicolateral portions of the lungs.

5. Pneumothorax is treated by immediate placement of a chest tube to decompress the lungs and drain the air.

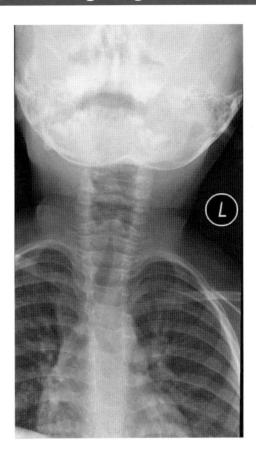

1. What is the name of the sign demonstrated in the image?

2. What is the most common etiology of this case?

3. What is the differential diagnosis?

4. What is the pathophysiology of this case?

5. What are the treatment options?

Case ranking/difficulty: 🌰

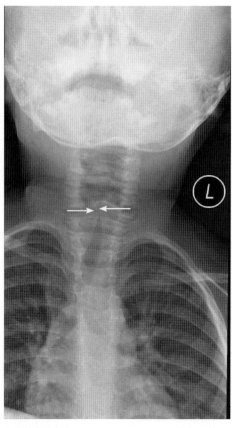

Frontal radiograph of the neck demonstrates narrowing of the subglottic trachea (*arrows*). There is loss of the lateral covexities of the trachea with steepling (called the steeple sign).

4. The viral infection that causes croup leads to swelling of the larynx, trachea, and large bronchi due to infiltration of white blood cells. Swelling produces airway obstruction, which, when significant, leads to increased work of breathing and the characteristic turbulent, noisy airflow known as stridor.

5. Antibiotics are not most commonly indicated as most of the cases are due to viral infection. Treatment includes racemic epinephrine, oxygen, corticosteroids, and cool mist administration.

Pearls

- Croup is a laryngotracheobronchitis.
- It is characterized by a loud cough.
- Viral etiology is most common.
- Steeple sign is seen on frontal view of the neck.
- Treatment commonly includes corticosteroids and racemic epinephrine.

Suggested Readings

Salour M. The steeple sign. *Radiology.* 2000;216(2):428-429.

Sammer M, Pruthi S. Membranous croup (exudative tracheitis or membranous laryngotracheobronchitis). *Pediatr Radiol.* 2010;40(5):781.

Zoorob R, Sidani M, Murray J. Croup: an overview. *Am Fam Physician.* 2011;83(9):1067-1073.

Answers

1. The steeple sign. There is loss of the lateral convexities of the subglottic trachea or loss of the normal shoulders of the subglottic larynx.

2. The etiology of croup is most commonly viral. In 75% of the cases, croup is due to parainfluenza virus.

3. The differential diagnosis includes acute epiglottitis, foreign body aspiration, angioneurotic edema, spasmodic croup, and laryngeal mass such as hemangioma.

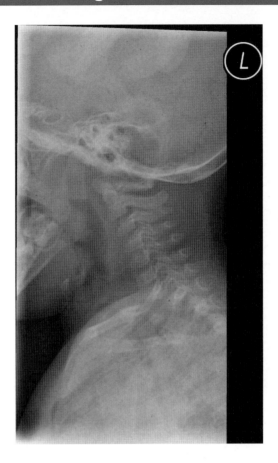

1. What are the findings?

2. What are the clinical symptoms of this case?

3. What is the imaging modality of choice for the diagnosis?

4. What are the microorganisms that can be cultured in this entity?

5. What are the indications for surgical treatment?

4. The microorganisms that can be cultured from enlarged adenoids include *Haemophilus influenzae*, Group A beta-hemolytic Streptococcus, *Staphylococcus aureus*, *Moraxella catarrhalis*, and *Streptococcus pneumoniae*.

5. Usually the adenoids involute. The indications for surgical adenoidectomy are enlargement causing nasal airway obstruction, recurrent or persistent otitis media in children aged 3-4 years and older, and recurrent and/or chronic sinusitis.

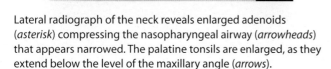

Pearls

- Adenoids are lymphoid tissue located at the back of the nose.
- Pathologic enlargement may cause narrowing of the nasopharyngeal airway and difficulty breathing.
- Complications include recurrent otitis media and sinusitis.
- Enlargement may be idiopathic or caused by bacterial growth.
- Enlarged adenoids usually involute after the age of 6 years.
- Treatment includes antibiotics or surgical adenoidectomy if there are recurrent complications.

Lateral radiograph of the neck reveals enlarged adenoids (*asterisk*) compressing the nasopharyngeal airway (*arrowheads*) that appears narrowed. The palatine tonsils are enlarged, as they extend below the level of the maxillary angle (*arrows*).

Answers

1. There is enlargement of the adenoids with narrowing of the nasopharyngeal airway. The palatine tonsils are mildly enlarged. There is no prevertebral soft tissue swelling.

2. The clinical symptoms of the shown case are nasal congestion, mouth breathing, snoring, painful swallowing, sleep apnea, and chronic or recurrent otitis media due to their proximity to the eustachian tubes.

3. The modality of choice is neck radiograph in lateral view.

Suggested Readings

Feres MF, Hermann JS, Cappellette M Jr, Pignatari SS. Lateral x-ray view of the skull for the diagnosis of adenoid hypertrophy: a systematic review. *Int J Pediatr Otorhinolaryngol.* 2011;75(1):1-11.

Kolo ES, Salisu AD, Tabari AM, Dahilo EA, Aluko AA. Plain radiographic evaluation of the nasopharynx: do raters agree? *Int J Pediatr Otorhinolaryngol.* 2010;74(5):532-534.

4-year-old male with fecal soiling

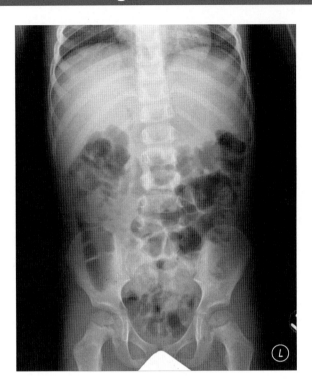

1. What are the findings?

2. What is the prevalence of this case in children less than 10 years old?

3. What is the gender ratio of this case?

4. How most patients with this entity present?

5. What are the treatment options?

Case ranking/difficulty:

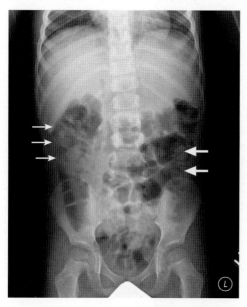

Frontal radiograph of the abdomen demonstrate bubbly appearance inside the colon with filling defects representing fecal material (*arrows*).

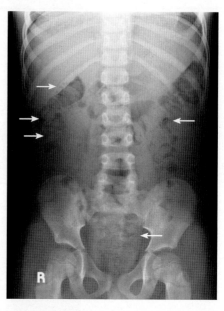

Abdominal radiograph of another patient reveals a large amount of bubbly appearance representing fecal material in the ascending colon, the descending colon, and the rectosigmoid (*arrows*).

Answers

1. The frontal radiograph of the abdomen demonstrates bubbly appearance inside the colon with filling defects representing fecal material.

2. An estimated 1 to 2% of children younger than 10 years have encopresis.

3. The male:female ratio is 6:1.

4. Approximately 80 to 90% of children with encopresis have a history of constipation or painful defecation.

5. Long-term laxatives may play a role in the treatment. Behavioral education for frequent evacuation, biofeedback training to teach the child to relax, and external anal sphincter also play a role in the treatment. There is no role for diet and surgery in the treatment.

- Fecal retention in encopretic children can be assessed from a plain abdominal roentgenogram.
- Images demonstrate a large amount of fecal material in the colon that has a bubbly appearance.
- Treatment is usually with laxatives and behavioral therapy.

Suggested Readings

Griffiths DM. The physiology of continence: idiopathic fecal constipation and soiling. *Semin Pediatr Surg.* 2002;11(2):67-74.

Nissen G, Menzel M, Friese HJ, Trott GE. Encopresis in children. Preliminary report of new therapeutic and diagnostic aspects. *Z Kinder Jugendpsychiatr.* 1991;19(3):170-174.

Rockney RM, McQuade WH, Days AL. The plain abdominal roentgenogram in the management of encopresis. *Arch Pediatr Adolesc Med.* 1995;149(6):623-627.

Pearls

- Encopresis is involuntary "fecal soiling" in adults and children who have usually already been toilet trained.
- Chronic constipation results in progressive rectal distention and stretching of the anal sphincters.
- The prevalence of encopresis in childhood: An estimated 1 to 2% of children younger than 10 years have encopresis.

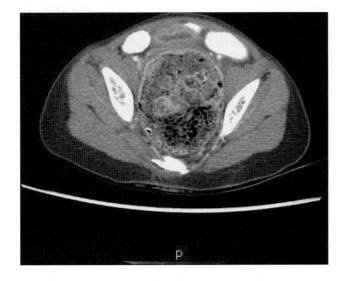
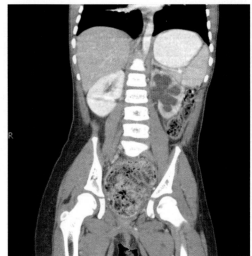
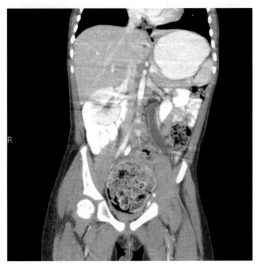
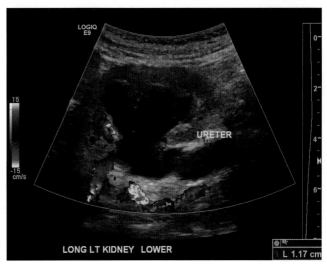

1. What is the diagnosis?

2. How can obstructive hydronephrosis be differentiated from nonobstructive hydronephrosis?

3. What is the radiopharmaceutical most commonly used during nuclear renal scintigraphy for evaluation of hydronephrosis?

4. What is the definition of constipation?

5. Describe the findings of the left ureter.

Case ranking/difficulty:

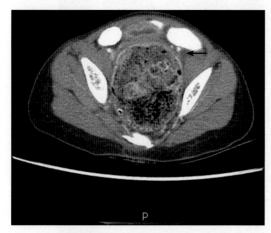

Axial CT of the pelvis reveals the rectum with fecal impaction compressing and displacing the bladder anteriorly. The dilated left ureter is seen (*arrow*).

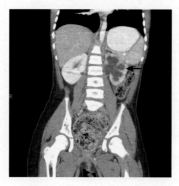

Coronal CT of the abdomen demonstrates hydronephrosis of the left kidney (*arrow*).

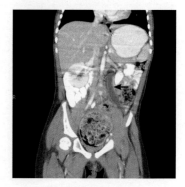

Coronal CT of the pelvis demonstrates left ureter that is severely dilated (*arrow*).

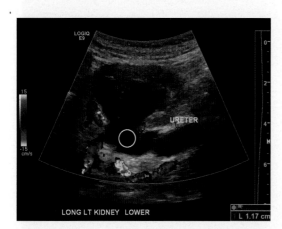

Longitudinal sonogram of the left kidney demonstrates that the left ureter is severely dilated. The *circle* demonstrates dilated renal pelvis. Left renal hydronephrosis is noted.

Answers

1. The diagnosis is fecal impaction with distended rectum compressing and displacing the bladder anteriorly. There is bilateral hydronephrosis and left hydroureter.

2. Dynamic nuclear scintigraphy can differentiate between obstructive and nonobstructive hydronephrosis. If furosemide is administered during the study, and there is complete excretion of the radiopharmaceutical from a hydronephrotic kidney, then the hydronephrosis is nonobstructive.

3. The radiopharmaceutical is Tc-99m-MAG3 (Mercaptoacetyltriglycine).

4. The definition of constipation includes the following: infrequent bowel movements (typically <3 times per wk), difficulty during defecation (straining during more than 25% of bowel movements or a subjective sensation of hard stools), or the sensation of incomplete bowel evacuation.

5. Left patent hydroureter that is not obstructed and does not abut the rectum.

Pearls

- There are few reports of obstructive uropathy due to constipation.
- There is no evidence in our case that the constipation induced the hydronephrosis. The uropathy persisted after cleansing.
- It might have been that the long-term bladder compression caused the hydronephrosis that damaged the left kidney.
- Renal scintigraphy performed 2 weeks following bowel cleaning demonstrates decreased function and excretion of the left kidney. The obstruction is partial and functional with no anatomic cause.

Suggested Readings

Chute DJ, Cox J, Archer ME, Bready RJ, Reiber K. Spontaneous rupture of urinary bladder associated with massive fecal impaction (fecaloma). *Am J Forensic Med Pathol.* 2009;30(3):280-283.

Gonzalez F. Obstructive uropathy caused by fecal impaction: report of 2 cases and discussion. *Am J Hosp Palliat Care.* 2010;27(8):557-559.

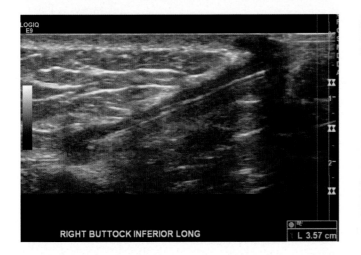

RIGHT BUTTOCK INFERIOR LONG

L 3.57 cm

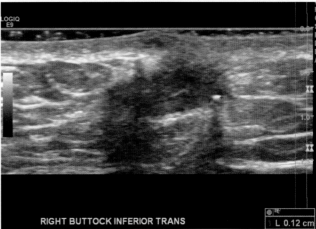

RIGHT BUTTOCK INFERIOR TRANS

L 0.12 cm

1. What are the findings?

2. What are the complications of this entity?

3. What is the most likely microorganism that may complicate this entity?

4. What is the differential diagnosis?

5. What are the treatment options?

Case ranking/difficulty:

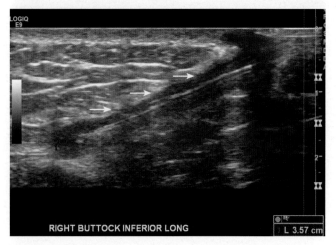

RIGHT BUTTOCK INFERIOR LONG   L 3.57 cm

Longitudinal sonogram of the right inferior buttock reveals that a linear, long, thin foreign body (*arrows*) enters deep the buttock. The tip is seen at 1.6 cm depth. Edema surrounds the foreign body.

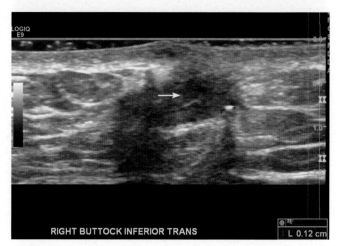

RIGHT BUTTOCK INFERIOR TRANS   L 0.12 cm

Transverse sonogram of the right inferior buttock reveals a foreign body entering deep into the buttock (*arrow*). Edema surrounds the foreign body.

Answers

1. In the right inferior buttock, there is a linear, thin foreign body surrounded by edema.

2. Complications may include infection, inflammation, and abscess formation.

3. The most likely microorganism that may complicate the case and cause infection is *Staphylococcus aureus*.

4. The entity shown is an obvious foreign body in the subcutaneous tissue of the buttock and no differential diagnosis is included.

5. The treatment options are antibiotics and tetanus prophylaxis. Surgical removal should be performed.

Pearls

- Subcutaneous foreign body due to sharp objects penetrating the skin is a common occurrence in children.
- A foreign body in the subcutaneous tissue may irritate and cause infection, inflammation, and an abscess.
- Surgical removal should be performed immediately to avoid complications.
- Not all foreign bodies are radio-opaque and can be visualized on plain radiographs.
- Sonogram is an excellent imaging modality to visualize foreign bodies and guide surgical removal.

Suggested Reading

Ludin M. Foreign body in buttock. *Radiol Clin.* 1951;20(3):185-186.

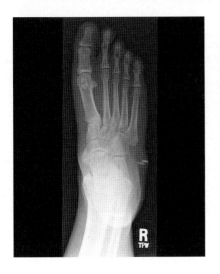 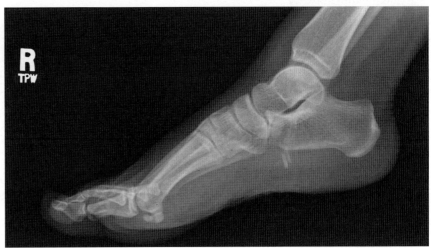

1. What are the findings?

2. What are the complications of this entity?

3. What is the least sensitive modality for detection of foreign body in the foot?

4. What is the most common microorganism that causes infection in this case?

5. What are the treatment options?

Case ranking/difficulty:

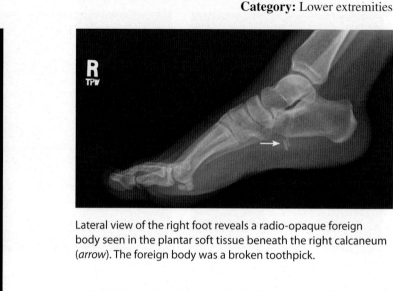

Lateral view of the right foot reveals a radio-opaque foreign body seen in the plantar soft tissue beneath the right calcaneum (*arrow*). The foreign body was a broken toothpick.

Frontal view of the right foot reveals a radio-opaque foreign body seen in the soft tissue medial to the right calcaneum (*arrow*). The foreign body was a broken toothpick.

Answers

1. Foreign body is seen in the soft tissue of the foot below the calcaneum.

2. Complications may include inflammation, infection, abscess formation around the foreign body, and scarring.

3. MRI (58%) and CT (63%) scan have higher sensitivity to detect foreign body than the radiographs (29%).

4. The most common microorganism that can complicate and causes infection of foreign body in soft tissue is *Staphylococcus aureus.*

5. Treatment options include removal of foreign body, tetanus prophylaxis, and antibiotics if infection is present.

Pearls

- Foreign bodies may enter the soft tissues through the skin. There may or may not be obvious entry wound.
- Radio-opaque foreign bodies can be identified on the radiograph. Radiolucent foreign body may only show soft tissue swelling on radiograph.
- Wood can be seen using ultrasound or CT scan.
- MRI (58%) and CT (63%) scans have higher sensitivity to detect foreign body than the radiographs (29%).
- Foreign body may initiate foreign body reaction or get infected and develop cellulitis or abscess. Infection may spread to adjacent bone leading to osteomyelitis.
- *Staphylococcus aureus* is the most common cause of infection related to foreign body.
- Treatment consists of removal of foreign body, tetanus prophylaxis, and antibiotic treatment if infection is present.

Suggested Readings

Gregori D, Foltran F, Passali D. Foreign body injuries in children: need for a step forward against an old yet neglected epidemic. *Paediatr Perinat Epidemiol.* 2011;25(2):98-99.

Pattamapaspong N, Srisuwan T, Sivasomboon C, et al. Accuracy of radiography, computed tomography and magnetic resonance imaging in diagnosing foreign bodies in the foot. *Radiol Med.* 2013;118(2):303-310.

Pogorelić Z, Biočić M, Bekavac J. An unusual foreign body in the foot: traumatic implantation of a human tooth. *J Foot Ankle Surg.* 2011;50(2):225-226.

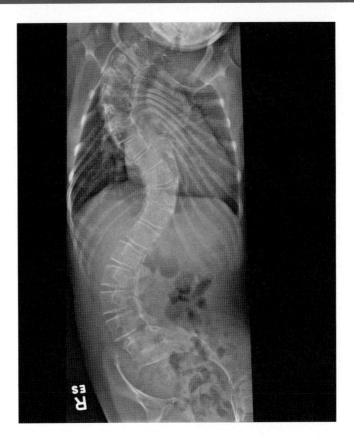

1. What is the pattern of the deformity seen in the thoracolumbar spine?

2. What is the most common spinal anomaly that causes such a case?

3. What is the incidence of spinal cord abnormalities associated with congenital scoliosis?

4. What are the associated anomalies?

5. What are the treatment options?

Case ranking/difficulty: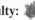

Category: Spine

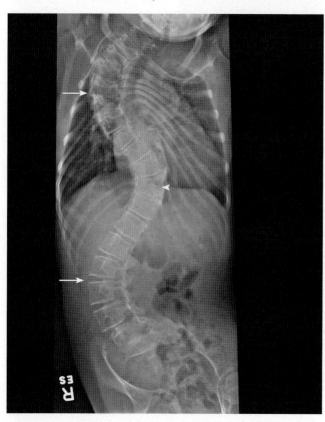

Frontal view of the thoracolumbar spine demonstrates severe scoliosis. The *arrows* demonstrate right-sided convexities, and the *arrowhead* demonstrates left-sided convexity.

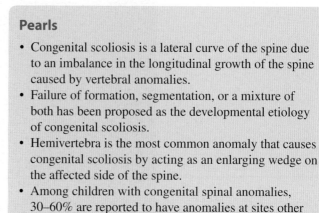

Pearls

- Congenital scoliosis is a lateral curve of the spine due to an imbalance in the longitudinal growth of the spine caused by vertebral anomalies.
- Failure of formation, segmentation, or a mixture of both has been proposed as the developmental etiology of congenital scoliosis.
- Hemivertebra is the most common anomaly that causes congenital scoliosis by acting as an enlarging wedge on the affected side of the spine.
- Among children with congenital spinal anomalies, 30–60% are reported to have anomalies at sites other than the spine.

Suggested Readings

Jog S, Patole S, Whitehall J. Congenital scoliosis in a neonate: can a neonatologist ignore it? *Postgrad Med J.* 2002;78:469-472.

McMaster MJ, David CV. Hemivertebra as a cause of scoliosis. A study of 104 patients. *J Bone Joint Surg Br.* 1986;68:588-595.

Oestreich AE, Young LW, Poussaint TY. Scoliosis circa 2000: radiologic imaging perspective 1. Diagnosis and pretreatment evaluation. *Skeletal Radiol.* 1998;27:591-605.

Answers

1. Scoliosis is noted. There is right-sided convexity centered on the mid thoracic spine. Left-sided convexity is noted centered on T11. There is right-sided convexity centered on the mid lumbar spine. Lateral wedging of the vertebral body T11 is seen.

2. Hemivertebra is the most common anomaly that causes congenital scoliosis by acting as an enlarging wedge on the affected side of the spine. The degree of scoliosis produced by hemivertebra depends on their type/site/ number/relationship to each other and the patient's age.

3. The incidence of spinal cord abnormalities associated with congenital scoliosis is reported to range from 20% to over 50% in most of the series.

4. The most common of anomaly sites are genitourinary tract, cardiac system, the spinal cord, and the cervical spine. Many are part of VACTREL association, and also incidence of Klippel–Feil syndrome is high.

5. Braces, orthopedic spinal fusion and, in some cases, hemiarthrodesis are treatment options.

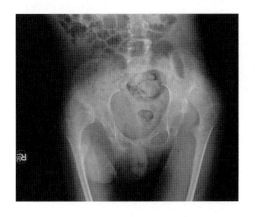 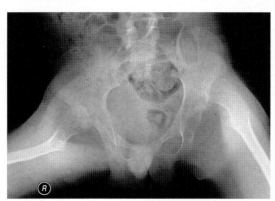 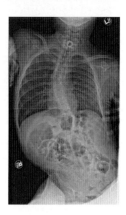

1. What are the findings?

2. What is the Hilgenreiner line?

3. What is the Perkin's line?

4. What is the normal acetabular angle?

5. In which quadrant formed by the intersection of the Hilgenreiner and Perkin's lines should the normal femoral head project?

Case ranking/difficulty:

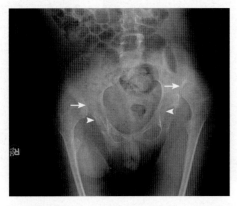

Pelvis x-ray in a frontal view reveals superior dislocation of both femoral heads. Both acetabula are shallow (*arrowheads*); pseudoacetabulum has been formed bilaterally (*arrows*) secondary to molding of the displaced femoral heads with the iliac bones.

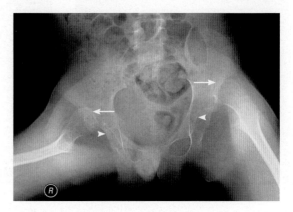

Pelvis radiograph in abduction view reveals superior dislocation of both femoral heads. Both acetabula are shallow (*arrowheads*); pseudoacetabulum has been formed bilaterally (*arrows*) secondary to molding of the displaced femoral heads with the iliac bones.

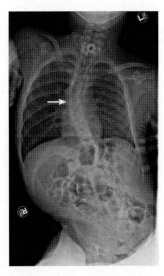

Frontal radiograph of the thoracolumbar spine reveals scoliosis. There is curvature with right-sided convexity. The scoliosis is centered on T6 (*arrow*).

Answers

1. There is bilateral dislocation of the femoral heads superiorly with formation of bilateral pseudoacetabulum. Scoliosis is seen. The patient has tracheostomy tube.

2. Hilgenreiner line is a horizontal line between the two triradiate cartilages.

3. The Perkin's line is drawn at the outer acetabular margin and is perpendicular to the Hilgenreiner line.

4. The normal acetabular angle measures slightly less than 30 degrees.

5. Both femoral heads should project in the inner lower quadrants formed by the intersection of the Hilgenreiner and Perkin's lines.

Pearls

- Line measurements made on the antero-posterior radiograph help in determining the relationship of the femoral head with the acetabulum.
- The Hilgenreiner and the Perkin's lines are two perpendicular lines to each other that help determine the position of the femoral head in relation to the acetabulum.
- Shenton arc and acetabular angle are measurements that help determine the presence of developmental hip dysplasia.
- Dislocation of the femoral head is usually posteriorly and superiorly.
- Pseudoacetabulum may be formed by molding of the displaced femoral head with the pelvic bones.

Suggested Readings

Kirks DR, Griscom NT. *Practical Pediatric Imaging Diagnostic Radiology of Infants and Children*. Philadelphia, PA: Lippincott-Raven; 1998.

Ozonoff MB. *Pediatric Orthopedic Radiology*. 2nd ed. Philadelphia, PA: WB Saunders; 1992.

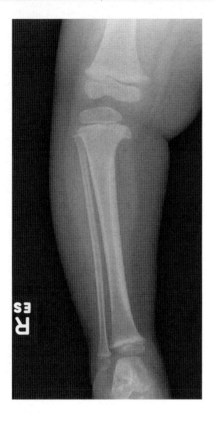
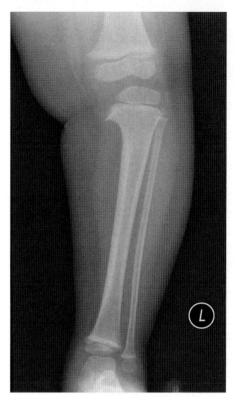

1. What is the diagnosis?

2. What are the imaging findings?

3. What is the possible etiology of this entity?

4. What is the normal metaphyseal-diaphyseal angle in an infant less than 2 years?

5. What should be the main differential diagnosis of this entity in a toddler less than 2 years?

Case ranking/difficulty:

Category: Lower extremities

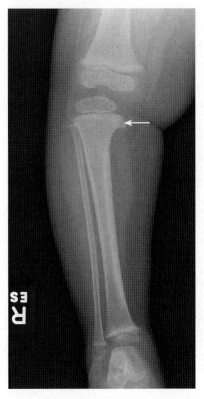

Frontal radiograph of the right leg reveals medial beaking of the proximal tibial metaphysis (*arrow*) Tibia vara noted.

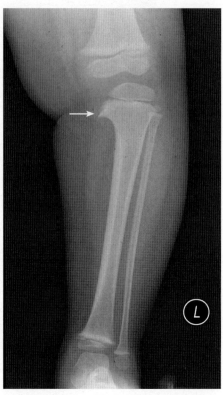

Frontal radiograph of the left leg reveals medial beaking of the proximal tibial metaphysis (*arrow*) Tibia vara noted.

Answers

1. The diagnosis is Blount's disease or tibia vara.

2. Imaging findings include varus deformity of the lower extremities (tibia vara), medial beaking, and fragmentation of the proximal tibial metaphysis.

3. Blount's disease is a developmental disease caused by excessive forces on the proximal metaphyses of the tibia in toddlers when they start to walk. During the growth period, altered endochondral bone formation may be a contributing factor for the development of this entity.

4. The normal metaphyseal-diaphyseal angle in an infant less than 2 years is less than 11 degrees.

5. The main differential diagnosis of Blount's disease in a toddler less than 2 years is physiologic bowing of the lower extremities.

Pearls

- Blount's disease is a deformity that manifests by varus deformity and internal rotation of the proximal tibia.

- Plain radiographs demonstrate tibia vara with beaking and fragmentation of the medial aspect of the proximal tibial metaphyses.
- The disease is ususally bilateral.
- Tibia vara and osteochondrosis deformans tibiae are two other terms that have been used to describe the deformity of Blount's disease.
- In toddlers, the normal bowing of the legs should disappear by the age of 2 years. Persistence of bowing is suspicious of the disease and plain radiographs of the lower extremities demonstrate the characteristic finding.
- A metaphyseal-diaphyseal angle of more than 11 degrees is considered diagnostic.

Suggested Readings

Hofmann A, Jones RE, Herring JA. Blount's disease after skeletal maturity. *J Bone Joint Surg Am.* 1982;64(7): 1004-1009.

Iwasawa T, Inaba Y, Nishimura G, Aida N, Kameshita K, Matsubara S. MR findings of bowlegs in toddlers. *Pediatr Radiol.* 1999;29(11):826-834.

Sabharwal S. Blount's disease. *J Bone Joint Surg Am.* 2009;91(7):1758-1776.

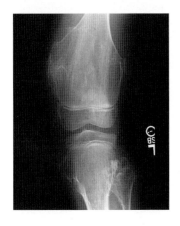 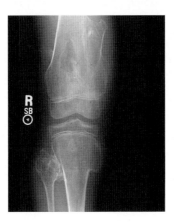 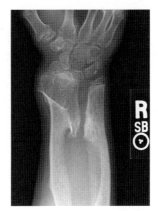 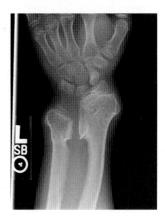

1. What is the diagnosis?

2. What are the complications of this case?

3. What are the findings?

4. What is the sign of malignant degeneration in MRI?

5. What is the percentage risk for malignant degeneration?

Case ranking/difficulty:

Category: Generalized diseases

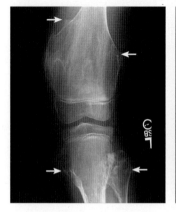

The left knee demonstrates multiple bony excrescences arising from the metaphyses of the bones. These excrescences have extension of the periosteum and form an obtuse angle with the bone (*arrows*).

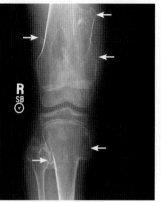

The right knee demonstrates multiple bony excrescences arising from the metaphyses of the bones. These excrescences have extension of the periosteum and form an obtuse angle with the bone (*arrows*).

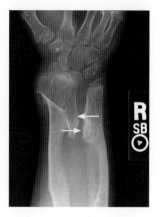

The right wrist demonstrates multiple bony excrescences arising from the metaphyses of the bones. These excrescences have extension of the periosteum and form an obtuse angle with the bone (*arrows*).

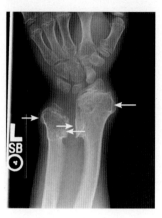

The left wrist demonstrates multiple bony excrescences arising from the metaphyses of the bones. These excrescences have extension of the periosteum and form an obtuse angle with the bone (*arrows*).

Answers

1. The diagnosis is hereditary multiple osteochondromatosis or hereditary multiple exostosis.

2. Tendons, nerves, or blood vessels may be trapped around osteochondromas, leading to symptoms. Symmetric or asymmetric impaired body growth is seen. Malignant degeneration can occur in about 1 to 20% of the cases.

3. There are bone excrescences arising from the metaphyses of long bones. The periosteum is in continuation with the excrescence. The pattern of these excrescences in hereditary multiple exostosis is being sessile. In most patients with single exostosis, the excrescence is pedunculated.

4. The MRI sign of malignant degeneration is cartilage cap thickness of more than 1 cm.

5. The risk for malignant degeneration is 1 to 20%.

Pearls

- An osteochondroma or exostosis is a cartilage-covered bony excrescence that arises from the surface of a parent bone.
- Hereditary multiple osteochondromatosis is an autosomal dominant condition where multiple osteochondromas are seen.
- In the hereditary form, most osteochondromas are sessile.
- Most of the osteochondromas are seen in the metaphyses of long bones.
- Osteochondromas do not grow after closure of the growth plates.

Suggested Readings

Kitsoulis P, Galani V, Stefanaki K, Paraskevas G, Karatzias G, Agnantis NJ, Bai M. Osteochondromas: review of the clinical, radiological and pathological features. *In Vivo*. 2008;22(5):633-646.

Reijnders CM, Waaijer CJ, Hamilton A, et al. No haploinsufficiency but loss of heterozygosity for EXT in multiple osteochondromas. *Am J Pathol*. 2010;177(4):1946-1957.

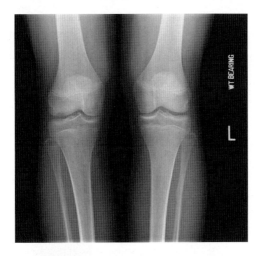
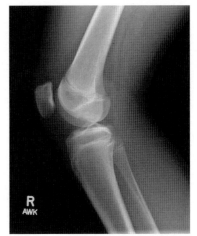
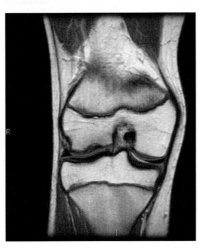
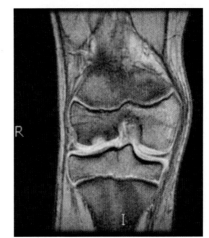

1. What is the diagnosis?

2. What is the most common location of this entity?

3. What is the second most common location of the entity shown?

4. What are the symptoms of focal chondral lesion?

5. What are the treatment options?

Case ranking/difficulty: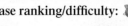

Category: Lower extremities

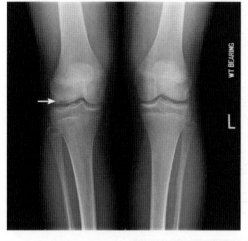

Frontal radiograph of the knees reveals a lucent defect in the lateral condyle of the right knee (*arrow*).

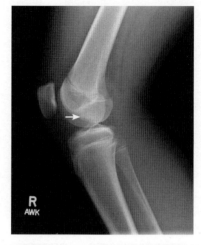

Lateral radiograph of the right knee reveals a lucent defect in the lateral condyle (*arrow*).

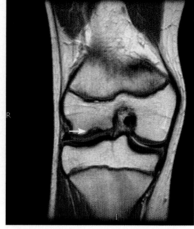

Coronal MRI T2 of the right knee reveals a low signal seen in the lateral condyle (*arrow*).

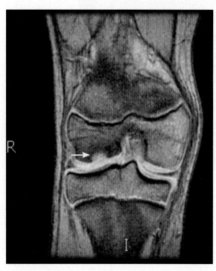

Coronal MRI, MPGR of the right knee reveals a high signal in the lateral condyle, representing cartilage (*arrow*).

Pearls

- Chondral and osteochondral injuries are commonly seen in today's clinical practice as a result of direct trauma, and typically affect a young athletic male population.
- Medial femoral condyle and patellar defects are more common than lateral femoral condyle and trochlear defects.
- Symptomatic focal chondral lesions present as pain, swelling, locking, and athletic dysfunction.
- Plain radiographs are typically normal unless there is an osseous component to the injury.
- The modality of choice for the diagnosis is MRI.

Answers

1. The diagnosis is osteochondral defect.

2. The most common location is femoral condyle.

3. The second most common location is the dome of the talus.

4. Symptomatic focal chondral lesions present as pain, swelling, locking, and athletic dysfunction.

5. Treatment options are arthroscopic surgery, conservative therapy, autologous chondrocyte implantation, allografts implantation, and microfracture surgical technique.

Suggested Readings

Gilley JS, Gelman MI, Edson DM, Metcalf RW. Chondral fractures of the knee. Arthrographic, arthroscopic, and clinical manifestations. *Radiology*. 1981;138(1):51-54.

Lindfors DP, Balart JT, Neitzschman HR. Radiology case of the month. Knee pain and swelling in a man. Osteochondral defect. *J La State Med Soc*. 2007;159(2):66-68.

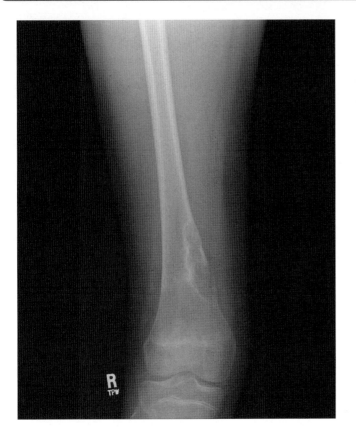
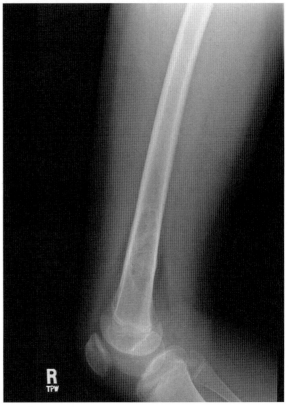

1. What are the names of this entity?

2. How will you radiographically characterize
   the lesion seen in the images?

3. What would the finding be on nuclear medicine
   bone scan?

4. What is the treatment for this entity?

5. What diseases have multiple such lesions?

Case ranking/difficulty: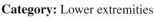

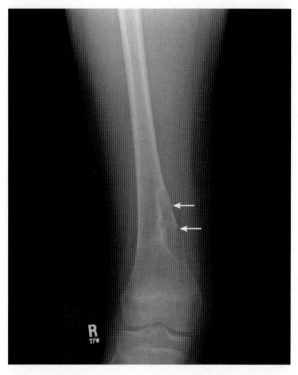

Frontal radiograph of the femur reveals a lytic lesion of the distal femur (*arrows*). The lesion is eccentric, well-circumscribed, with septations, and with sclerotic margins.

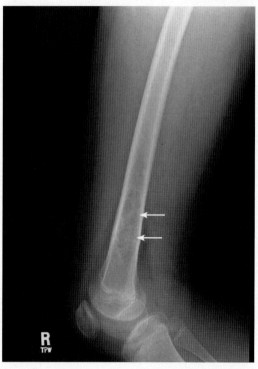

Lateral radiograph of the femur reveals a lytic lesion of the distal femur (*arrows*). The lesion is eccentric, well-circumscribed, with septations, and with sclerotic margins.

Answers

1. Smaller lesions that are less than 3 cm are epicentered at the cortex and are called fibrous cortical defect. Larger lesions more than 3 cm involve medulla and are called non ossifying fibroma or fibroxanthoma.

2. Radiographically, the lesion is lytic, metaphyseal, eccentric, well-circumscribed with surrounding sclerosis.

3. NOF shows normal or mildly increased radiotracer uptake. Significantly increased radiotracer uptake is seen if there is pathologic fracture.

4. No treatment is necessary as the lesion spontaneously regresses and is ususaly asymptomatic. It is also known as "No touch lesion." Only very large lesions or pathologic fracture need treatment.

5. Neurofibromatosis type I and Jaffe Campanacci syndrome show multiple NOFs. Both these conditions show cafe au lait spots on the skin.

Pearls

- A non ossifying fibroma, also called fibroxanthoma, is a benign fibrous lesion of the bone that is usually asymptomatic and detected as an incidental finding on radiographs.
- NOF is the most common benign bone tumor in children and adolescents.
- Most common location is around the knee, ie, distal femur and proximal tibia.
- Radiographically, NOFs are well marginated, eccentric, metaphyseal lesions with narrow zone of transition and sclerotic margin. They may be unilocular or multilocular with septae within it.
- NOF regresses spontaneously over time. Surgery is only required for very large lesions or pathologic fracture.
- Multiple NOFs are seen in neurofibromatosis type I and Jaffe Campanacci syndrome. Patients with both these disorders show cafe au lait spots.

Suggested Reading

Hetts SW, Hilchey SD, Wilson R, Franc B. Case 110: Nonossifying fibroma. *Radiology*. 2007;243(1):288-292.

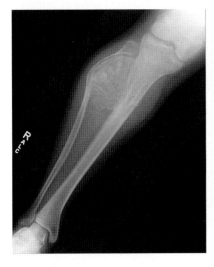 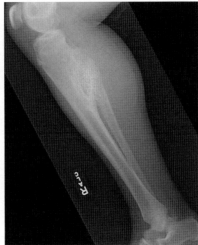 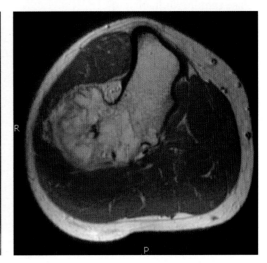

1. What are the findings?

2. What is the most common malignant degeneration that can complicate this lesion?

3. What disease presents with multiple such lesions?

4. What imaging finding is associated with increased risk for transformation to malignancy?

5. What are the treatment options?

Case ranking/difficulty:

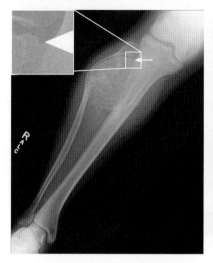

Frontal radiograph of the right tibia shows a mass arising from the proximal right tibia. The periosteum of the tibia is in contiguity with the margins of the mass (*arrow*). There is deformity of the fibula due to the compressive force of the mass.

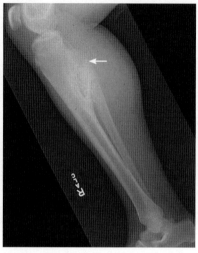

Lateral radiograph of the right tibia shows a mass arising from the proximal right tibia. The perisoteum of the tibia is in contiguity with the margins of the mass (*arrow*). There is a deformity of the fibula due to the compressive force of the mass.

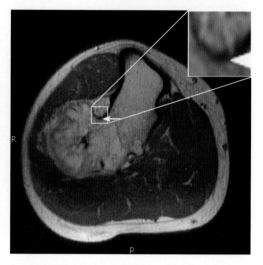

Axial MRI T2 demonstrates a mass arising from the proximal tibia. There is a periosteum around the mass in continuity with the periosteum of the tibia (*arrow*).

Answers

1. There is a mass arising from the proximal right tibia. The cortex of the tibia is in contiguity with the margins of the mass and there is deformity of the fibula.

2. The most common malignant degeneration that can complicate osteochondroma is chondrosarcoma.

3. Multiple lesions as shown in the image are associated with hereditary multiple exostosis (HME).

4. Cartilage cap thickness more than 1 cm has higher association with chondrosarcoma.

5. Symptomatic lesions require resection, which should include perichondrium resection to avoid recurrence. Asymptomatic lesions may be observed. Usually, resection is performed if the cartilage cap measures more than 1 cm as thicker cartilage caps are associated with transformation to chondrosarcoma.

- When osteochondroma involve the long bone, it is located at the metaphysis and tends to grow away from the nearest joint.
- Sudden development of pain or sudden increase in size after skeletal maturation is suspicious for transformation to chondrosarcoma.
- Osteochondroma may present as a lump, pain from nerve impingement, limited motion, or may be asymptomatic.
- Most lesions are solitary. Multiple lesions are seen in HME.
- The cartilaginous cap does not enhance and appear hyperintense on T2-weighted MRI with surrounding thin hypointense perichondrium. The cartilagenous cap may show calcification. Calcific areas are hypointense on T2.
- Resection is performed if the cartilage cap measures more than 1 cm as thicker cartilage caps are associated with transformation to chondrosarcoma.

Pearls

- Osteochondroma or exostosis is a benign cartilage capped exophytic growth of the bone where the cortex and medulla of the lesion are continuous with that of the parent bone.
- Osteochondroma can be sessile or pedunculated.
- Most common location is around the knee, but can also be seen in the humerus, vertebra, and other bones.

Suggested Readings

Ramos-Pascua LR, Sanchez-Herraez S, Alonso-Barrio JA, Alonso-Leon A. Solitary proximal end of femur osteochondroma. An indication and result of the en bloc resection without hip luxation. *Rev Esp Cir Ortop Traumatol*. 2012;56(1):24-31.

Stoller DW, Tirman PF, Bredella MA, Branstetter R, Blease S, Beltran S. *Diagnostic Imaging: Orthopaedics*. Salt Lake City, Utah, USA: Amirsys; 2003.

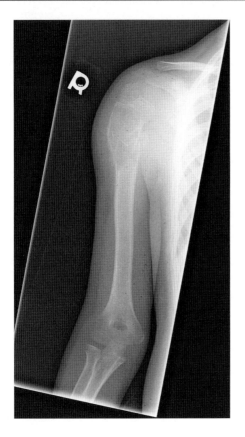 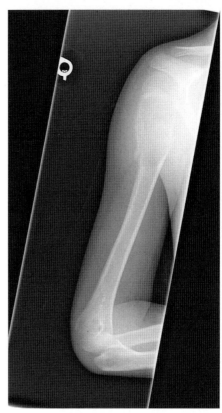

1. What are the findings?

2. What is the most common location of this lesion?

3. What is the etiology of this case?

4. What is the linear bone density noted inside the lesion?

5. What are the treatment options?

Case ranking/difficulty: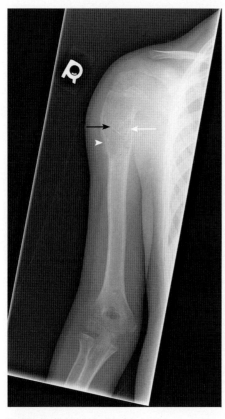

Category: Upper extremities

Frontal radiograph of the right humerus shows a septated lytic lesion in the proximal humerus. Fracture of the medial aspect of the lesion noted (*white arrow*). The *black arrow* points to the fallen fragment sign. *White arrowhead* points to healing of a fracture in the lateral aspect of the lesion.

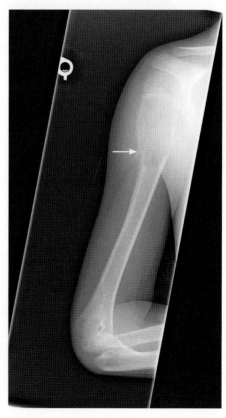

Frontal radiograph of the right humerus shows a lytic septated lesion in the proximal humerus. There is a healing fracture in the lateral aspect of the lesion (*arrow*).

Answers

1. There is a lytic lesion in the proximal humerus. The lesion has septations. Pathologic fracture is seen.

2. In 90% of cases, unicameral bone cyst is found in the proximal humerus.

3. The etiology is not known.

4. The fallen fragment sign is seen as a bony fragment floating inside the fluid-filled cyst. It appears following a pathologic fracture.

5. Treatment may include observation in the absence of trauma and the patient is asymptomatic. It may include analgesics if pain occurs. Curettage and packing with bone allograft material, and subtotal resection with or without grafting may be considered.

Pearls

- A unicameral bone cyst is a benign, fluid-filled lesion found in children.
- In the absence of a fracture through the cyst, unicameral bone cysts are asymptomatic.
- On plain radiograph, the lesion appears as a lytic, concentric, septated with cortical thinning.
- The lesion is prone to pathologic fractures.
- The fallen-fragment sign is found in approximately 20% of patients who present with a pathologic fracture secondary to a unicameral bone cyst. The fallen fragment is seen because the unicameral bone cyst is filled with fluid and is not a solid.

Suggested Reading

Lokiec F, Wientroub S. Simple bone cyst: etiology, classification, pathology, and treatment modalities. *J Pediatr Orthop B*. 1998;7(4):262-273.

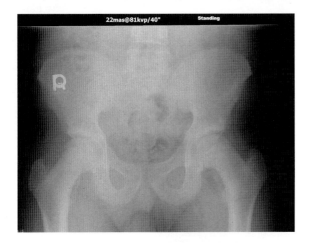
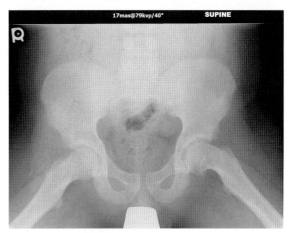
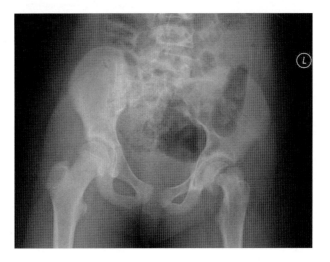

1. What is the early radiographic sign of this case?

2. Why the treatment of this case is urgent?

3. What are the characteristic imaging features of this entity?

4. Which side of this entity is more commonly affected?

5. In younger patients, this entity may be associated with which disorders?

Case ranking/difficulty: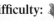

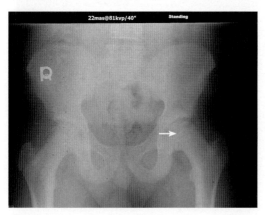

The finding in the frontal radiograph of the pelvis is very subtle. There is minimally widening of the growth plate in the left femur (*arrow*) when compared to the right growth plate.

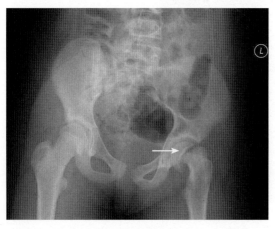

Frontal radiograph of the pelvis and hips shows medial displacement of the left femoral head (*arrow*). If a line is drawn along the lateral surface of the left femoral neck, it will not intersect with the femoral head. The left growth plate is severely widened when compared to the right.

Answers

1. The early radiographic sign of slipped capital femoral epiphysis is widening of the proximal femoral growth plate.

2. Treatment of this entity is urgent to prevent avascular necrosis of the affected femoral head.

3. Characteristic imaging features are widening of the growth plate and the femoral head is displaced medially and posteriorly in relation to the femoral neck. In MRI, joint effusion may be seen.

4. The left side is more commonly affected than the right.

5. In children less than 10 years old, the disease may be associated with hypothyroidism, hypogonadism, renal osteodystrophy, panhypopituitarism, and growth hormone abnormalities.

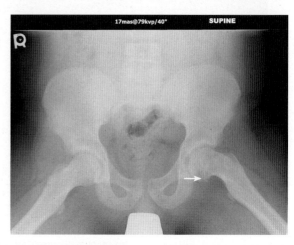

Frontal radiograph in abduction view of the pelvis and hips shows medial displacement of the left femoral head (*arrow*). If a line is drawn along the lateral surface of the left femoral neck, it will not touch or intersect with the lateral aspect of the left femoral head.

Pearls

- Slipped capital femoral epiphysis is one of the most important pediatric and adolescent hip disorders encountered in medical practice.
- The left hip is affected more commonly than the right.
- In patients younger than 10 years, slipped capital femoral epiphysis is associated with metabolic endocrine disorders (eg, hypothyroidism, panhypopituitarism, hypogonadism, renal osteodystrophy, growth hormone abnormalities).
- Bilateral slipped capital femoral epiphysis is more common in younger patients.
- On plain radiographs, the femoral head is seen displaced, posteriorly and inferiorly in relation to the femoral neck and within the confines of the acetabulum.
- Slippage must be suspected if a straight line drawn along the lateral surface of femoral neck does not touch the femoral head (Klein's line sign).

Suggested Readings

Katz DA. Slipped capital femoral epiphysis: the importance of early diagnosis. *Pediatr Ann*. 2006;35(2):102-111.

Lehmann CL, Arons RR, Loder RT, Vitale MG. The epidemiology of slipped capital femoral epiphysis: an update. *J Pediatr Orthop*. 2006;26(3):286-290.

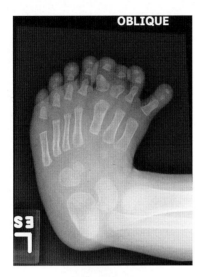 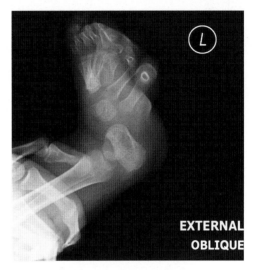

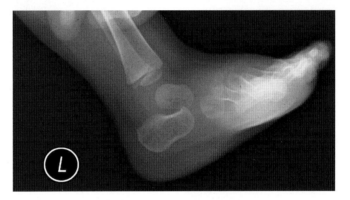

1. What are the findings?

2. What can be etiology of this entity?

3. What are the syndromes that this entity may be associated with?

4. What are the imaging modalities for the diagnosis of this entity?

5. What is the approximate age that corrective surgery should be performed?

Case ranking/difficulty: 🎋

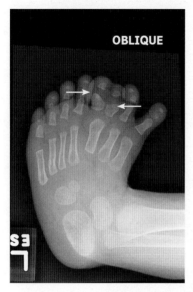

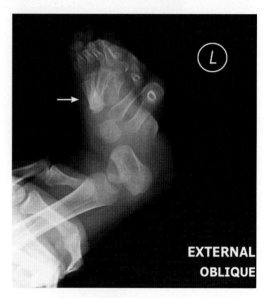

Oblique radiograph of the left foot reveals seven metatarsals and eight sets of phalanges. The third metatarsal has two sets of phalanges; each of them has only two phalanges (*arrows*).

Oblique radiograph of the left foot (*arrow*) reveals seven metatarsals. The 3rd metatarsal has two sets of phalanges.

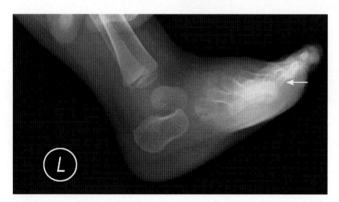

Lateral radiograph of the left foot (*arrow*) reveals seven metatarsals. The third metatarsal has two sets of phalanges.

5. Surgery is indicated to improve the appearance of the foot and to improve foot-wear. It is usually performed when the patient is aged approximately 1 year, so the effect on development and walking is minimal.

Pearls

- Polydactyly can be isolated or part of a syndrome.
- Most commonly occurs in the lateral ray.
- Polydactyly may occur as a duplication of a digit or duplication of multiple digits.
- Radiographs are essential prior to surgery, so that the anatomy can be understood.
- Delaying treatment until ossification centers are developed is recommended.

Answers

1. There are seven metatarsals and eight sets of phalanges. The third metatarsal has two sets of phalanges; each of them contains only two phalanges.

2. The etiology of polydactyly is congenital. It can be a feature of a syndrome of congenital anomalies or self-entity without association with a syndrome.

3. The syndromes with which polydactyly has been associated include Ellis-van Creveld syndrome, trisomy 13, tibial hemimelia, and trisomy 21.

4. Plain radiography is usually adequate. In complicated cases, CT and MRI may be performed to evaluate the anatomy.

Suggested Readings

Turra S, Gigante C, Bisinella G. Polydactyly of the foot. *J Pediatr Orthop B*. 2007;16(3):216-220.

Venn-Watson EA. Problems in polydactyly of the foot. *Orthop Clin North Am*. 1976;7(4):909-927.

Yucel A, Kuru I, Bozan ME, Acar M, Solak M. Radiographic evaluation and unusual bone formations in different genetic patterns in synpolydactyly. *Skeletal Radiol*. 2005;34(8):468-476.

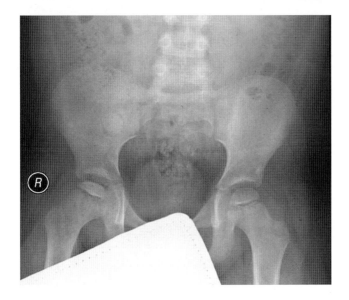 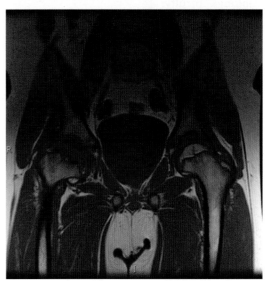

1. What is the pathophysiology of this entity?

2. What are the clinical features of this entity?

3. What are the radiographic features of this entity?

4. What are the magnetic resonance imaging features of the chronic phase of this entity?

5. What is the age range that this entity most likely develops?

Case ranking/difficulty:

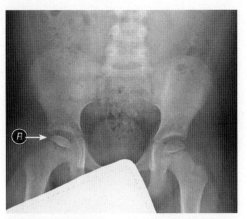

Frontal radiograph of the pelvis demonstrates sclerosis and decrease in height of the right femoral head (*arrow*). This is the chronic phase of the disease.

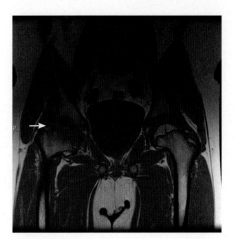

Coronal MRI T1 demonstrates low signal and decrease in height of the right femoral head (*arrow*). This is the chronic phase of the disease.

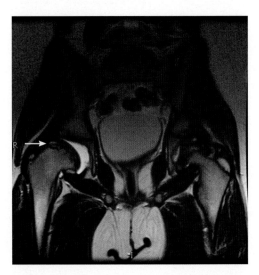

Coronal MRI T2 demonstrates low signal and decrease in height of the right femoral head (*arrow*). Small amount of fluid noted in the right hip. This is the chronic phase of the disease.

and in T2-weighted sequences. During the acute phase, there may be edema in the femoral head and T2-weighted sequence may show high signal. The femoral head may show contrast enhancement during the healing phase.

5. The age range that this entity most likely develops is between 2 and 12 years.

Answers

1. The diagnosis is avascular necrosis of the femoral head, and the blood supply to the femoral head is interrupted.

2. The clinical features are pain, gait disturbance, decreased range of motion of the affected hip, and muscle spasm.

3. The radiographic features of this entity are subchondral lucencies, fragmentation of the femoral head, sclerosis of the femoral head, and decrease in height of the femoral head. The findings vary according to the time interval following the event (interruption of blood supply to the femoral head).

4. Magnetic resonance imaging features of the chronic phase of this entity are low signal in T1-weighted sequence

Pearls

- Legg-Calvé-Perthes disease is the name given to idiopathic osteonecrosis of the capital femoral epiphysis, the femoral head.
- The blood supply to the femoral head is interrupted.
- Patients have pain, gait disturbance, and decreased range of motion of the affected hip. Muscle spasm and atrophy may occur.
- Radiographically, there is cessation of growth at the capital femoral epiphysis; larger and wider femoral head epiphysis (coxa magna), and widening of articular space on the affected side.
- Magnetic resonance imaging demonstrates low signal in T1- and T2-weighted images. Small amount of joint effusion may be seen.

Suggested Readings

Kaniklides C. Diagnostic radiology in Legg-Calve-Perthes disease. *Acta Radiol Suppl.* 1996;406:1-28.

Roy DR. Current concepts in Legg-Calve-Perthes disease. *Pediatr Ann.* 1999;28(12):748-752.

Thompson GH, Salter RB. Legg-Calve-Perthes disease. *Clin Symp.* 1986;38(1):2-31.

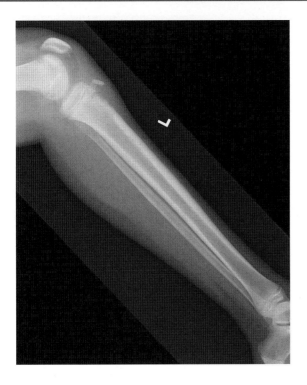 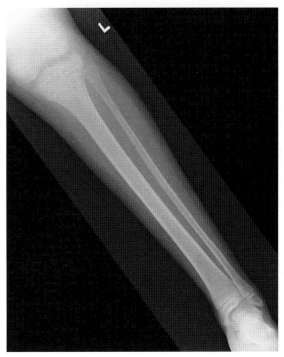

1. What are the findings?

2. What is the most common clinical presentation of this case?

3. What is age range that the disease occurs?

4. What is the cause of the disease?

5. What are the treatment options?

Case ranking/difficulty: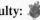

Category: Lower extremities

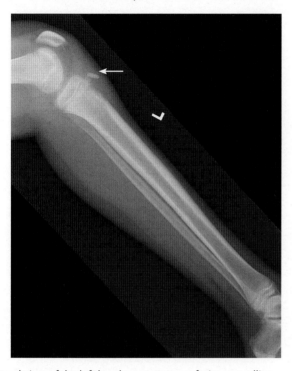

Lateral view of the left leg demonstrates soft tissue swelling adjacent to the tibial tuberosity. Avulsion of a fragment of the tibial tuberosity noted (*arrow*).

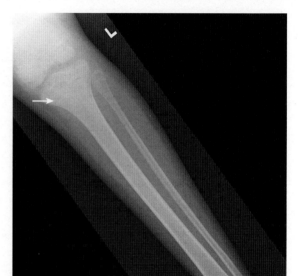

Frontal view of the left leg demonstrates a lucent line (*arrow*) that represents the normal tibial tuberosity. The avulsed fragment could not be visualized.

Answers

1. There is a soft tissue swelling adjacent to the tibial tuberosity, fragmented tibial tuberosity with avulsed fragment.

2. Pain is the most common presenting complaint.

3. The age range that Osgood Schlatter's disease occurs is between 9 and 16 years.

4. Osgood-Schlatter's disease occurs due to a period of rapid growth, combined with a high level of sporting activity. It is associated with traction apophysitis of the tibial tubercle due to repetitive strain on the secondary ossification center of the tibial tubercle.

5. Treatment is conservative. Recommended conservative treatments are ice, analgesics, activity restriction, stretching, strengthening, or anti-inflammatory medications.

Pearls

- Osgood-Schlatter's disease is generally a benign, self-limited disease of the knee.
- Relief of symptoms occurs with rest or restriction of activities.
- The Osgood-Schlatter's lesion is best seen on the lateral radiograph with the knee in slight internal rotation of 10 to 20 degrees. Irregular ossification of the proximal tibial tuberosity and soft tissue edema proximal to the tibial tuberosity are seen.

Suggested Readings

Gottsegen CJ, Eyer BA, White EA, Learch TJ, Forrester D. Avulsion fractures of the knee: imaging findings and clinical significance. *Radiographics*. 2008;28(6):1755-1770.

Rosenberg ZS, Kawelblum M, Cheung YY, Beltran J, Lehman WB, Grant AD. Osgood-Schlatter lesion: fracture or tendinitis? Scintigraphic, CT, and MR imaging features. *Radiology*. 1992;185(3):853-858.

Smith JB. Knee problems in children. *Pediatr Clin North Am*. 1986;33(6):1439-1456.

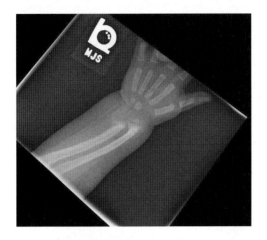
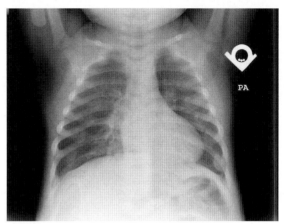
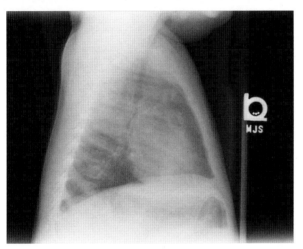
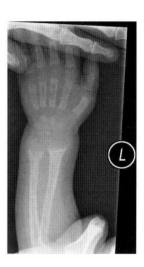

1. What is the active form of vitamin D?

2. What are the findings in the shown images?

3. In which part of the body is the pattern of rachitic rosary seen?

4. What is the most common risk factor for the entity shown in the images?

5. How is this condition treated?

Case ranking/difficulty: 🔥

Category: Generalized diseases

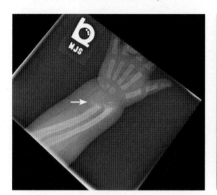

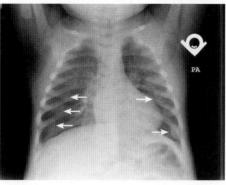

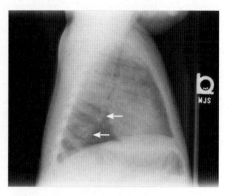

Frontal radiograph of the wrist shows widening and cupping of the metaphysis of the radius and ulna (*arrow*) with irregular calcification. There is decreased zone of the provisional calcification.

Frontal radiograph of the chest shows prominent knobs of bone at the costochondral joints that resembles string of beads, known as rachitic rosary (*arrows*).

Lateral radiograph of the chest shows prominent knobs of bone at the costochondral joints that resembles string of beads, known as rachitic rosary (*arrows*).

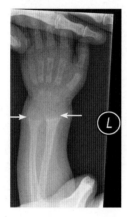

Frontal radiograph of the wrist shows widening and cupping of the metaphysis of the radius and ulna (*arrows*) with irregular calcification. There is decreased zone of the provisional calcification.

Answers

1. The active form of vitamin D is 1,25-dihydroxycholecalciferol.

2. The radiographic findings of the entity shown include flaring and cupping of the metaphysis of long bones, decreased zone of provisional calcifications, irregular calcifications of the metaphysis of long bones, and string of beads appearance of the costo-chondral junctions.

3. The pattern of rachitic rosary is seen in the chest. The chest radiograph demonstrates widened costo-chondral junctions that resemble a string of beads.

4. Malnutrition is the most common risk factor for developing the entity shown in the image. Hepatic and renal disease and malabsorption are also risk factors, but are less common.

5. The entity described above is treated with vitamin D supplementation.

Pearls

- Rickets is a disorder caused by a lack of vitamin D, calcium, or phosphate.
- It leads to softening and weakening of the bones. Infants who are only breast-fed may develop vitamin D deficiency.
- The active form of the vitamin D 1,25-dihydroxycholecalciferol is responsible for the regulation of the calcium and phosphor in the body.
- Intestinal mal-absorption of fat and diseases of the liver or kidney may produce the clinical and the secondary biochemical picture of nutritional rickets.

Suggested Readings

Chapman T, Sugar N, Done S, Marasigan J, Wambold N, Feldman K. Fractures in infants and toddlers with rickets. *Pediatr Radiol*. 2010;40(7):1184-1189.

Harrison HE, Harrison HC. *Disorders of Calcium and Phosphate Metabolism in Childhood and Adolescence*. Philadelphia: WB Saunders Co; 1979.

Zmora E, Gorodischer R, Bar-Ziv J. Multiple nutritional deficiencies in infants from a strict vegetarian community. *Am J Dis Child*. 1979;133(2):141-144.

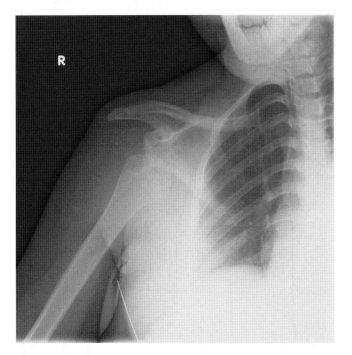
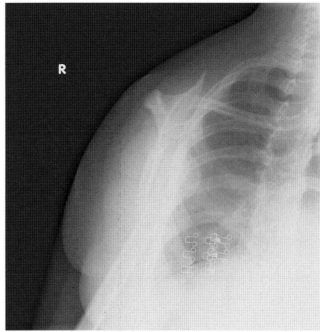

1. What is the etiology of this case?

2. What is the approximate percentage of this type of dislocation when compared to all types of shoulder dislocations?

3. What is the mechanism of the ocurrence of this entity in children?

4. What are the structures that maintain the integrity of the shoulder?

5. What is the management of the case?

Case ranking/difficulty:

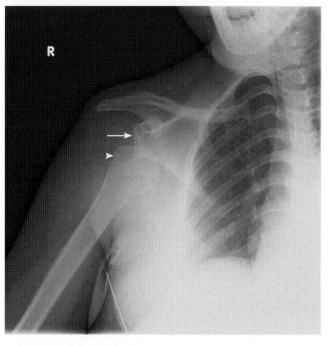

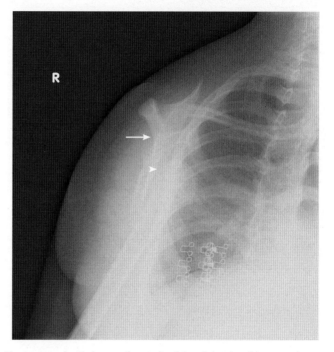

Frontal radiograph of the right shoulder reveals malalignment between the glenoid (*arrow*) and the humeral head (*arrowhead*). The humeral head is seen inferiorly and medially relative to the glenoid fossa.

Trans-scapular Y view radiograph of the right shoulder reveals that the humeral head (*arrowhead*) is inferior and anterior relative to the junction of the coracoid process and the acromion (*arrow*).

Answers

1. The etiology of anterior shoulder dislocation is traumatic.

2. 98% of all shoulder dislocations are anterior.

3. The mechanism of anterior shoulder dislocation is abduction, extension, and external rotation.

4. The structures that maintain the integrity of the shoulder are glenohumeral joint capsule, cartilaginous glenoid labrum, and muscles of the rotator cuff.

5. Management of the case include analgesics to decrease pain, pre-reduction and post reduction radiographs, immobilization of the shoulder after reduction, placement of a pillow between the patient's arm and torso to increase comfort, and treatment of associated trauma as indicated.

Pearls

- The shoulder is the most frequently dislocated joint.
- Anterior dislocations occur in as many as 98% of cases.
- Anterior shoulder dislocations usually result from abduction, extension, and external rotation, such as when preparing for a volleyball spike.
- The humeral head is forced out of the glenohumeral joint, rupturing or detaching the anterior capsule from its attachment to the head of the humerus or from its insertion to the edge of the glenoid fossa. This occurs with or without lateral detachment.
- Plain radiographs are the modality of choice for diagnosis.
- Three views should be obtained: Frontal view, trans-scapular Y view, and, if the patient can cooperate, an axillary view.

Suggested Readings

Rubin SA, Gray RL, Green WR. The scapular "Y": a diagnostic aid in shoulder trauma. *Radiology*. 1974;110(3):725-726.

Vastamaki M. Recurrent anterior shoulder dislocation. A review. *Ann Chir Gynaecol*. 1996;85(2):133-136.

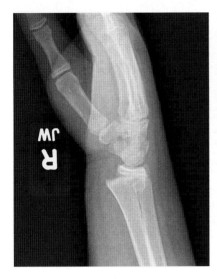 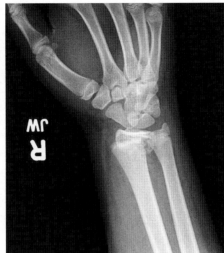 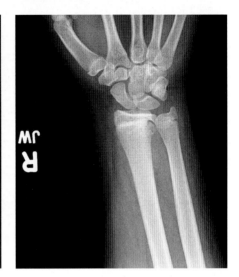

1. What are the findings?

2. What is the definition of Salter-Harris fracture?

3. What is the most common type of fractures
   in the Salter-Harris classification?

4. Which type in the Salter-Harris classification
   involves only the physis?

5. Which type in the Salter-Harris classification
   involves the metaphysis and the epiphysis?

Case ranking/difficulty:

Category: Upper extremities

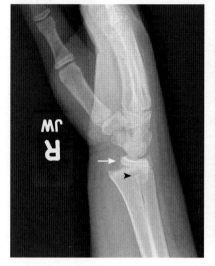

Lateral radiograph of the right hand shows Salter-Harris type I fracture (*arrow*) with displacement of the epiphysis dorsally. Salter-Harris type II fracture is seen (*arrowhead*).

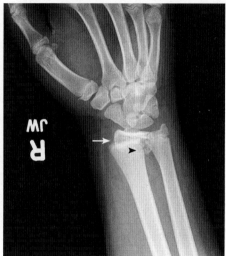

Oblique radiograph of the right hand shows Salter-Harris type I fracture (*arrow*) with displacement of the epiphysis dorsally. Salter-Harris type II fracture is seen (*arrowhead*).

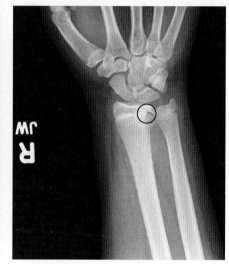

Frontal radiograph of the right hand shows Salter-Harris type II fracture (*circle*).

Answers

1. There is fracture of the distal radial physis with fracture of the distal radial metaphysis that abuts the growth plate (Salter-Harris II). The epiphysis is displaced dorsally.

2. Salter-Harris fracture is a fracture that involves through the growth plate.

3. Type II is the most common type of fractures that involves the physis. This fracture involves the metaphysis and the physis.

4. Type I is a transverse fracture of the physis without involvement of the metaphysis or the epiphysis. Type V is a complete crush injury of the physis without involvement of the metaphysis and the epiphysis.

5. Type IV in the Salter-Harris classification involves the metaphysis and the epiphysis. By definition of Salter-Harris fracture, the physis is always involved.

Pearls

- Salter-Harris fracture is a fracture through the growth plate of a pediatric patient.
- Occurs in 15% of childhood long bone fractures.
- Classified by types I to V.
- The classification is important as it affects treatment.

Suggested Readings

Lemburg SP, Lilienthal E, Heyer CM. Growth plate fractures of the distal tibia: is CT imaging necessary? *Arch Orthop Trauma Surg.* 2010;130(11):1411-1417.

Peart O. Detecting a Salter-Harris fracture. *Radiol Technol.* 2012;83(4):395.

White PG, Mah JY, Friedman L. Magnetic resonance imaging in acute physeal injuries. *Skeletal Radiol.* 1994;23(8):627-631.

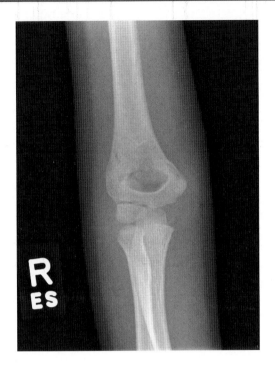 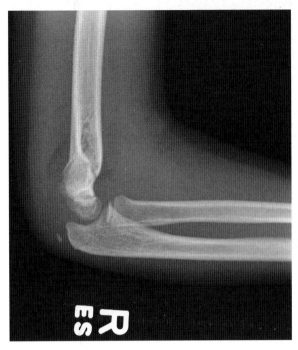

1. What are the findings?

2. What is the clinical significance of elevation of the dorsal fat pad in distal humerus?

3. What are possible complications of the shown entity?

4. What is the mechanism of injury of this entity?

5. What are the treatment options?

Case ranking/difficulty: 🐾

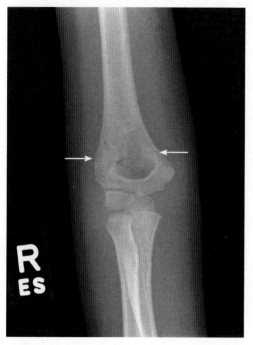

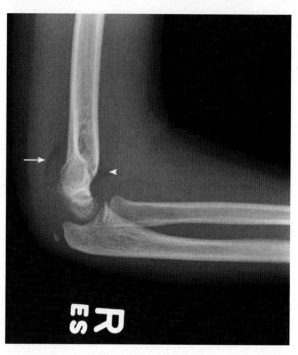

Frontal radiograph of the right elbow demonstrates a lucent line in the distal humerus, supracondylar region (*arrows*) representing a fracture.

Lateral radiograph of the right elbow demonstrates elevation of the posterior fat pad (*arrow*). The ventral fat pad is also elevated (*arrowhead*). The lucent line representing the fracture still noted (between the two fat pads). The distal humerus is dorsally angulated.

Answers

1. There is supracondylar fracture with elevation of the dorsal and the ventral fat pads of the distal humerus. The distal humerus is dorsally angulated.

2. Elevation of the dorsal fat pad of the distal humerus is significant only for joint effusion. It is not significant for a fracture. However, with a fracture there is secondary joint effusion, most likely traumatic effusion such as hemarthrosis. The effusion causes the elevation of the fat pad and not the fracture. Elevation of the fat pads can be seen in other conditions such as arthritis with joint effusion. Elevation of the dorsal fat pad is always pathologic. The ventral fat pad can be normally elevated without pathologic condition.

3. Complications of supracondylar fracture may include neurovascular injuries, post-traumatic periarticular calcification, myositis ossificans, avascular necrosis, and/ or intra-articular loose bodies.

4. The fracture is caused by fall on an outstretched hand in 70% of cases. As the hands hits the ground, the elbow is hyperextended, resulting in fracture above the condyles.

5. In mild cases, immobilization with cast is adequate to facilitate healing. K-wires fixation device often used. In severe cases with displacement of intra-articular fragments, surgery is needed.

Pearls

- A supracondylar fracture is a fracture of the distal humerus above the epicondyles.
- Mechanism of injury is fall on an outstretched hand with hyperextended elbow in 70% of the cases.
- The fracture is mostly extra-articular.
- The fracture is difficult to identify on radiographs.
- Plain radiographs demonstrate lucent line above the epicondyles. Dorsal fat pad is usually elevated. Angulation and usually dorsal displacement may occur.

Suggested Readings

Allen SR, Hang JR, Hau RC. Review article: paediatric supracondylar humeral fractures: emergency assessment and management. *Emerg Med Australas.* 2010;22(5): 418-426.

Bryan RS, Morrey BF. Fractures of the distal humerus. In: Morrey BF, ed. *The Elbow and Its Disorders.* Philadelphia: WB Saunders Co; 1985:302-339.

Pollock JW, Faber KJ, Athwal GS. Distal humerus fractures. *Orthop Clin North Am.* 2008;39(2):187-200, vi.

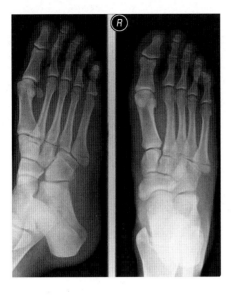 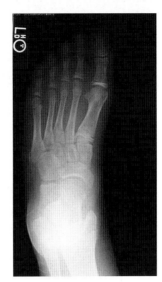 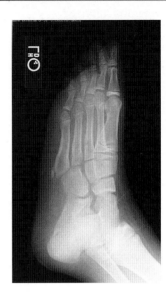

1. What are the findings?

2. What is the orientation of normal apophyseal line of the base of the fifth metatarsal?

3. In the provided images, what is the orientation of the abnormality in relation to the axis of the fifth metatarsal?

4. What is the differential diagnosis?

5. What is the most common treatment of this entity?

Case ranking/difficulty: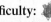

Category: Lower extremities

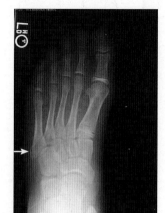

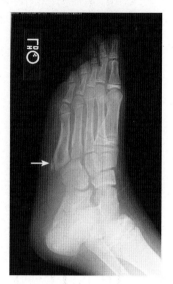

Frontal (right) and oblique (left) radiographs of the right foot demonstrate a fracture of the base of the fifth metatarsal (*arrow*). The fracture line is perpendicular to the shaft.

X-ray of the left foot of another patient demonstrates the normal apophyseal line, which is parallel to the shaft of the metatarsal (*arrow*).

X-ray of the left foot of another patient demonstrates the normal apophyseal line, which is parallel to the shaft of the metatarsal (*arrow*).

Answers

1. Fracture line seen in the base of the fifth metatarsal.

2. The apophyseal line of the base of the fifth metatarsal is parallel to the long axis of the shaft.

3. The fracture of the base of the fifth metatarsal is oriented perpendicular to the shaft of the fifth metatarsal, while normal apophysis is parallel to the axis of the fifth metatarsal and should not be mistaken for a fracture.

4. The differential diagnosis include normal apophysis, os peroneum, and stress fracture.

5. The most common way to treat a non displaced Jones fracture is casting.

Pearls

- Jones fracture is a fracture of the base of the fifth metatarsal.
- The fracture is perpendicular to the shaft of the fifth metatarsal.
- Frequently confused with normal apophysis, in which the apolyseal line is oriented parallel to the shaft of the fifth metatarsal.
- Diagnosis is simple by plain foot radiograph.
- Treatment is usually made by casting.

Suggested Readings

Rhim B, Hunt JC. Lisfranc injury and Jones fracture in sports. *Clin Podiatr Med Surg*. 2011;28(1):69-86.

Sethuraman U, Grover SK, Kannikeswaran N. Tarsometatarsal injury in a child. *Pediatr Emerg Care*. 2009;25(9):594-596.

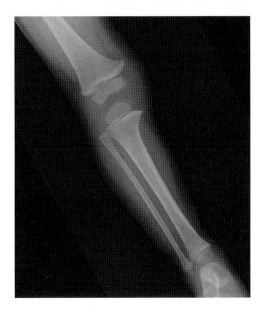 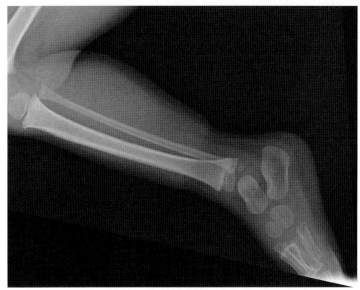

1. What are the findings?

2. What is the most common location of this entity?

3. What is the mechanism for the appearance of this entity?

4. What is the typical age that this entity occurs?

5. What is the management of this case?

Case ranking/difficulty: 🌑

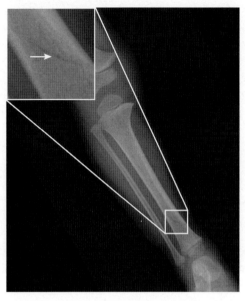

Frontal radiograph of the right tibia demonstrates a lucent line (*arrow*) in the distal tibial diaphysis representing a fracture.

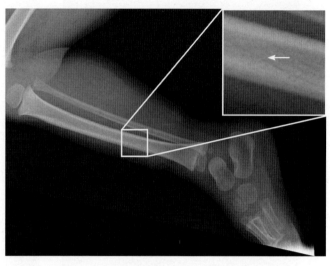

Lateral radiograph of the right tibia demonstrates a lucent line in the distal tibial diaphysis (*arrow*) representing a fracture.

Answers

1. There is a lucent line in the distal tibial diaphysis. Based on the history and the age of the patient, this is consistent with the Toddler's fracture.

2. Toddler's fracture is most commonly seen in the tibia.

3. Shear stress and minor trauma is the mechanism for Toddler's fracture.

4. Peak incidence of the Toddler's fracture is between 1 and 2 years of age. Usually, minor stress leads to this type of fracture when toddlers start walking.

5. Casting for 3 weeks.

Pearls

- Toddler's fracture is a spiral, non displaced fracture of the distal tibia usually seen in children when they start to walk.
- It is common between 1 to 3 years of age.
- It is a stress fracture.
- Initial radiograph may show a subtle oblique lucency or may not show the fracture. Follow-up radiograph after 1 to 2 weeks shows sclerotic linear density at the site of fracture due to callus formation.

- Toddler's fracture is very common and usually not due to child abuse. However, fracture of tibia in a child who is not yet walking should raise suspicion of child maltreatment.
- Although other modalities like CT scan, MRI, and nuclear medicine bone scan can demonstrate Toddler's fracture, these studies are usually not required for diagnosis.
- The clinical presentation is a toddler who has recently started walking, refusing to walk and bearing weight.

Suggested Readings

Halsey MF, Finzel KC, Carrion WV, Haralabatos SS, Gruber MA, Meinhard BP. Toddler's fracture: presumptive diagnosis and treatment. *J Pediatr Orthop*. 2001;21(2): 152-156.

Mellick LB, Milker L, Egsieker E. Childhood accidental spiral tibial (CAST) fractures. *Pediatr Emerg Care*. 1999;15(5):307-309.

Sarmah A. Toddler's fracture? A recognised entity. *Arch Dis Child*. 1995;72(4):376.

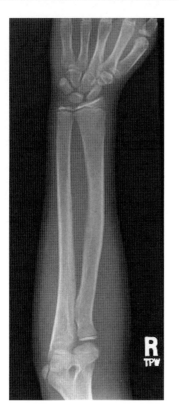 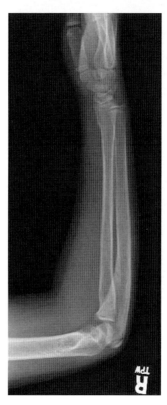

1. What type of fracture is seen?

2. Which bone is most commonly affected in this entity?

3. What is the mechanism contributing to this entity?

4. Describe the findings that may present in this entity.

5. What are the treatment options?

Case ranking/difficulty: 🏵️

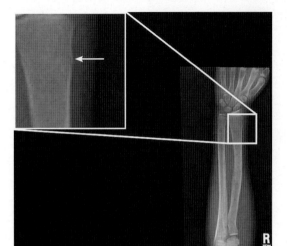

Frontal radiograph of the right forearm shows outward bulging of the lateral aspect of the distal radial cortex (*arrow*).

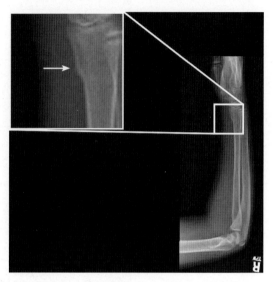

Lateral radiograph of the right forearm shows outward bulging of the anterior aspect of the distal radial cortex (*arrow*).

Answers

1. The diagnosis is Torus fracture (or Buckle fracture).

2. The most common bone affected in this entity is the distal radius.

3. The mechanisms contributing to this entity include axial loading, compression forces, fall on outstretched hands, and hyperextension.

4. The findings may include unilateral outward bulging of the bony cortex, bulging of the bony cortex in either end of the metaphysis, inward bulging with angulation of the bony cortex, or only inward bulging.

5. Casting is the only treatment for noncomplicated Buckle fracture.

Pearls

- Buckle fracture (or Torus fracture) are very common in children.
- The mechanism of injury is forces distributed evenly across the metaphysis of the bone; the cortex bends resulting in unilateral or bilateral outward bulging of the bone.
- Because children have softer bones, one side of the bone may buckle upon itself without disrupting the other side.
- The most common bone affected is the distal radius.

Suggested Readings

Bozentka DJ, Beredjiklian PK, Westawski D, Steinberg DR. Digital radiographs in the assessment of distal radius fracture parameters. *Clin Orthop Relat Res.* 2002;397:409-413.

Reed MH. Fractures and dislocations of the extremities in children. *J Trauma.* 1977;17:351-354.

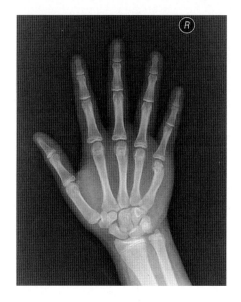 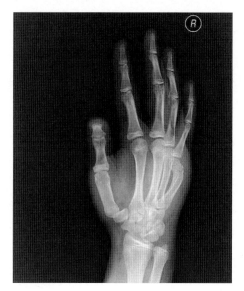 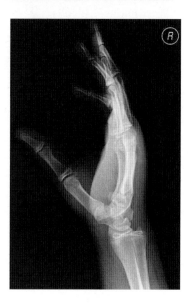

1. What is the finding?

2. What metacarpals may be involved in this entity?

3. What is the mechanism that contributes to this case?

4. In what direction does the apex of the angulation of the case point to?

5. What are the other names for this fracture?

Case ranking/difficulty: 🖑

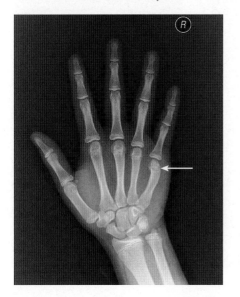

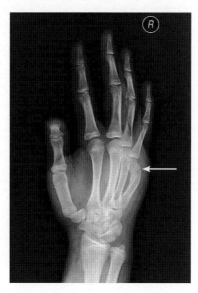

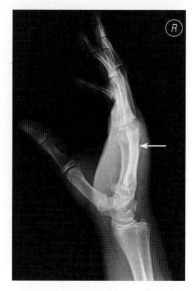

Frontal radiograph of the right wrist reveals fracture of the fifth metacarpal neck with apex ulnar angulation (*arrow*).

Oblique radiograph of the right wrist reveals fracture of the fifth metacarpal neck with apex ulnar angulation (*arrow*).

Lateral radiograph of the right wrist reveals fracture of the fifth metacarpal neck with apex dorsal angulation (*arrow*).

Answers

1. Fracture of fifth metacarpal neck called Boxer's fracture.

2. The fifth or fourth metacarpals may be involved in Boxer's fracture.

3. Striking a solid object with a clenched fist can lead to Boxer's fracture.

4. The apex of the angulation in Boxer's fracture is usually ulnar and dorsal.

5. Brawler's fracture and bar room fracture.

Pearls

- Boxer's fractures occur in the fourth and fifth metacarpal bones.
- The fracture usually occurs at the neck of the fifth metacarpal, which forms the knuckle of the little finger.
- It usually results from striking a solid object with a clenched fist.

Suggested Readings

Ashkenaze DM, Ruby LK. Metacarpal fractures and dislocations. *Orthop Clin North Am.* 1992;23(1):19-33.

Cornwall R. Finger metacarpal fractures and dislocations in children. *Hand Clin.* 2006;22(1):1-10.

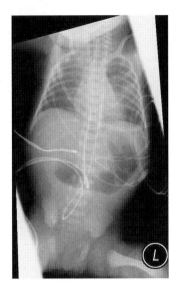 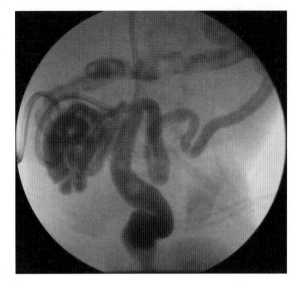

1. What are the findings?

2. What is the etiology of this entity?

3. What may cause this entity?

4. What are the entities that may be associated with the case?

5. What is the most commonly required treatment?

Case ranking/difficulty:

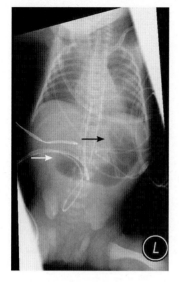

Frontal radiograph of the chest and abdomen reveals air in the stomach (*black arrow*) and air in the proximal duodenum (*white arrow*). Otherwise, the abdomen is gasless and no air is seen distally.

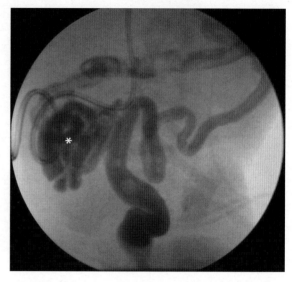

Water-soluble contrast enema reveals a colon small in caliber. Reflux to the distal ileum noted (*asterisk*).

Answers

1. The colon is noted to be small in caliber, consistent with the microcolon.

2. The etiology is congenital.

3. Microcolon is caused by a non-used colon during the fetal life. Reasons can be: ileal atresia, jejunal atresia, total colonic aganglionosis, meconium plug ileus, and cystic fibrosis that can lead to meconium ileus.

4. The entity shown is associated with cystic fibrosis. Also, it can be associated with megacystis-microcolon-intestinal hypoperistalsis syndrome.

5. Most commonly surgery is required, depending on the etiology.

Pearls

- Microcolon is a radiological finding of a colon of small caliber on barium enema examination.
- Differential diagnosis includes mecomium plug ileus in patients with cystic fibrosis. Viscous meconium is trapped in the small bowel and does not move into the colon. The colon remains empty of material and does not distend.
- Microcolon can be due to functional immaturity. In this case, small amount of meconium can be found in the colon, but not enough to cause distension.
- Treatment depends on the etiology. If ileal atresia is present, immediate surgery is necessary. If the cause is functional, the treatment is conservative with multiple enemas that can lead to colonic dilation and normal function.
- In this case, the cause was due to proximal jejunal atresia.

Suggested Readings

LeQuesne G, Reilly B. Functional immaturity of the large bowel in the newborn infant. *Radiol Clin North Am.* 1975;13:331-342.

Loening-Baucke V, Kimura K. Failure to pass meconium: diagnosing neonatal intestinal obstruction. *Am Fam Physician.* 1999;60(7):2043-2050.

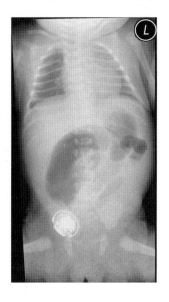 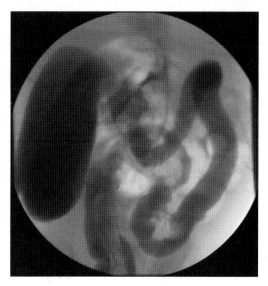

1. Describe the findings.

2. What are the predisposing factors of the case?

3. What is the presumed pathophysiology
   of the case?

4. What are the clinical symptoms?

5. What are the treatment options?

Case ranking/difficulty:

Category: Gastrointestinal

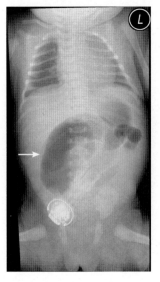

Frontal abdominal radiograph shows a dilated loop of bowel suggestive of obstruction (*arrow*).

Fluoroscopic contrast enema demonstrates narrowed left and transverse colon (*black arrows*) with significantly dilated right colon (*arrowhead*). Transitional zone is noted in the region of the hepatic flexure (*white arrow*).

Answers

1. In the plain abdominal radiograph, a loop of bowel appears dilated suggestive of obstruction. The contrast enema demonstrates that the left colon and the transverse colon are small when compared to the dilated right colon. Transitional zone is noted at the level of the hepatic flexure.

2. Predisposing factors for neonatal small left colon syndrome include a diabetic mother, cystic fibrosis with development of meconium plug, hypermagnesemia, and aganglionosis of the entire left colon (Hirshprung's disease).

3. The presumed pathophysiology of the case is neurohumoral imbalance between the autonomic nervous system and glucagon.

4. All patients do not pass meconium within the first 24 hours of life, and they all develop abdominal distension with bilious vomiting or nasogastric aspirates.

5. Treatment varies depending on the etiology. Initially repeats of enema relieve obstruction from meconium plug (if exists). Later, the treatment depends on the etiology. Cystic fibrosis requires medical management, while Hirshprung's disease requires surgical intervention.

Pearls

- Neonatal small left colon syndrome is a functional disease of the lower colon that produces typical signs and symptoms of intestinal obstruction.

- Approximately 50% have a history of maternal diabetes mellitus, and other maternal comorbidities (usually eclampsia), which contribute to neonatal stress, may also be present.

- A small number of infants develop progressive distension leading to perforation, typically in the cecum, within the first 24 to 36 hours of life.

- Plain abdominal radiograph demonstrates dilated bowel loops suggestive of obstruction.

- Contrast enema demonstrates small caliber of the left colon and normal caliber of the ascending colon.

Suggested Readings

Berdon WE, Slovis TL, Campbell JB, et al. Neonatal small left colon syndrome: its relationship to aganglionosis and meconium plug syndrome. *Radiology*. 1977;125(2): 457-462.

Ellerbroek C, Smith WL. Neonatal small left colon in an infant with cystic fibrosis. *Pediatr Radiol*. 1986;16(2):162-163.

Stewart DR, Nixon GW, Johnson DG, Condon VR. Neonatal small left colon syndrome. *Ann Surg*. 1977;186(6):741-745.

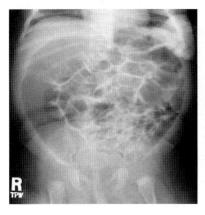 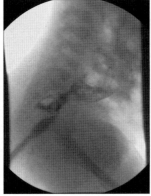 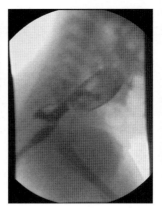 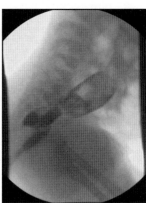

1. What are the findings?

2. What is the diagnosis?

3. What are few of the differential diagnoses
   of this case?

4. What are diseases associated with this entity?

5. What are the treatment options?

Case ranking/difficulty:    **Category:** Gastrointestinal

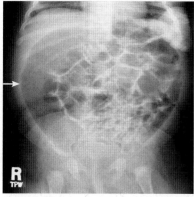
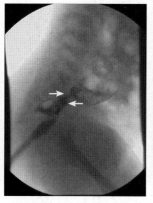
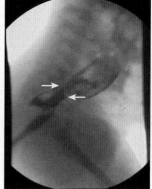
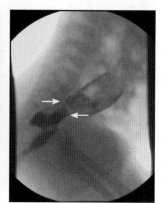

Frontal radiograph of the abdomen reveals dilated colon filled with air (*arrow*).

Lateral view of a contrast enema reveals that the rectosigmoid ratio is less than one. Transitional zone is noted (*arrows*).

Answers

1. The plain frontal radiograph reveals dilated air-filled colon.

   Contrast enema: Lateral view of the first pass of the rectal contrast in the recto-sigmoid area reveals that the diameter ratio of the rectum to the sigmoid is less than one. There is transitional zone. Proximal to the transitional zone, the sigmoid and the left colon are dilated. Distal to the transitional zone, the rectum is narrowed.

2. The diagnosis is Hirshprung's disease.

3. Few of the differential diagnoses include constipation, hypothyroidism, and megacolon.

4. Among the diseases associated with Hirshprung's disease are Down syndrome, neurocristopathy syndromes, multiple endocrine neoplasia type II, Waardenburg-Shah syndrome, and congenital central hypoventilation syndrome.

5. Treatment includes surgical resection of the abnormal section of the colon and reanastomosis.

Pearls

- Hirschsprung's disease, also called congenital aganglionic megacolon, consists of an aganglionic segment of bowel that starts at the anus and progresses proximally.
- Both the myenteric (Auerbach) plexus and the submucosal (Meissner) plexus are absent, resulting in reduced bowel peristalsis and function.
- An enlarged section of the bowel is found proximally, while the narrowed, aganglionic section is found distally.
- Treatment of Hirschsprung's disease consists of surgical removal (resection) of the abnormal section of the colon, followed by reanastomosis.

Suggested Readings

Heanue TA, Pachnis V. Enteric nervous system development and Hirschsprung's disease: advances in genetic and stem cell studies. *Nat Rev Neurosci.* 2007;8(6):466-479.

Russell MB, Russell CA, Niebuhr E. An epidemiological study of Hirschsprung's disease and additional anomalies. *Acta Paediatr.* 1994;83(1):68-71.

Ryan ET, Ecker JL, Christakis NA, Folkman J. Hirschsprung's disease: associated abnormalities and demography. *J Pediatr Surg.* 1992;27(1):76-81.

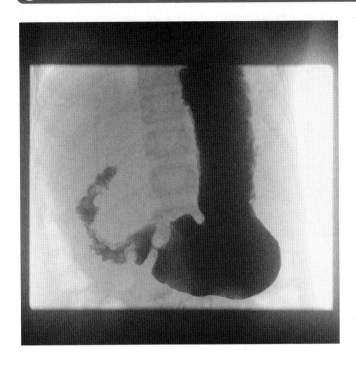 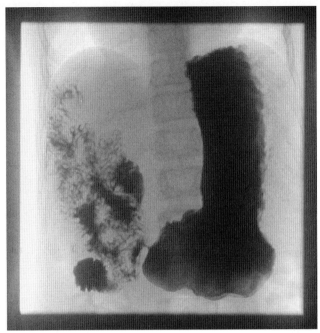

1. What are the findings?

2. Where is the normal anatomic location of the ligament of Treitz?

3. What is the normal relation between the superior mesenteric artery (SMA) and the superior mesenteric vein (SMV)?

4. What is the major risk of intestinal malrotation?

5. What is the treatment option?

Case ranking/difficulty: 🏅

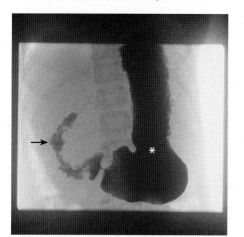

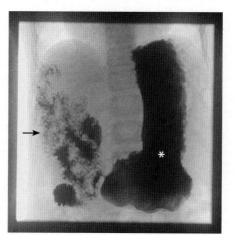

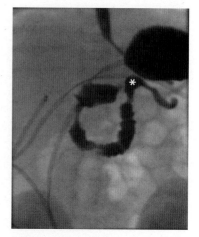

Early image of an upper GI study demonstrates the second portion of the duodenum in the right side of the abdomen, extending upwards (*arrow*). Normally, the second portion of the duodenum extends in the right abdomen downwards. The *asterisk* represents the stomach.

Late image of an upper GI study demonstrates the entire duodenum in the right side of the abdomen (*arrow*). The normal C-loop of the duodenum did not form. The duodenum did not cross the midline to the left. The ligament of Treitz is in the right upper quadrant of the abdomen. The *asterisk* represents the stomach.

Normal upper GI study. C-loop of the duodenum is formed. The duodenum crossed the midline to the left. The ligament of Treitz (junction between the fourth portion of the duodenum and proximal jejunum) noted to be in its normal position, left of the spine and same level of the duodenal bulb. The *asterisk* points to the ligament of Treitz.

Answers

1. The diagnosis is intestinal malrotation. The C-loop of the duodenum did not cross midline to the left, and the ligament of Treitz is in the right upper quadrant of the abdomen.

2. The normal position of the ligament of Treitz is left of the spine and at the same level of the duodenal bulb.

3. Normally SMA is on the left side of SMV.

4. The major risk of intestinal malrotation is development of midgut volvulus.

5. Surgical treatment of malrotation consists of placement and fixation of small bowel on the right side of the abdomen and the large bowel on the left side of the abdomen. This is known as Ladd's procedure.

- Upper GI study is the modality of choice for the diagnosis.
- Low-lying ligament of Treitz or failure of the duodenum to cross the midline is diagnostic of intestinal malrotation.
- Reversal of the normal relation between superior mesenteric artery and superior mesenteric vein is diagnostic of malrotation.
- Ladd's procedure is the corrective surgical treatment for malrotation–fixation of small bowel in the right side of the abdomen and large bowel in the left side of the abdomen.

Pearls

- Intestinal malrotation involves anomalies of intestinal fixation due to malrotation or nonrotation around the superior mesenteric artery.
- This condition predisposes to midgut volvulus that occurs most commonly during infancy.
- Intestinal malrotation can be asymptomatic and discovered during upper GI study performed for other reasons.

Suggested Readings

Draus JM Jr, Foley DS, Bond SJ. Laparoscopic Ladd procedure: a minimally invasive approach to malrotation without midgut volvulus. *Am Surg.* 2007;73(7):693-696.

Estrada RL. *Anomalies of Intestinal Rotation and Fixation.* Springfield, IL: Charles C Thomas; 1958.

Irish MS, Pearl RH, Caty MG, Glick PL. The approach to common abdominal diagnosis in infants and children. *Pediatr Clin North Am.* 1998;45(4):729-772.

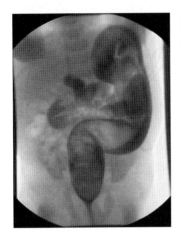 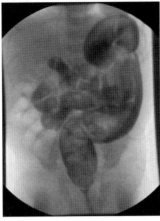 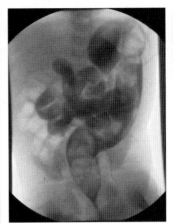 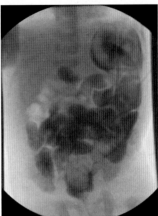

1. How many degrees of normal intestinal rotation occur during the embryonic life?

2. What are the conditions associated with the case?

3. Around which vessel the normal intestinal rotation occurs during the embryonic life?

4. What is the differential diagnosis of the enema shown in this case?

5. What are the treatment options of gastroschisis?

Case ranking/difficulty:

Category: Gastrointestinal

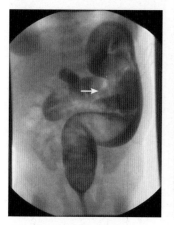 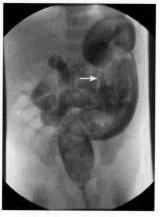 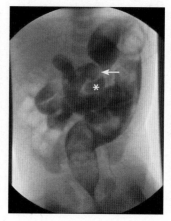 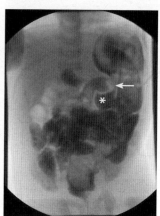

Fluoroscopic enema performed with water-soluble contrast demonstrates the entire colon in the left hemi-abdomen and the small bowel in the right hemi-abdomen. The *arrow* points to the distal ileum.

Fluoroscopic enema performed with water-soluble contrast demonstrates the entire colon in the left hemi-abdomen and the small bowel in the right hemi-abdomen. The *arrow* points to the distal ileum. The *asterisk* points the cecum.

Answers

1. The normal intestinal rotation during the embryonic life is 270 degrees counterclockwise.

2. Most infants with gastroschisis, omphalocele, or congenital diaphragmatic hernia present with intestinal malrotation. Intestinal malrotation occurs in association with Hirschsprung's disease, persistent cloaca, imperforate anus, duodenal atresia, and extrahepatic anomalies.

3. Normal intestinal rotation takes place around the superior mesenteric artery.

4. Differential diagnosis of the shown enema includes Hirschsprung's disease, intestinal nonrotation, colonic stricture, and bowel obstruction.

5. After birth, the lower body will be placed in a sterile bag to prevent infection in the exposed intestines. A silo, a special kind of sac, is wrapped around the intestines, holding them above the abdomen. Over the course of a week or more, the effects of gravity gently push most of the intestines into the abdominal cavity. When the intestines are level with the abdomen, surgery will be used to place the remainder of the intestines in the abdomen and close the opening. Surgical fixation of the bowel in the abdomen is performed in cases of malrotation or nonrotation.

Pearls

- Intestinal nonrotation is the extreme end of the spectrum of intestinal malrotation, where the rotation of the intestine does not happen.
- Normal rotation occurs during the embryonic life when the midgut undergoes rotation of 270 degrees counterclockwise. If rotation does not occur, the large bowel remains in the left side of the abdomen and the small bowel remains in the right side of the abdomen.
- Nonrotation is an arrest in development at stage I of the rotation, between 5 and 10 weeks of gestational age.
- Intestinal nonrotation and malrotation may be associated with gastroschisis, omphalocele, congenital diaphragmatic hernia, and duodenal atresia.
- Treatment of choice of gastroschisis associated with nonrotation is a silo with gradual pressure to push the bowel to the abdominal cavity. In cases of nonrotation, surgical fixation may be prophylactically necessary.

Suggested Readings

Ford KL 3rd. Aunt Minnie's corner. Nonrotation of the bowel. *J Comput Assist Tomogr*. 1997 Apr;20(4):693.

McLennan MK. Radiology rounds. Malrotation of the midgut with a nonrotation pattern. *Can Fam Physician*. 1998;44(44):271, 277-279.

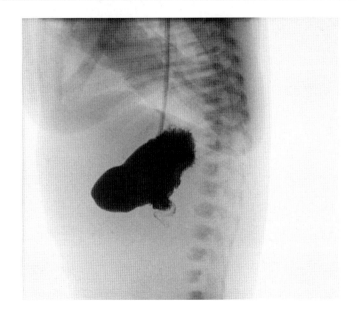 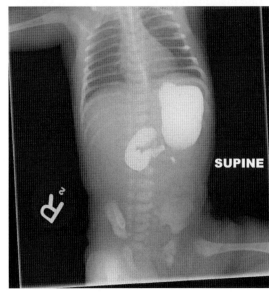

1. What is the clinical presentation of this case?

2. What is the risk factor of this entity?

3. What is the radiographic appearance of this case?

4. What is the age range that this condition is most commonly seen?

5. Why is the surgical treatment urgent?

Case ranking/difficulty:

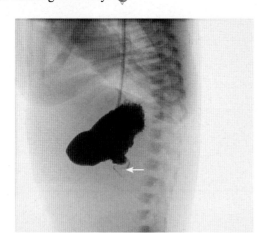

Lateral image of upper GI study demonstrates obstruction at the level of the third portion of the duodenum with corkscrew tapering of the contrast; appearance (*arrow*) that represents midgut volvulus.

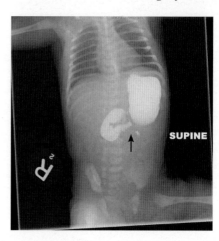

Frontal radiograph obtained immediately following an upper GI study demonstrates obstruction at the level of the third portion of the duodenum with corkscrew tapering of the contrast; appearance (*arrow*) that represents midgut volvulus.

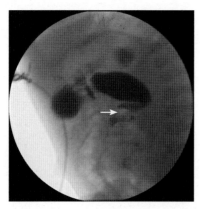

Upper GI study performed on another 5-week-old male with bilious vomiting demonstrates the corkscrew appearance of the duodenum (*arrow*) consistent with midgut volvulus.

Pearls

- Midgut volvulus refers to twisting of the entire midgut around the axis of the superior mesenteric artery.
- Midgut volvulus develops most commonly in infants with intestinal malrotation.
- Upper GI study is the diagnostic modality of choice.
- Upper GI demonstrates obstruction at the level of the third portion of the duodenum. There is a corkscrew pattern of tapering of the contrast.
- Treatment is emergent surgery as lack of vascular supply may cause a gangrenous bowel. Nonviable bowel should be resected.
- Ladd procedure is the surgical treatment of choice. The small bowel is placed and fixed on the right side of the abdomen and the large bowel on the left.

Answers

1. The clinical presentation of midgut volvulus is bilious vomiting (green vomiting).

2. The risk factor for the development of midgut volvulus is intestinal malrotation.

3. The radiographic appearance of this entity in upper GI fluoroscopic study is corkscrew tapering of the contrast at the level of the third portion of the duodenum.

4. The condition shown above is most commonly seen during infancy.

5. Surgical treatment is urgent due to lack of vascular supply to the bowel. Affected bowel becomes gangrenous.

Suggested Readings

Andrassy RJ, Mahour GH. Malrotation of the midgut in infants and children: a 25-year review. *Arch Surg.* 1981;116(2):158-160.

Kealey WD, McCallion WA, Brown S. Midgut volvulus in children. *Br J Surg.* 1996;83(1):105-106.

Seashore JH, Touloukian RJ. Midgut volvulus. An ever-present threat. *Arch Pediatr Adolesc Med.* 1994;148(1):43-46.

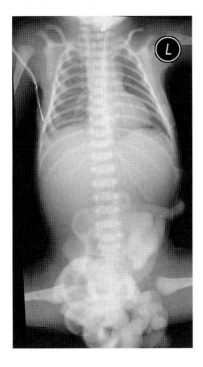
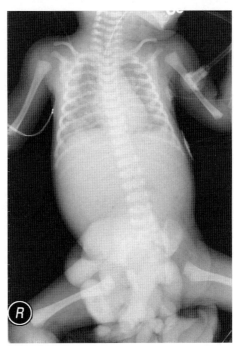
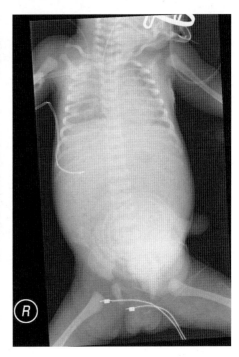

1. What is the diagnosis?

2. What may be included in the differential diagnosis?

3. What is the serum marker that may be seen in the mother and the newborn in this case?

4. What is being postulated on the pathogenesis of the shown case?

5. What is the frequency of the shown entity?

Case ranking/difficulty: 🔥

Category: Abdomen

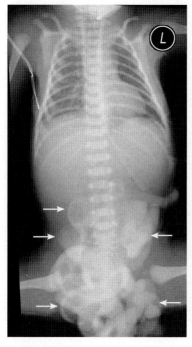

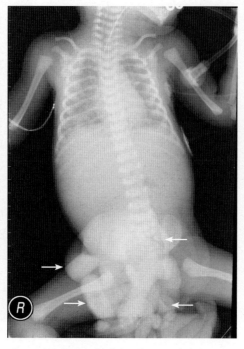

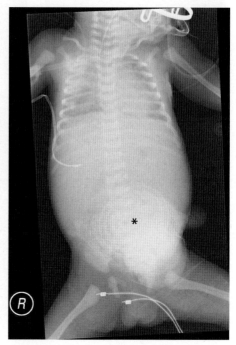

Chest and abdomen radiograph demonstrates bowel loops protruding beyond the contour of the abdomen (*arrows*).

Frontal radiograph of the chest and abdomen of another patient shows bowel loops (*arrows*) outside the abdomen consistent with gastroschisis.

Frontal radiograph of the chest and abdomen shows that the gastroschisis was treated with a silo (*asterisk*).

Answers

1. The diagnosis is gastroschisis.

2. Prune belly syndrome, omphalocele, and umbilical hernia may be included in the differential diagnosis.

3. Serum alpha-feto-protein may be elevated in the mother and the newborn.

4. The pathogenesis may involve defective mesenchymal development at the junction of the body stalk and the abdominal wall, resulting in increased abdominal pressure that may cause the dysplastic abdominal wall to rupture. There may be an abnormal involution of the right umbilical vein or a vascular accident involving the omphalomesenteric artery that may cause a localized weakness and subsequent rupture. It was also postulated that there may be a rupture of a small omphalocele, absorption of the sac, and growth of skin between the resultant opening and the umbilical cord.

5. The frequency is 1 in 10,000.

Pearls

- Gastroschisis is herniation of abdominal contents through a paraumbilical abdominal defect.
- Bowel loops are not covered by a membrane.
- It is associated with malrotation or nonrotation.
- Other gastrointestinal anomalies may be associated.
- Mother and fetus may have elevated serum alpha-feto-protein.
- Treatment consists of placing a silo around the herniated bowel. The silo is being gradually squeezed to bring the herniated bowel back to the body through the open abdominal wall defect.
- Surgical repair may also be performed after delivery to avoid infection.

Suggested Readings

Emanuel PG, Garcia GI, Angtuaco TL. Prenatal detection of anterior abdominal wall defects with US. *Radiographics.* 1995;15(3):517-530.

Khati NJ, Enquist EG, Javitt MC. Imaging of the umbilicus and periumbilical region. *Radiographics.* 1998;18(2):413-431.

Vermeij-Keers C, Hartwig NG, van der Werff JF. Embryonic development of the ventral body wall and its congenital malformations. *Semin Pediatr Surg.* 1996;5(2):82-89.

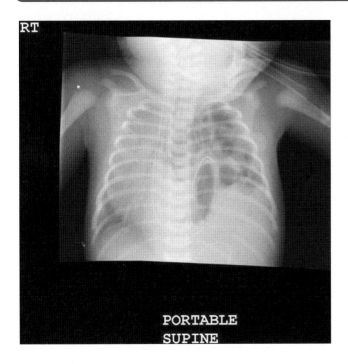

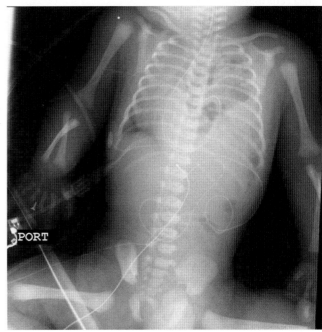

1. What are the findings?

2. What is the most common location in the chest that this entity occurs?

3. Where is Morgagni type of this entity usually seen?

4. Enumerate at least three differential diagnoses of the shown entity.

5. What are the treatment options?

Case ranking/difficulty: 🌰

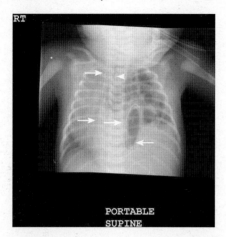

Frontal radiograph of the chest shows bowel loops in the left hemi thorax. The stomach is in the left chest. Nasogastric tube is shown (*arrows*) and its distal tip coils in the stomach, inside the chest. The mediastinum is shifted to the right. The *arrowhead* points to the distal tip of the endotracheal tube.

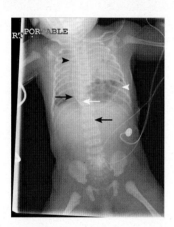

Frontal radiograph of the chest shows bowel loops and stomach in the left lower hemi thorax. The distal tip of the nasogastric tube (*white arrowhead*) is in the chest. The *black arrowhead* points to the distal tip of the endotracheal tube. *White arrow* points to the distal tip of the umbilical arterial line, and the *black arrows* point to the umbilical venous line. The mediastinum and the tubes and lines are displaced to the right. Low lung volume of the right lung is noted. There is no aeration of the left lung, and the abdomen shows no bowel gas.

Answers

1. The stomach with bowel loops are in the left hemi thorax, and the mediastinum is deviated to the right.

2. Eighty-five percent of the cases are Bochdalek type and they appear in the diaphragmatic defect, which is located in the left posterolateral aspect of the diaphragm.

3. In the Morgagni type of congenital diaphragmatic hernia, the diaphragmatic defect is usually seen in the right anteromedial aspect of the diaphragm.

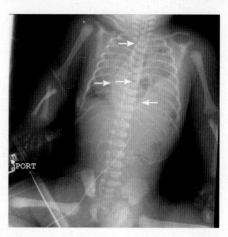

Frontal radiograph of the chest and abdomen shows bowel loops in the left hemi thorax. The stomach is in the left chest. Nasogastric tube is shown (*arrows*) and its distal tip coils in the stomach, inside the chest. The mediastinum is shifted to the right. The abdomen demonstrates paucity of bowel gas.

4. Differential diagnosis of the entity shown in the image may include bronchopulmonary sequestration, congenital cystic adenomatoid malformation, and congenital lobar emphysema.

5. Treatment may include surgical repair, extracorporeal membranous oxygenation (ECMO), stabilizing vital signs, and decreasing pulmonary hypertension.

Pearls

- Diaphragmatic hernia is a defect in the diaphragm that allows the abdominal contents to move into the chest cavity.
- Newborns usually present with respiratory distress and scaphoid abdomen.
- Congenital diaphragmatic hernia is associated with lung hypoplasia and increased persistent pulmonary hypertension of the newborn.
- Treatment consists of improving oxygenation, stabilizing patient's vital signs, reducing the pulmonary hypertension, and surgical repair. Usually patients are placed on ECMO in order to allow the lungs to mature properly before the corrective surgery.

Suggested Readings

Gross RE. Congenital hernia of the diaphragm. *Am J Dis Child.* 1946;71:579-592.

Lally KP. Extracorporeal membrane oxygenation in patients with congenital diaphragmatic hernia. *Semin Pediatr Surg.* 1996;5(4):249-255.

Nobuhara KK, Wilson JM. Pathophysiology of congenital diaphragmatic hernia. *Semin Pediatr Surg.* 1996;5(4): 234-242.

4-day-old male in the neonatal intensive care unit on ventilator with abdominal distension

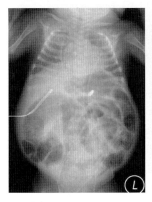 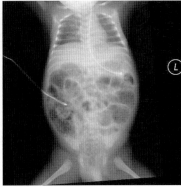 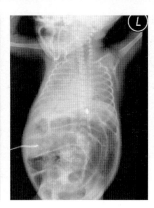 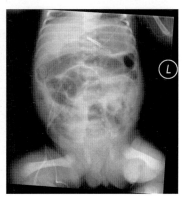

1. What is the imaging modality of choice for the diagnosis of this case?

2. What are the complications of this case?

3. What is the radiographic appearance of portal venous gas?

4. What are the major risk factors for the development of this entity?

5. What is the approximate mortality rate of the shown case?

Case ranking/difficulty:

Category: Gastrointestinal

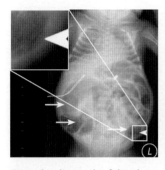

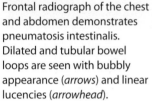

Frontal radiograph of the chest and abdomen demonstrates pneumatosis intestinalis. Dilated and tubular bowel loops are seen with bubbly appearance (*arrows*) and linear lucencies (*arrowhead*).

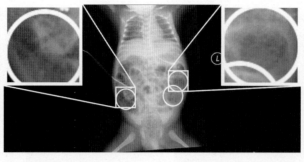

Frontal radiograph of the chest and abdomen demonstrates pneumatosis intestinalis. Dilated and tubular bowel loops are seen with bubbly appearance (*circles*).

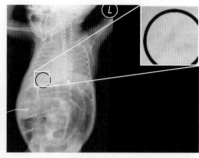

Frontal radiograph of the abdomen demonstrates pneumatosis intestinalis. Bubbly appearance and linear lucencies of bowel loops are noted. In addition, branching lucencies are noted in the right upper quadrant of the abdomen (*circle*) representing portal venous gas (a complication of necrotizing enterocolitis).

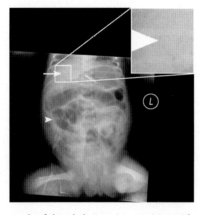

Frontal radiograph of the abdomen in a patient with necrotizing enterocolitis demonstrates branching lucencies in the right upper quadrant of the abdomen, consistent with portal venous gas (*arrow*). Pneumatosis intestinalis noted as linear bowel wall lucency (*arrowhead*).

Pearls

- NEC is an idiopathic necrosis of the intestinal mucosa seen primarily in premature infants in the neonatal intensive care units (NICU) who sustain ischemia and hypoxia.
- This leads to breakdown of the intestinal mucosal barrier allowing normal flora of the GI tract to invade.
- Abdominal distension, dilated and tubular bowel loops, and pneumatosis intestinalis (air in bowel wall) are diagnostic in plain abdominal radiograph.

Suggested Readings

Donnelly LF. Gastrointestinal tract. *Fundamentals of Pediatric Radiology*. Philadelphia, PA: Saunders; 2001;97-98.

Epelman M, Daneman A, Navarro OM, et al. Necrotizing enterocolitis: review of state-of-the-art imaging findings with pathologic correlation. *Radiographics*. 2007;27(2):285-305.

Muchantef K, Epelman M, Darge K, Kirpalani H, Laje P, Anupindi SA. Sonographic and radiographic imaging features of the neonate with necrotizing enterocolitis: correlating findings with outcomes. *Pediatr Radiol*. 2013;43(11):1444-1452.

Slovis TL, Caffey J. *Necrotizing Enterocolitis. Caffey's Pediatric Diagnostic Imaging*. 11th ed. Vol. 1. Philadelphia, PA: Mosby/Elsevier; 2008:257-263.

Answers

1. The best imaging modality for the diagnosis of necrotizing enterocolitis (NEC) in a pre-term infant is abdominal radiograph that demonstrates abdominal distension, dilated bowel loops, and pneumatosis intestinalis.

2. Complications of NEC include intestinal perforation and portal venous gas. Mortality is high.

3. The radiographic appearance of portal venous gas is branching lucencies in the right upper quadrant of the abdomen.

4. The major risk factors of the development of NEC are prematurity and hypoxia.

5. The mortality rate of NEC is between 15 and 30 percent.

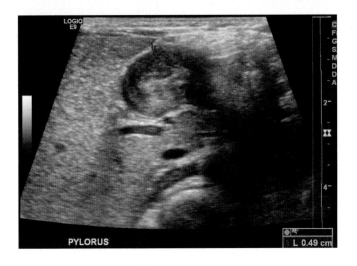 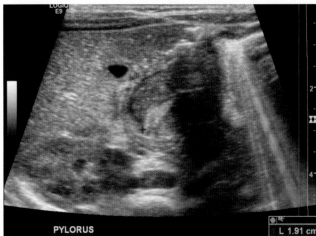

1. What is the structure that is shown in the images?

2. What is the usual age of presentation of this entity?

3. What are the clinical features of this case?

4. What are the sonographic signs of this entity?

5. What are the signs seen on barium upper GI study in this entity?

Case ranking/difficulty:  **Category:** Gastrointestinal

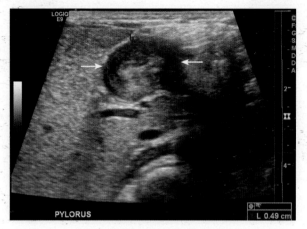

Transverse sonographic view of the pylorus (*between arrows*) demonstrates thickened pyloric muscular wall (above 3 mm).

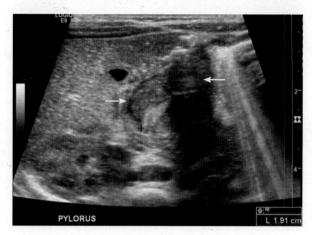

Longitudinal sonographic view of the pylorus (*between arrows*) demonstrates long pylorus (above 1.7 cm).

Answers

1. This is the pylorus and is consistent with hypertrophic pyloric stenosis. Wall thickness is more than the cut-off level of 3 mm. The length is increased (normal to below 14 mm).

2. Hypertrophic pyloric stenosis is usually seen between 3 to 12 weeks of age.

3. Clinical presentation of hypertrophic pyloric stenosis includes non-billious, projectile vomiting, dehydration, and hypokalemic alkalosis.

4. Ultrasonography is the imaging modality of choice as it is nearly 100% sensitive and specific. During the study, the infant is usually fed with water or electrolyte solution. Real-time ultrasound shows lack of movement of gastric contents through the pyloric channel. Over-distended stomach may displace the pylorus dorsally, making it difficult to visualize. Gastric decompression by enteric tube is helpful in such cases. Hypertrophied pyloric channel resembles uterine cervix on longitudinal view on ultrasound, called the "cervix sign."

   Measurements are preferred on longitudinal view. Measurement criteria for making the diagnosis include pyloric muscle thickness greater than 3 mm and pyloric channel length greater than 14 mm. Gastric hyperperistalsis may be visible on real-time ultrasound. Redundant, hypertrophied, echogenic mucosa is seen in the pyloric channel. Morphology of the pyloric channel and lack of passage of gastric content through the pyloric channel on real-time ultrasound are more important than absolute measurements. Pyloric channel length criteria vary. Visualization of fluid-filled distended duodenum excludes the diagnosis of hypertrophic pyloric stenosis.

5. String sign is presence of barium within the narrowed pyloric channel. Beak sign or teat sign is beak of barium trying to enter the pyloric channel. Shoulder sign is impression of hypertrophied pyloric muscle on the antrum. Mushroom sign is indentation of duodenal bulb by hypertrophied pyloric muscle.

Pearls

- The exact etiology of hypertrophic pyloric stenosis is unknown. Male: Female ratio is 4:1. First-born males are much more likely to be affected. Although familial cases are common, environmental factors also play some role.
- Ultrasonography is the imaging modality of choice as it is nearly 100% sensitive and specific.
- Measurement criteria for making the diagnosis include pyloric muscle thickness greater than 3 mm and pyloric channel length greater than 14 mm.
- Visualization of fluid-filled distended duodenal bulb excludes the diagnosis of hypertrophic pyloric stenosis.
- Radiograph of abdomen shows caterpillar stomach due to gastric hyperperistalsis.
- The definitive treatment is Ramstedt pyloromyotomy, where underlying antro-pyloric mass is split longitudinally.

Suggested Readings

Cogley JR, O'Connor SC, Houshyar R, Al Dulaimy K. Emergent pediatric US: what every radiologist should know. *Radiographics*. 2012;32(3):651-665.

Maheshwari P, Abograra A, Shamam O. Sonographic evaluation of gastrointestinal obstruction in infants: a pictorial essay. *J Pediatr Surg*. 2009;44(10):2037-2042.

Vasavada P. Ultrasound evaluation of acute abdominal emergencies in infants and children. *Radiol Clin North Am*. 2004;42(2):445-456.

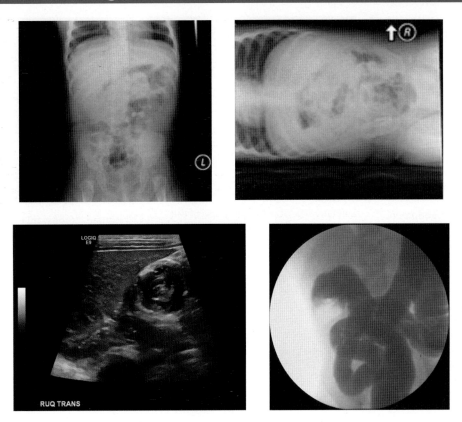

1. What is the most common type of this case in children?

2. What is the age that this case is most commonly seen?

3. What are the steps in the evaluation of this case?

4. What is the most common etiology?

5. What is the reason for obtaining a left lateral decubitus radiograph as part of the evaluation?

Case ranking/difficulty: 🌶   **Category:** Gastrointestinal

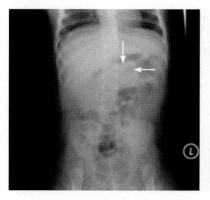

Frontal radiograph of the abdomen demonstrates mass effect in the upper abdomen, in the transverse colon, that has a crescent appearance (*arrows*), representing the intussusceptum.

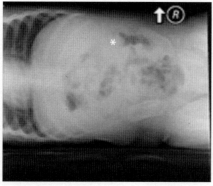

Left lateral decibitus radiograph of the abdomen demonstrates no evidence of intraperitoneal free air. The intussusceptum is shown (*asterisk*).

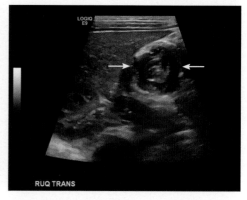

Sonogram of the right upper quadrant of the abdomen demonstrates the target sign (loop of bowel within a loop) (*arrows*) representing intussusception.

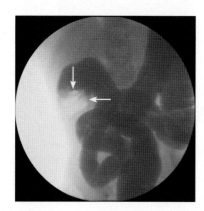

Fluoroscopic enema with water-soluble contrast was performed to diagnose and treat intussusception. The intussusceptum is encountered in the right upper quadrant of the abdomen, near the hepatic flexure (*arrows*). The intussusceptum has a coiled string appearance.

Answers

1. Ileocolic intussusception is the most common type of intussusception in children.

2. Ileocolic intussusception is most commonly seen between 5 months to 5 years of age with a peak incidence between 1 and 2 years.

3. Ultrasound and/or contrast enema are the steps in evaluating suspicion for intussusception.

4. Viral illness may trigger the process. Meckel's diverticulum or a mass of different etiologies may be a lead point. Most of the time, the etiology is unknown and the case is considered as idiopathic. In older children beyond 5 years, lead point like lymphoma is more likely.

5. The reason is to exclude possibility of free air. If there is a free air, contrast enema for diagnosis confirmation and reduction should not be performed. The patient should go directly for surgery.

Pearls

- Most common in children younger than 5 years old.
- Intussusception should be considered in the differential diagnosis and be excluded in any restless child with abdominal pain and blood in stool.
- Ultrasound is an excellent modality to diagnose intussusception without radiating a child.
- Contrast enema either with water-soluble contrast or air contrast is diagnostic as well as therapeutic.
- Intussusception is an emergency. Immediate treatment by enema or surgery is necessary to avoid necrosis of the affected bowel.

Suggested Readings

Bhisitkul DM, Todd KM, Listernick R. Adenovirus infection and childhood intussusception. *Am J Dis Child.* 1992;146:1331.

Byrne AT, Goeghegan T, Govender P, Lyburn, ID, Colhoun E, Torreggiani WC. The imaging of intussusceptions. *Clin Radiol.* 2005;60(1):39-46.

Winslow BT, Westfall JM, Nicholas RA. Intussusception. *Am Fam Physician.* 1996;54(1):213-217, 220.

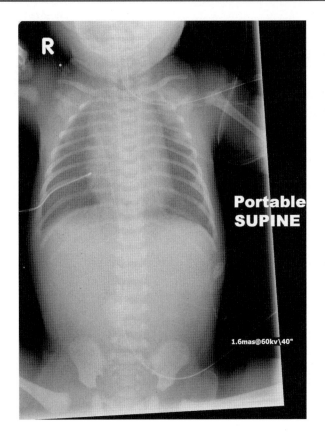
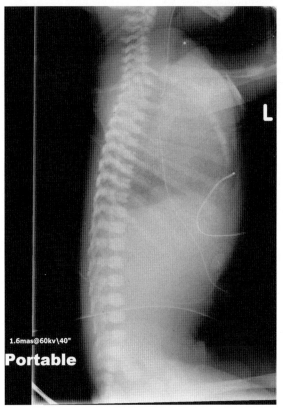

1. What are the findings?

2. What is the most common type of this entity?

3. Which type of this entity is present in the provided images?

4. What are the clinical presentations of this case?

5. What are the treatment options?

Case ranking/difficulty:

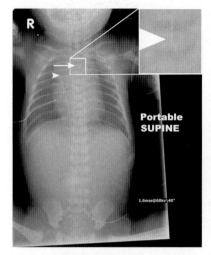

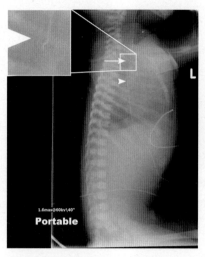

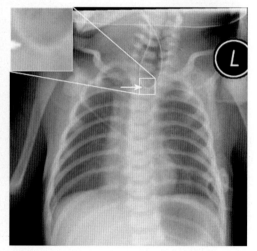

Frontal radiograph of the chest and abdomen demonstrates an enteric tube with its distal tip in the proximal third of the esophagus (*arrow*). The abdomen is gasless. Note is made of umbilical venous line with its distal tip in the region of the superior vena cava (*arrowhead*), which is high in position.

Lateral radiograph of the chest and abdomen demonstrates an enteric tube with its distal tip in the proximal third of the esophagus (*arrow*). The abdomen is gasless. Note is made of umbilical venous line with its distal tip in the region of the superior vena cava (*arrowhead*), which is high in position.

Frontal radiograph of the chest of another newborn with esophageal atresia demonstrates an enteric tube with its distal tip coils in the proximal third of the esophagus (*arrow*). In this case gas is seen in the stomach, due to the presence of distal tracheoesophageal fistula (TEF).

Answers

1. There is gasless abdomen, and the distal tip of the enteric tube is in the proximal esophagus.

2. Esophageal atresia with distal tracheoesophageal fistula (TEF) represents 82% of the cases.

3. Only esophageal atresia with proximal TEF or atresia without TEF can be present. There is no gas in bowel loops. Other types include communication between the trachea and the distal esophagus and connection to bowel loops.

4. Clinical presentation of the disease may include excessive oral and pharyngeal secretions, chocking, coughing during feeding attempts, and cyanosis.

5. Treatment is surgical. Anastomosis of the esophageal segments and excision of the tracheoesophageal fistula if exists.

Pearls

- Esophageal atresia is a congenital anomaly of the esophagus.
- This condition may be associated with tracheoesophageal fistula (TEF) and with other anomalies (VACTERL).
- There is a risk of aspiration if the newborn is fed.

- There are five types of esophageal atresia:
  a. Esophageal atresia without TEF (9% of cases).
  b. Esophageal atresia with proximal TEF (1% of cases).
  c. Esophageal atresia with distal TEF (82% of cases).
  d. Esophageal atresia with proximal and distal TEF (2%).
  e. H-type TEF without atresia (6% of cases).
- Plain radiograph with insertion of enteric tube demonstrates that the tube cannot be advanced into the stomach and the distal tip remains in the proximal esophagus.
- Plain radiograph of the abdomen is gasless if there is no TEF or if the fistula is distal to the atretic portion.
- The diagnosis is confirmed by upper gastrointestinal series that demonstrates that the contrast ends as blind pouch in the proximal esophagus.

Suggested Readings

Donnelly LF. *Diagnostic Imaging. Pediatrics*. 4-44-47. Amirsys; 2005.

Orenstein S, Peters J, Khan S, Youssef N, Hussain SZ. Congenital anomalies: esophageal atresia and tracheoesophageal fistula. In: Kliegman RM, Behrman RE, Jenson HB, Stanton BF, eds. *Nelson Textbook of Pediatrics*.18th ed. Philadelphia, PA: Saunders Elsevier; 2007 [chapter 316].

Newborn with bilious vomiting

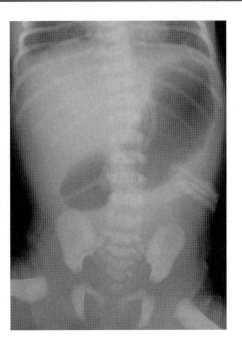

1. What are the findings?

2. One-third of the cases of this entity are associated with:

3. The triple bubble sign in abdominal radiograph is consistent with:

4. Name at least four entities in the differential diagnosis.

5. What is the surgical procedure that is performed to treat this entity?

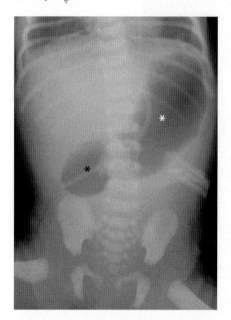 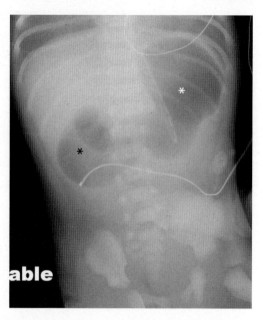

Frontal radiographs of the chest and abdomen in a newborn demonstrates the double bubble sign. The first air bubble (*white asterisk*) represents the stomach. The second air bubble (*black asterisk*) represents the duodenum. There is no bowel gas distally.

Answers

1. The frontal view of the chest and abdomen demonstrates the "double bubble sign" consistent with duodenal atresia.

2. One-third of the cases of this entity are associated with trisomy 21.

3. The triple bubble sign in abdominal radiograph is consistent with jejunal atresia. The third bubble represents distended proximal portion of the jejunum.

4. Differential diagnosis includes duodenal atresia, annular pancreas, midgut volvulus, and pyloric stenosis.

5. The surgical procedure that is performed to treat duodenal atresia is duodenoduodenostomy.

Pearls

- Presenting symptoms and signs are the result of high intestinal obstruction.
- Usually clinical signs present in the first few hours of life.
- While vomitus is most often bilious, it may be nonbilious because 15% of defects occur proximal to the ampulla of Vater.
- Abdominal radiograph in frontal view shows the "double bubble" sign.
- Treatment is urgent.

Suggested Readings

Aubrespy P, Derlon S, Seriat-Gautier B. Congenital duodenal obstruction: a review of 82 cases. *Prog Pediatr Surg.* 1978;11:109-124.

Fonkalsrud EW, DeLorimier AA, Hays DM. Congenital atresia and stenosis of the duodenum: a review compiled from the members of the Surgical Section of the American Academy of Pediatrics. *Pediatrics.* 1969;43(1):79-83.

Freeman SB, Torfs CP, Romitti PA, et al. Congenital gastrointestinal defects in Down syndrome: a report from the Atlanta and National Down Syndrome Projects. *Clin Genet.* 2009;75(2):180-184.

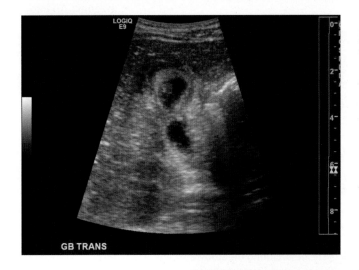

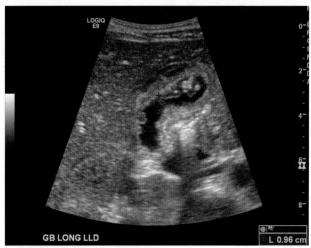

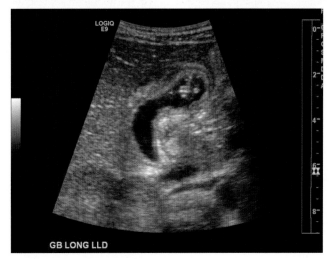

1. What is the diagnosis?

2. Enumerate few diseases in the differential.

3. What are the sonographic findings of this entity?

4. What is the finding of this entity in hepatobiliary scintigraphy?

5. What are the risk factors?

Case ranking/difficulty: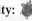

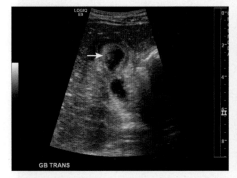

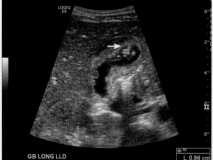

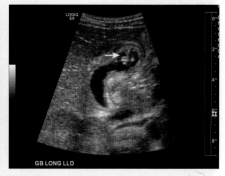

Transverse sonogram of the right upper quadrant of the abdomen reveals nonshadowing gallstones in the nondependent aspect of the gallbladder (*arrow*), thickening wall of the gallbladder, and anechoic sleeve around the gallbladder representing pericholecystic fluid. During the study, the patient was tender on touching the right upper quadrant of the abdomen, representing the sonographic Murphy's sign.

Longitudinal sonogram of the right upper quadrant of the abdomen reveals nonshadowing gallstones in the nondependent aspect of the gallbladder (*arrow*), thickening wall of the gallbladder, and anechoic sleeve around the gallbladder representing pericholecystic fluid. During the study the patient was tender on touching the right upper quadrant of the abdomen, representing the sonographic Murphy's sign.

Answers

1. The diagnosis is acute calculous cholecystitis. Gallstones are seen.

2. Diseases in the differential include cholangitis, gastritis, pancreatitis, and biliary colic.

3. Sonographic findings include increase thickness of the gallbladder wall, pericholecystic fluid, and sonographic Murphy's sign. Gallstones may be present.

4. The sign of acute cholecystitis in hepatobiliary scintigraphy is nonvisualization of the gallbladder. The rim sign may be seen.

5. Risk factors for this entity may include gallstones, obesity, sickle cell disease, and spherocytosis.

Pearls

- Acute cholecystitis is acute inflammation of the gallbladder that causes severe abdominal pain.
- Acute calculous cholecystitis is caused by obstruction of the cystic duct, leading to distention of the gallbladder.
- Hemolytic anemia such as sickle cell disease may facilitate the production of gallstones that can indirectly lead to cholecystitis.
- Ultrasonographic findings that are suggestive of acute cholecystitis include the following: pericholecystic fluid, gallbladder wall thickening greater than 4 mm, and sonographic Murphy sign. The presence of gallstones also helps to confirm the diagnosis.
- Laparoscopic cholecystectomy is the standard of care for the surgical treatment of cholecystitis.

Suggested Readings

Irizarry K, Rossbach HC, Ignacio JR, et al. Sickle cell intrahepatic cholestasis with cholelithiasis. *Pediatr Hematol Oncol.* 2006;23(2):95-102.

Rao VM, Mapp EM, Wechsler RJ. Radiology of the gastrointestinal tract in sickle cell anemia. *Semin Roentgenol.* 1987;22(3):195-204.

Rescorla FJ, Grosfeld JL. Cholecystitis and cholelithiasis in children. *Semin Pediatr Surg.* 1992;1(2):98-106.

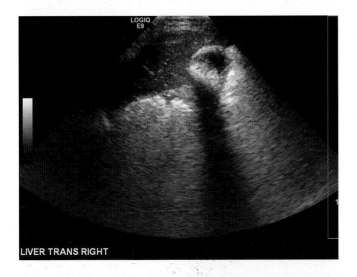

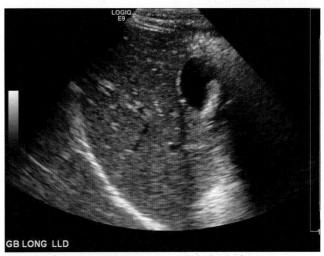

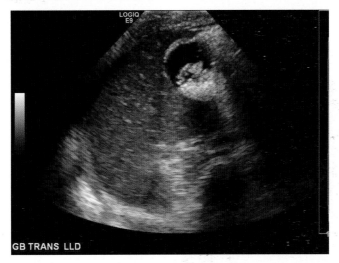

1. What are the findings?

2. What is the most common type of this case
   in children?

3. What are the predisposing factors that can lead
   to this entity?

4. What are the complications of this case?

5. What is the imaging modality of choice for the
   diagnosis of this entity in children?

Case ranking/difficulty:

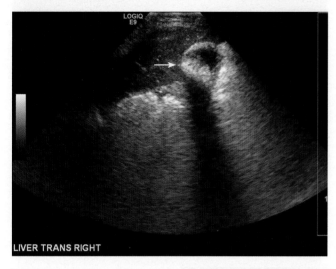

LIVER TRANS RIGHT

Transverse sonogram of the gallbladder demonstrates intraluminal echogenic shadowing structure (*arrow*) representing gallstone.

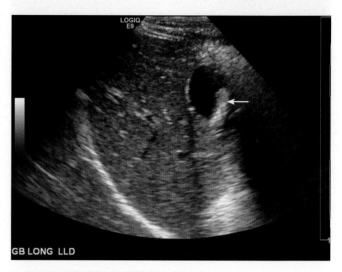

GB LONG LLD

Longitudinal sonogram of the gallbladder demonstrates intraluminal echogenic shadowing structure (*arrow*) representing gallstone.

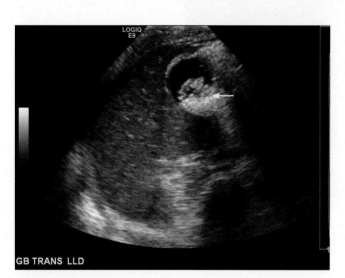

GB TRANS LLD

Transverse sonogram of the gallbladder demonstrates intraluminal echogenic shadowing structure (*arrow*) representing gallstone.

Answers

1. The gallbladder has an intraluminal mass that is echogenic and is shadowing. The biliary ducts are not dilated. The spleen is not visualized in the three provided images.

2. Black pigment stones are the most common gallstone type that makes up 48% of gallstones in children.

3. Hemolytic disease, hepatobiliary disease, obesity, prolonged parenteral nutrition, abdominal surgery, trauma, sepsis, and pregnancy–all may lead to an increased incidence of gallstones in the pediatric population.

4. Complications of gallstones in the pediatric population are similar to gallstone complications in adults. The complications include acute cholecystitis, cholangitis, pancreatitis, and biliary obstruction.

5. Ultrasound is the imaging modality of choice for the diagnosis of gallstones. Its sensitivity is high and there is no radiation exposure.

Pearls

- Black pigment is the most common type of gallstones in the pediatric population.
- The frequency of cholelithiasis in children with sickle cell disease is almost double than that of the general population.
- Ultrasound is the imaging modality of choice for the diagnosis of cholelithiasis.
- Ultrasound demonstrates echogenic intraluminal structures in the gallbladder that are mobile and shadow.

Suggested Readings

Lobe TE. Cholelithiasis and cholecystitis in children. *Semin Pediatr Surg*. 2000;9(4):170-176.

Poddar U. Gallstone disease in children. *Indian Pediatr*. 2010;47(11):945-953.

Stringer MD, Taylor DR, Soloway RD. Gallstone composition: are children different? *J Pediatr*. 2003;142(4):435-440.

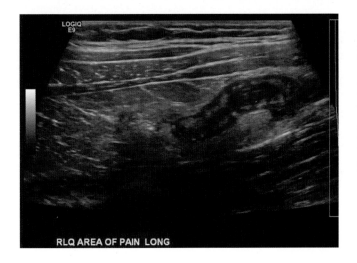

RLQ AREA OF PAIN LONG

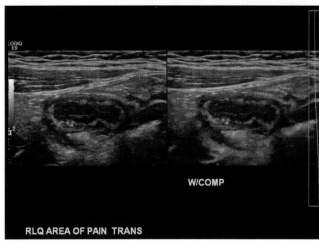

W/COMP

RLQ AREA OF PAIN TRANS

1. What is the structure seen in the sonographic images?

2. What are the sonographic findings of this entity?

3. What are the CT findings of this entity?

4. What is the differential diagnosis?

5. What are the treatment options?

Case ranking/difficulty: 🏮

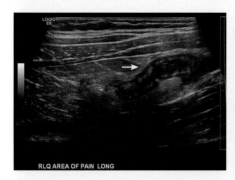

Longitudinal sonogram of abdominal right lower quadrant shows the appendix (*arrow*) which is dilated and measures 9 mm in its outer wall diameter.

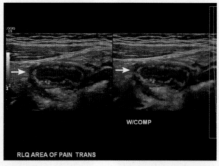

Transverse sonogram of abdominal right lower quadrant reveals dilated appendix (*left image*). The right image demonstrates a non compressible appendix (*arrows*).

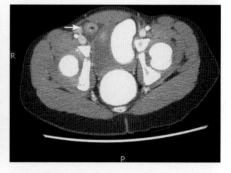

CT of the abdomen in axial view demonstrates dilated and enhancing appendix (*arrow*).

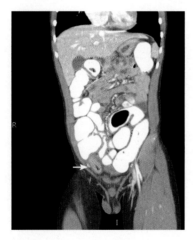

CT of the abdomen in coronal view demonstrates dilated and enhancing appendix (*arrow*).

Answers

1. The structure seen in the sonographic images is the appendix.

2. Sonographic findings of the shown entity may include diameter of the appendix more than 6 mm, the appendix is noncompressible, and filled with periappendicular fluid.

3. CT findings of acute appendicitis may include diameter of the appendix more than 6 mm, peri-appendicular fluid, stranding of the periappendicular fat, and an enhanced appendicular wall.

4. Differential diagnosis may include diverticulitis, ovarian torsion in females, mesenteric adenitis, and pelvic inflammatory disease.

5. Treatment may include appendectomy, intravenous antibiotics, and drainage if there is a periappendicular abscess.

Pearls

- The appendix is an anatomic blind pouch branching from the cecum.
- Patients present with abdominal pain and tenderness in the abdominal right lower quadrant. Nausea and vomiting may be present.
- Major risk of acute appendicitis is perforation and peritonitis.
- Most of the time there is periappendicular inflammation that can turn to phlegmon and abscess.
- It is preferable to start evaluating the patients and mostly children with sonography to avoid excessive radiation to children. If the diagnosis cannot be made on sonography, then CT is most of the time diagnostic.
- Sonography demonstrates a dilated appendix (more than 6 mm) and is non-compressible. There is tenderness during the exam.
- Non visualization of the appendix on sonography without tenderness on graded compression favors normal appendix.
- CT demonstrates dilated appendix, periappendicular stranding of the fat, and appendicular wall enhancement.

Suggested Readings

Birnbaum BA, Wilson SR. Appendicitis at the millennium. *Radiology*. 2000;215:337-348.

Oto A, Ernst RD, Mileski WJ, et al. Localization of appendix with MDCT and influence of findings on choice of appendectomy incision. *AJR Am J Roentgenol*. 2006;187(4):987-990.

Sivit CJ, Siegel MJ, Applegate KE, Newman KD. When appendicitis is suspected in children. *Radiographics*. 2001;21:247-262.

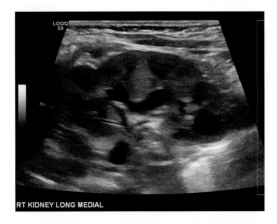
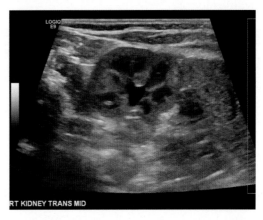
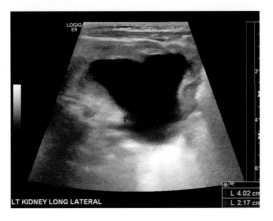
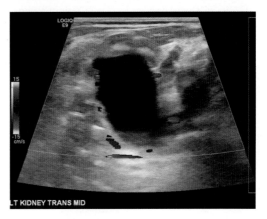

1. What is grade 1 hydronephrosis as described by the grading system of the society of fetal urology?

2. What is grade 2 hydronephrosis as described by the grading system of the society of fetal urology?

3. What is grade 3 hydronephrosis as described by the grading system of the society of fetal urology?

4. What is grade 4 hydronephrosis as described by the grading system of the society of fetal urology?

5. What is the grade of hydronephrosis of both kidneys in the provided images?

Case ranking/difficulty:

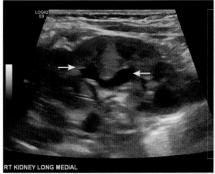

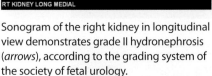

Sonogram of the right kidney in longitudinal view demonstrates grade II hydronephrosis (*arrows*), according to the grading system of the society of fetal urology.

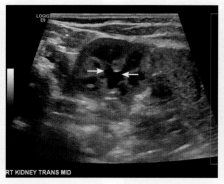

Sonogram of the right kidney in transverse view demonstrates grade II hydronephrosis (*arrows*), according to the grading system of the society of fetal urology.

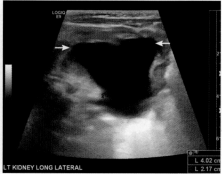

Sonogram of the right left in longitudinal view demonstrates grade IV hydronephrosis (*arrows*), according to the grading system of the society of fetal urology.

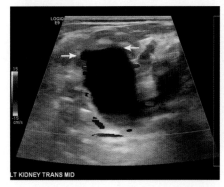

Sonogram of the right left in transverse view demonstrates grade IV hydronephrosis (*arrows*), according to the grading system of the society of fetal urology.

Pearls

- A system to grade upper tract dilatation or hydronephrosis imaged by ultrasound has been developed and is being used by the society of fetal urology.
- The appearance of the calices, renal pelvis and renal parenchyma is the key to determining the grade of hydronephrosis.
- The etiology of hydronephrosis varies. Obstructive etiology can be at different levels. It can be obstruction of the ureteropelvic junction or posterior urethral valve. Non-obstructive etiology can exist such as vesicoureteral reflux.
- Differential diagnosis should be made with multicystic dysplastic kidney disease that consists of non-communicating renal cysts.

Answers

1. In grade 1 hydronephrosis as described by the grading system of the society of fetal urology, there is slight separation of the central renal echo complex.

2. In grade 2 hydronephrosis as described by the grading system of the society of fetal urology, the renal pelvis is further dilated and a single or a few calices may be visualized.

3. In grade 3 hydronephrosis as described by the grading system of the society of fetal urology, the renal pelvis is dilated and there are fluid filled calices throughout the kidney. The renal parenchyma is of normal thickness.

4. In grade 4 hydronephrosis as described by the grading system of the society of fetal urology, the calices throughout the kidney are fluid filled and the renal parenchyma over the calices is thinned.

5. The images demonstrate right-sided hydronephrosis grade II and left-sided hydronephrosis grade IV.

Suggested Readings

Dighe M, Moshiri M, Phillips G, Biyyam D, Dubinsky T. Fetal genitourinary anomalies – a pictorial review with postnatal correlation. *Ultrasound Q*. 2011;27(1):7-21.

Fernbach SK, Maizels M, Conway JJ. Ultrasound grading of hydronephrosis: introduction to the system used by the Society for Fetal Urology. *Pediatr Radiol*. 1993;23:478.

Keays MA, Guerra LA, Mihill J, et al. Reliability assessment of Society for Fetal Urology ultrasound grading system for hydronephrosis. *J Urol*. 2008; 180(4 Suppl):1680-1682; discussion 1682-1683.

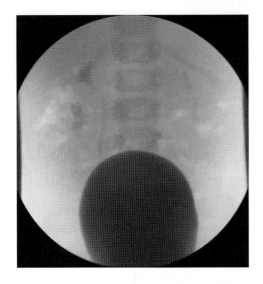
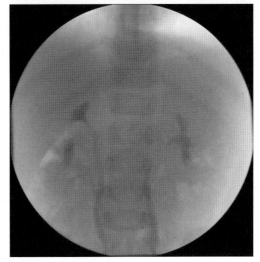
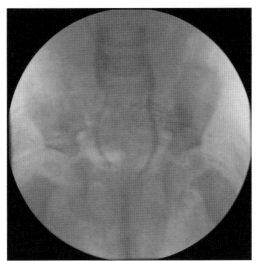

1. What is the diagnosis?

2. What are the complications of vesicoureteral reflux?

3. What are the causes of vesicoureteral reflux?

4. Describe the morphology of the right kidney in the present images.

5. What are the treatment options?

Case ranking/difficulty:

Category: Genitourinary

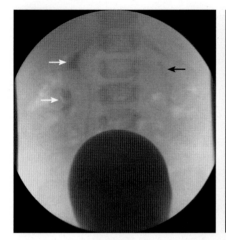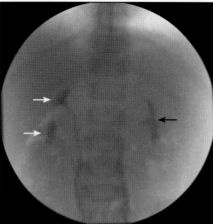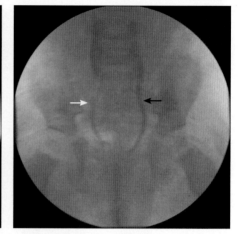

Voiding cystourethrography reveals bilateral vesicoureteral reflux. There is right renal duplication with two ureters that join distally to one ureter. The *white arrows* demonstrate right-sided reflux to both moieties. The *black arrow* demonstrates left-sided vesicoureteral reflux. There is no duplication on the left.

Voiding cystourethrography during the voiding phase demonstrate bilateral vesicoureteral reflux. *White arrow* points to the right-sided vesicoureteral reflux and *black arrow* points to the left-sided vesicoureteral reflux.

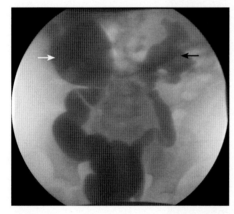

Voiding cystourethrography of another two-year-old male reveals severe right-sided vesicoureteral reflux, grade 5 (*white arrow*) and left-sided vesicoureteral reflux, grade 4 (*black arrow*). Bilateral tortuous ureters are noted.

5. Most cases resolve spontaneously and antibiotic prophylaxis is the only treatment to prevent urinary tract infections. More severe cases will be benefitted from the deflux procedure or ureteral reimplantation.

Answers

1. The diagnosis is bilateral vesicoureteral reflux.

2. Complications of vesicoureteral reflux include recurrent urinary tract infections, hydronephrosis, and renal damage such as scarring.

3. Causes of vesicoureteral reflux include short or absent intravesical ureter, absence of adequate detrusor backing, lateral displacement of the ureteral orifice, and paraureteral (Hutch) diverticulum.

4. Two ureters are seen emerging from the right kidney, which means that the right kidney has duplicated collecting system.

> **Pearls**
>
> - Vesicoureteral reflux is characterized by the retrograde flow of urine from the bladder to the kidneys.
> - Usually graded according to severity.
> - Complicated by recurrent urinary tract infection and hydronephrosis that can lead to renal damage.
> - Prophylactic antibiotics are necessary to prevent urinary tract infection and further renal damage.
> - Grade 1 to 3 usually resolve spontaneously.
> - Severe vesicoureteral reflux (grades 4 and 5) necessitates more aggressive treatment such as deflux procedure or ureteral reimplantation.

Suggested Readings

Feld LG, Mattoo TK. Urinary tract infections and vesicoureteral reflux in infants and children. *Pediatr Rev.* 2010;31(11):451-463.

Shaikh N, Ewing AL, Bhatnagar S, Hoberman A. Risk of renal scarring in children with a first urinary tract infection: a systematic review. *Pediatrics.* 2010;126(6):1084-1091.

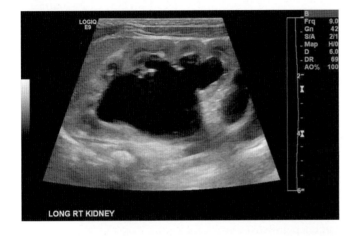

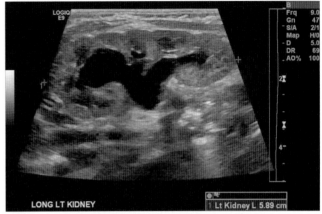

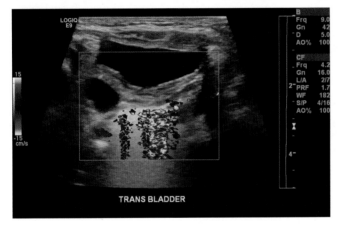

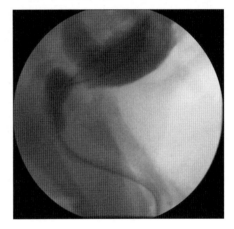

1. What is the diagnosis?

2. Enumerate at least three entities in the differential diagnosis.

3. What is the imaging modality of choice for the diagnosis?

4. What is the shape of the bladder as may be seen in the ultrasound of this entity?

5. What are the imaging modalities to assess renal function?

Case ranking/difficulty: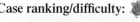

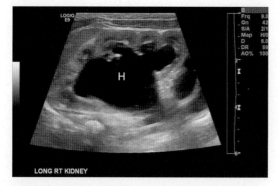

Longitudinal sonogram of the right kidney reveals severe hydronephrosis (H).

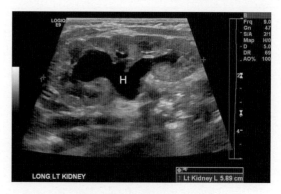

Longitudinal sonogram of the left kidney reveals severe hydronephrosis (H).

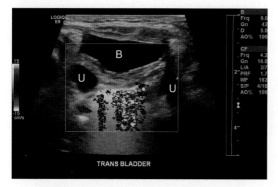

Transverse sonogram of the bladder (B) reveals the two dilated ureters (U) representing hydroureters bilaterally.

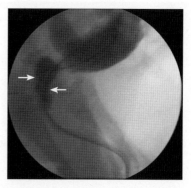

Voiding cystourethrogram reveals posterior dilatation of the urethra (*arrows*).

Answers

1. The diagnosis is posterior urethral valve which leads the bilateral vesicoureteral reflux, bilateral hydroureter, and bilateral hydronephrosis.

2. Differential diagnosis may include anterior urethral valve, urethral stricture, and hydronephrosis due to pyeloureteral obstruction.

3. The imaging modality of choice is voiding cystourethrogram (VCUG).

4. The bladder may assume the pattern of a key hole. The bladder is round with anechoic protrusion in its postero inferior aspect representing the dilated urethra.

5. Ultrasound gives us anatomical details of the kidney. Nuclear renogram with MAG3 is a study of renal function. Renal cortical scintigraphy with DMSA permits us to assess damage to the kidney and evaluate for scars.

- Severe forms may present with vesicoureteral reflux, hydroureter and hydronephrosis bilaterally.
- VCUG is the modality of choice for the diagnosis.
- Renal sonogram should be performed to assess the renal status for presence of hydronephrosis.
- A follow-up with nuclear renogram should be performed to assess renal function.
- Renal cortical scintigraphy should be performed later on to assess renal scarring.

Suggested Readings

Heikkilä J, Rintala R, Taskinen S. Vesicoureteral reflux in conjunction with posterior urethral valves. *J Urol.* 2009;182(4):1555-1560.

Taskinen S, Heikkilä J, Rintala R. Posterior urethral valves: primary voiding pressures and kidney function in infants. *J Urol.* 2009;182(2):699-702; discussion 702-703.

Uthup S, Binitha R, Geetha S, Hema R, Kailas L. A follow-up study of children with posterior urethral valve. *Indian J Nephrol.* 2010;20(2):72-75.

Pearls

- Posterior urethral valve is the most common cause of bladder outlet obstruction in male newborns.

5-month-old female with urinary tract infection

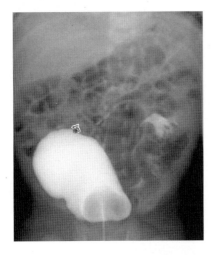
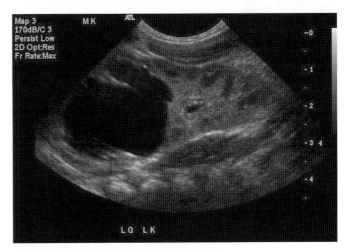
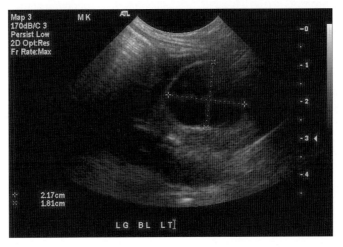

1. How are patients with this entity most likely to present clinically?

2. How will you characterize the upper and the lower poles of this case?

3. What is the Weigert-Meyer law?

4. What is the morphology of the lower pole of the left kidney as seen in the images?

5. What can be included in the differential diagnosis?

Case ranking/difficulty: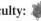

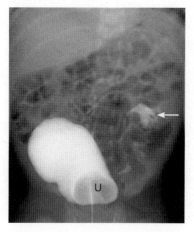

Fluoroscopic image obtained during a VCUG reveals left-sided vesicoureteral reflux. The left kidney is duplicated and the obstructed upper moiety displaces the refluxed lower moiety caudally (*arrow*), having the appearance of a "drooping lilly." Ureterocele seen (U).

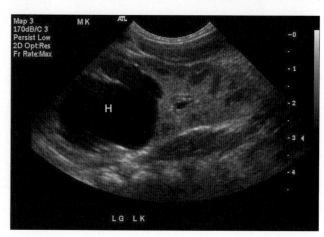

Longitudinal sonogram of the duplicated left kidney shows large hydronephrosis of the upper moiety (H).

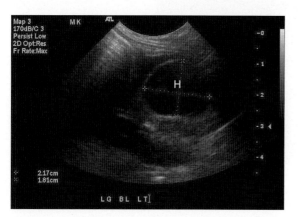

Longitudinal sonogram of the duplicated left kidney shows large hydronephrosis of the upper moiety (H).

Pearls

- Duplicated collecting system consists of a kidney with two pyelocaliceal systems.
- This system has two ureters that may drain into the bladder or fuse distally to a single ureter.
- Symptomatic patients usually have complete ureteric duplication in which the ureters are prone to developing obstruction, reflux, and infection.
- With a complete duplication system the ureter originating from the upper moiety inserts in the bladder medial and inferior to the lower moiety ureter. Most commonly, the upper moiety is obstructed and vesicoureteral reflux is seen in the lower moiety.
- Ureterocele is common.
- In VCUG, the "drooping lilly" sign may be seen, as the upper moiety displaces the refluxed lower moiety caudally.

Answers

1. Most patients are asymptomatic.

2. Most commonly, the upper moiety obstructs and lower moiety refluxes.

3. Weigert-Meyer law states that the ureter originating from the upper moiety of the duplicated kidney inserts in the bladder medial and inferior to the lower moiety ureter.

4. In VCUG, the "drooping lilly" sign is seen. The refluxed lower moiety is displaced caudally by the obstructed upper moiety.

5. Differential diagnosis may include ureteropelvic junction obstruction, ureterovesical junction obstruction, hydronephrosis, and multicystic dysplastic kidney.

Suggested Readings

Bisset GS, Strife JL. The duplex collecting system in girls with urinary tract infection: prevalence and significance. *AJR Am J Roentgenol.* 1987;148(3):497-500.

Callahan MJ. The drooping lily sign. *Radiology.* 2001;219(1):226-228.

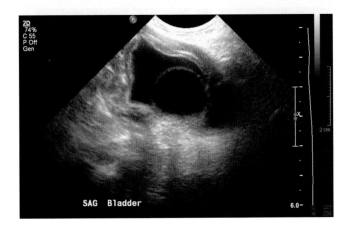

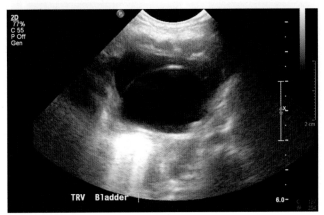

1. What is the anatomical abnormality of this case?

2. What are the possible complications of the case?

3. What is the appearance of the case in the images in voiding cystourethrography (VCUG)?

4. What are the sonographic findings?

5. What are the management options?

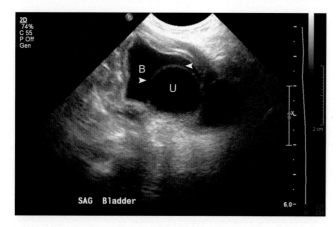

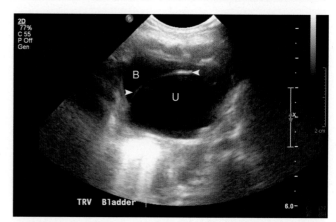

Sagittal sonogram of the bladder shows an echogenic regular and curvilinear structure (*arrowheads*) consistent with ureterocele. This is a fluid-filled cystic intravesical mass (U). B, bladder.

Transverse sonogram of the bladder shows an echogenic regular and curvilinear structure (*arrowheads*) consistent with ureterocele. This is a fluid-filled cystic intravesical mass (U). B, bladder.

Answers

1. Ureterocele is a saccular out-pouching of the distal ureter into the urinary bladder.

2. Complications may include urinary tract infection, ureteral calculus, vesicoureteral reflux, and hydronephrosis.

3. In VCUG, ureterocele appears as smooth, round filling defect along the base of the bladder.

4. In sonography, ureterocele appears as a fluid-filled cystic intravesical mass.

5. Management options may include control of urinary tract infections, preservation of renal function, maintenance of urinary continence, and surgical approach.

Pearls

- Ureteroceles arise from abnormal embryogenesis, with anomalous development of the intravesical ureter, the kidney, and the collecting system.
- Complications of ureteroceles in both pediatric and adult populations occur because of the obstructive nature of the ureterocele and its anatomic location.
- Due to the distal ureteral obstruction, the ipsilateral renal moiety is often hydronephrotic or dysplastic.
- The presence of ureterocele suggests the presence of a duplicated renal system.

Suggested Readings

Ayers E. Incidental sonographic finding of bilateral ureteroceles. *Journal of Diagnostic Medical Sonography*. 2006;22:123-126.

Uson AC, Lattimer JK, Melicow MM. Ureteroceles in infants and children: a report based on 44 cases. *Pediatrics*. 1961;27:971-983.

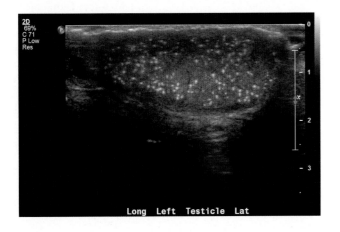
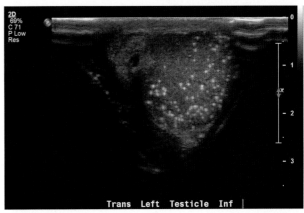

1. What is the frequency of this entity?

2. What are the sonographic findings of this entity?

3. Why periodic sonographic follow-up is necessary?

4. What are the clinical features of the case?

5. What are the treatment options?

Case ranking/difficulty: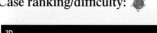

Category: Genitourinary

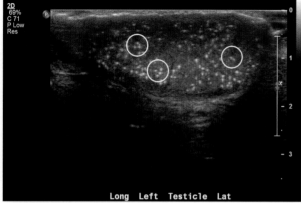

Longitudinal sonogram of the left testicle demonstrates multiple punctate echogenic foci (*circles*).

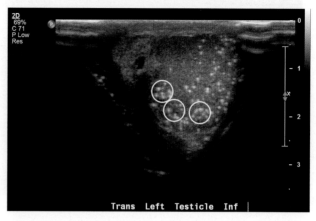

Transverse sonogram of the left testicle demonstrates multiple punctate echogenic foci (*circles*).

Answers

1. Testicular microlithiasis is an unusual condition found in up to 5% of normal males. The condition is found in up to 14% in African American males.

2. Sonography findings of this entity are small bilateral nonshadowing hyperechoic foci.

3. Interval sonographic follow-up is necessary to monitor development of malignant tumors. There is increased risk for malignancy. Two-thirds of the tumors are of the nonseminomatous type and only one-third are seminomas.

4. The condition is asymptomatic.

5. There is no treatment. Only periodic sonographic follow-up should be performed due to the risk of development of seminoma.

Pearls

- Testicular microlithiasis is usually asymptomatic.
- Found in up to 5% of normal males.
- Sonogram shows small nonshadowing hyperechoic foci ranging in diameter from 1 to 3 mm.
- The condition is bilateral.
- There is increased risk to develop malignant tumors. Two-thirds of the tumors are of the nonseminomatous type and only one-third are seminomas.
- No definite treatment.
- Needs interval follow-up to monitor malignant development (seminoma).

Suggested Readings

Janzen DL, Mathieson JR, Marsh JI, et al. Testicular microlithiasis: sonographic and clinical features. *AJR Am J Roentgenol*. 1992;158(5):1057-1060.

Kragel PJ, Delvecchio D, Orlando R, Garvin DF. Ultrasonographic findings of testicular microlithiasis associated with intratubular germ cell neoplasia. *Urology*. 1991;37(1):66-68.

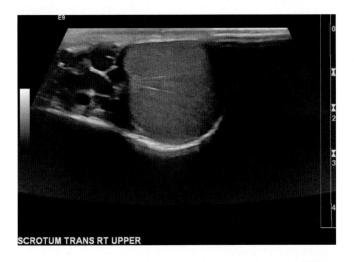

SCROTUM TRANS RT UPPER

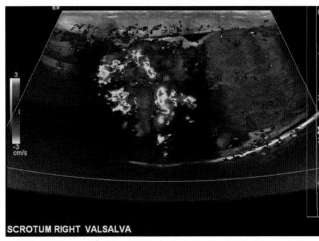

SCROTUM RIGHT VALSALVA

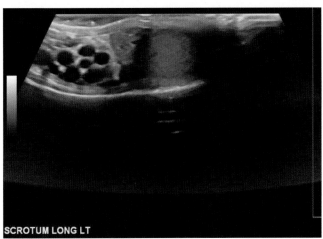

SCROTUM LONG LT

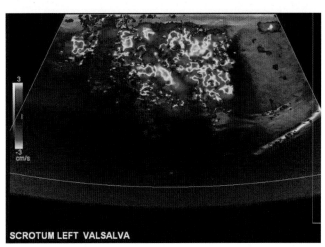

SCROTUM LEFT VALSALVA

1. What are the findings?

2. What is the most common side that this entity occurs?

3. What is the pampiniform plexus?

4. What is the complication of this entity?

5. What is the typical age range that this condition is mostly seen?

Case ranking/difficulty: 🌸

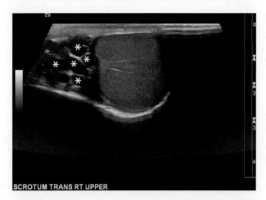

Sonogram of the right testicle reveals round and tubular anechoic structures (*asterisks*) representing the pampiniform plexus.

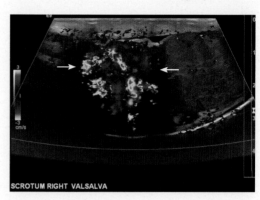

Sonogram of the right testicle with Doppler imaging during the Valsalva maneuver reveals that the pampiniform plexus fills with venous blood (*arrows*).

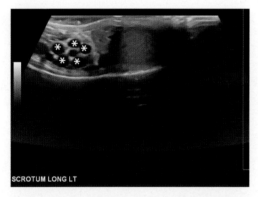

Sonogram of the left testicle reveals round and tubular anechoic structures (*asterisks*) representing the pampiniform plexus.

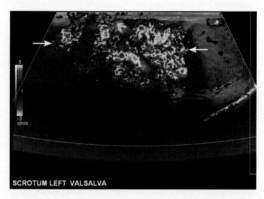

Sonogram of the left testicle with Doppler imaging during the Valsalva maneuver reveals that the pampiniform plexus fills with venous blood (*arrows*).

Answers

1. Both the testicles appear to be normal. There are dilated anechoic tubular structures in the scrotum, bilaterally representing the pampiniform plexus that fills with venous blood during the Valsalva maneuver.

2. Ninety-eight percent of cases of varicocele are seen in the left scrotum.

3. The pampiniform plexus is a network of many small veins found in the human male spermatic cord.

4. Varicocele has been associated with infertility.

5. Typical age range that varicocele is mostly seen is between 15 to 30 years of age.

- This results in the back flow of blood into the pampiniform plexus.
- A secondary varicocele is due to compression of the venous drainage from the testicle.
- Sonogram shows dilated anechoic tubular structures representing the veins in the pampiniform plexus.
- During Doppler sonography and Valsalva maneuver, these tubular structures fill with venous blood.

Pearls

- Varicocele is an abnormal enlargement of the scrotal venous system (pampiniform plexus).
- Idiopathic varicocele occurs when the valves within the veins along the spermatic cord do not work properly.

Suggested Readings

Das KM, Prasad K, Szmigielski W, Noorani N. Intratesticular varicocele: evaluation using conventional and Doppler sonography. *AJR Am J Roentgenol.* 1999;173(4):1079-1083.

de Castro JF, Fonseca D, Branco J. Intratesticular varicocele. *AJR Am J Roentgenol.* 1995;164(5):1302.

Simpson WL Jr, Rausch DR. Imaging of male infertility: pictorial review. *AJR Am J Roentgenol.* 2009;192(6 Suppl): S98-S107 (Quiz S108-S111).

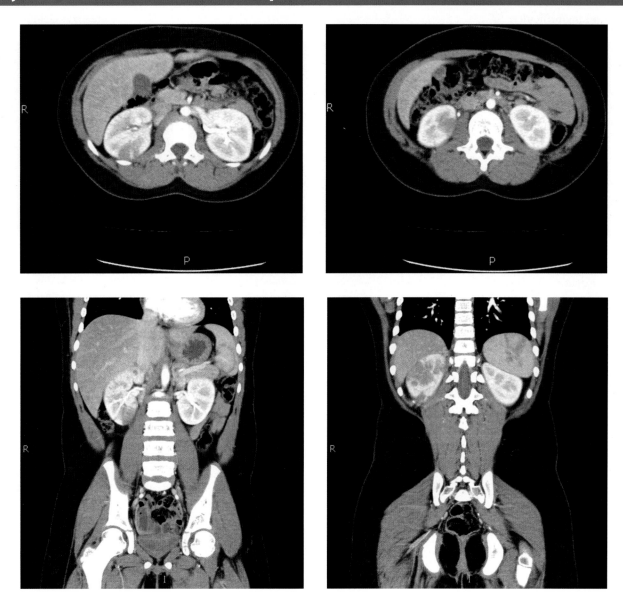

1. What are the findings?

2. What are the risk factors?

3. What are the usual organisms that cause this entity?

4. What is the most common gender that gets this entity in the neonatal period?

5. What are the clinical symptoms?

Case ranking/difficulty: **Category:** Genitourinary

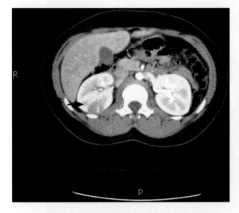

Contrast axial CT of the abdomen shows a wedge-shaped low attenuation in the upper pole of the right kidney (*arrow*).

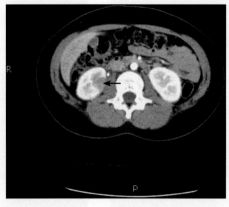

Contrast axial CT of the abdomen shows a wedge-shaped low attenuation in the lower pole of the right kidney (*arrow*).

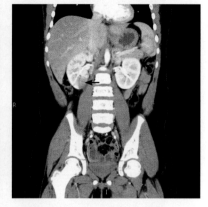

Contrast coronal CT of the abdomen shows a wedge-shaped low attenuation in the lower pole of the right kidney (*arrow*).

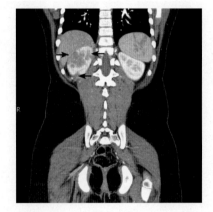

Contrast coronal CT of the abdomen shows multiple areas of wedge-shaped low attenuation in the right kidney (*arrows*).

Answers

1. There are few areas of wedge-shaped low attenuation in the right kidney.

2. Among the risk factors for acute pyelonephritis are structural renal abnormalities, diabetes mellitus, renal calculi, neurogenic bladder, and stents or drainage procedures.

3. The usual organisms are the same as for lower urinary tract infection: *Escherichia coli*, *Klebsiella* spp, *Proteus* spp, and *Enterococcus* spp.

4. In neonates, it is 1.5 times more common in boys and tends to be associated with abnormalities of the urinary tract. Uncircumcised boys tend to have a higher incidence than circumcised boys.

5. Clinical symptoms vary. Patient can be asymptomatic or can present with fever, chills dysuria, headache, or fatigue.

Pearls

- Pyelonephritis is infection within the renal pelvis, usually accompanied by infection within the renal parenchyma.
- The usual organisms are the same as for lower urinary tract infection (eg, *Escherichia coli*, *Klebsiella* spp, *Proteus* spp, *Enterococcus* spp).
- Acute pyelonephritis can occur at any age. In neonates, it is 1.5 times more common in boys and tends to be associated with abnormalities of the renal tract.
- Beyond that age, girls have a ten-fold higher incidence.
- Acute pyelonephritis is associated with diabetes mellitus, nephrolithiasis, and structural renal abnormalities.
- Contrast enhanced CT demonstrates low attenuation wedge-shaped areas in the periphery of the renal cortex.
- Renal cortical scintigraphy with Tc-99m DMSA shows photon deficient wedge-shaped defects.

Suggested Readings

Hitzel A, Liard A, Vera P, et al. Color and power Doppler sonography versus DMSA scintigraphy in acute pyelonephritis and in prediction of renal scarring. *J Nucl Med.* 2002;43(1):27-32.

Zorc JJ, Levine DA, Platt SL, et al. Clinical and demographic factors associated with urinary tract infection in young febrile infants. *Pediatrics.* 2005;116(3):644-648.

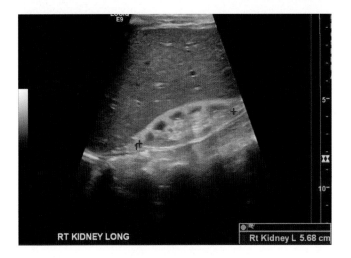
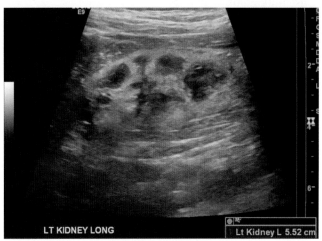

RT KIDNEY LONG — Rt Kidney L 5.68 cm

LT KIDNEY LONG — Lt Kidney L 5.52 cm

1. What are the findings?

2. What is the clinical significance of the echogenic pattern of the kidneys?

3. What is included in the etiology?

4. Enumerate few diseases that may represent the same echogenic pattern of the kidneys.

5. What is the treatment?

Case ranking/difficulty:

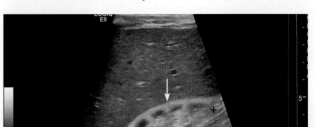

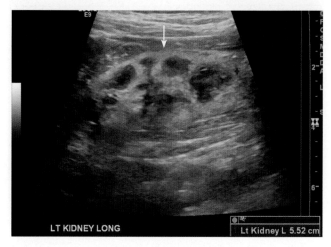

Sonogram of the right kidney reveals a very echogenic kidney (*arrow*). The size of the kidney is small for the patient's chronological age.

Sonogram of the left kidney reveals a very echogenic kidney (*arrow*). The size of the kidney is small for the patient's chronological age.

Answers

1. Small and echogenic kidneys.

2. The kidneys are small and echogenic. This represents chronic renal parenchymal disease and/or end-stage renal disease.

3. Etiology can be scarred kidneys due to recurrent urinary tract infections, glomerulosclerosis, hypoplastic or dysplastic kidneys.

4. Ecogenic kidneys in ultrasound are seen in autosomal recessive polycystic kidney disease, HIV, and may be seen in end-stage renal disease.

5. Treatment of end-stage renal disease is dialysis and renal transplant.

Pearls

- End-stage renal disease is a term that refers to severe kidney failure that necessitates the initiation of dialysis therapy or kidney transplantation to maintain life.
- Recurrent urinary tract infection leads to scarred kidneys and renal failure.
- Small and echogenic kidneys in ultrasound are nonspecific patterns that represent chronic renal parenchymal disease and renal failure.
- In the newborn period, until six months of age, the kidneys are normally echogenic in ultrasound and should not be mistaken for renal parenchymal disease.

Suggested Readings

Ardissino G, Dacco V, Testa S, et al. Epidemiology of chronic renal failure in children: data from the ItalKid project. *Pediatrics*. 2003;111(4 Pt 1):e382-e387.

Mak RH. Chronic kidney disease in children: state of the art. *Pediatr Nephrol*. 2007;22(10):1687-1688.

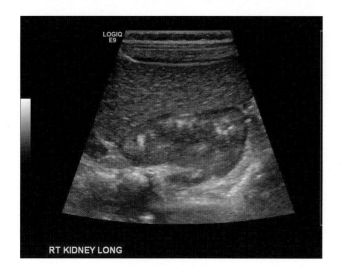

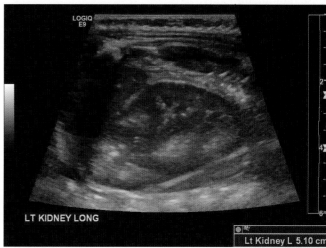

1. What is the finding?

2. What is the etiology of this entity?

3. What is the most common cause of this entity in neonatal intensive care newborns?

4. What is the most likely cause if this finding was unilateral?

5. What is the etiology of cortical nephrocalcinosis?

Case ranking/difficulty:

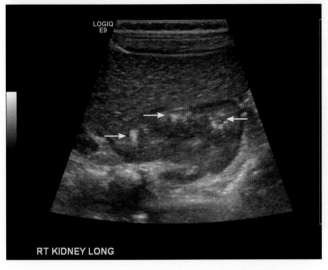

Longitudinal sonogram of the right kidney reveals echogenicity in the medullary pyramids (*arrows*) representing calcinosis.

Longitudinal sonogram of the left kidneys reveals echogenicity in the medullary pyramids (*arrows*) representing calcinosis.

Answers

1. Medullary nephrocalcinosis. Unlike renal calculi, the echogenic areas of nephrocalcinosis do not show posterior acoustic shadowing.

2. Etiology includes furosemide administration, renal tubular acidosis type I, milk alkali syndrome, hyperparathyroidism, and medullary sponge kidney.

3. Long-term furosemide administration is the most common cause of medullary nephrocalcibosis in newborns hospitalized in the intensive care unit.

4. Medullary sponge kidney may show unilateral or partial nephrocalcinosis of a kidney.

5. Cortical nephrocalcinosis is calcium deposition within the renal cortex. It is seen in chronic glomerulonephritis, renal cortical necrosis, and chronic transplant rejection.

Pearls

- Nephrocalcinosis is calcium deposited in the renal parenchyma.
- Ultrasound is the modality of choice for the diagnosis.
- Medullary nephrocalcinosis is seen in up to 60% of premature infants.
- Most common risk factor in a premature infant is furosemide administration.

Suggested Readings

Cranefield DJ, Odd DE, Harding JE, Teele RL. High incidence of nephrocalcinosis in extremely preterm infants treated with dexamethasone. *Pediatr Radiol.* 2004;34(2):138-142.

Daneman A, Navarro OM, Somers GR, Mohanta A, Jarrín JR, Jeffrey Traubici J. Renal pyramids: focused sonography of normal and pathologic processes. *Radiographics.* 2010;30:1287-1307.

Dyer RB, Chen MY, Zagoria RJ. Abnormal calcifications in the urinary tract. *Radiographics.* 1998;18:1405-1424.

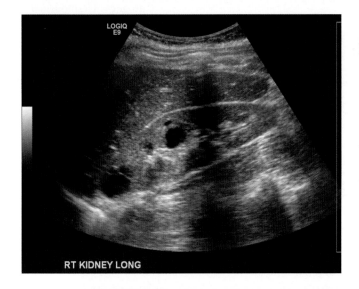

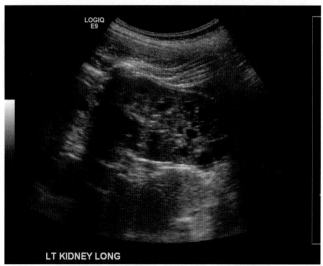

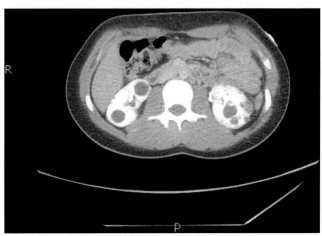

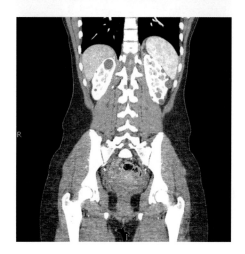

1. What are the findings?

2. What are the risk factors?

3. What are the clinically presenting signs?

4. What is the natural history of the disease?

5. What are the treatment options?

Case ranking/difficulty: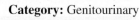

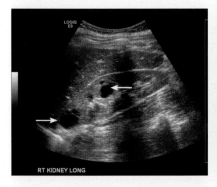

Longitudinal sonogram of the right kidney reveals multiple cystic structures (*arrows*).

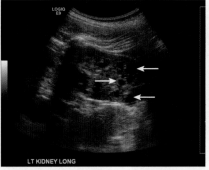

Longitudinal sonogram of the left kidney reveals multiple cystic structures (*arrows*).

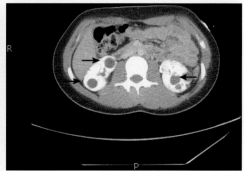

Contrast axial CT at the level of the kidneys reveals multiple renal cysts of various size (*arrows*).

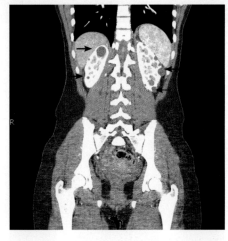

Contrast coronal CT reveals multiple renal cysts of various size (*arrows*).

Answers

1. There are bilateral multiple renal cysts of various size.

2. Risk factors for polycystic kidney disease include younger age at diagnosis, black race, male gender, presence of polycystin-1 mutation, and hypertension.

3. General presenting symptoms and signs include abdominal discomfort, hematuria, urinary tract infection, incidental discovery of hypertension, abdominal mass, elevated serum creatinine, or cystic kidneys on imaging studies, patients usually have renal pain, and develop renal insufficiency.

4. The disease is slowly progressive. Cysts enlarge and the disease progresses towards renal failure and end-stage renal disease.

5. Treatment is supportive. Hypertension should be controlled. Urinary tract infection should be treated with antibiotics and prophylaxis. When end-stage renal disease occurs, dialysis should be performed. Renal transplantation is an option.

Pearls

- Dominant polycystic kidney disease is the most common hereditary cystic disease of the kidney.
- It is characterized by progressive cyst development and bilaterally enlarged kidneys with multiple cysts.
- Risk factors for progressive kidney disease include male gender, presence of polycystine-1 maturation, hypertension, black race, and younger age at presentation.
- There are three genetic mutations in the PKD-1, PKD-2, and PKD3 gene with similar phenotypical presentations.
- The presenting signs may include abdominal discomfort, hematuria, abdominal mass, hypertension and urinary tract infection.
- Renal cysts are discovered on cross-sectional imaging. The cysts are simple, fluid-filled, but may have septations and mild enhancement.
- Imaging modalities include ultrasound, computed tomography and magnetic resonance images where cysts of various sizes are visualized.

Suggested Readings

Gabow PA. Autosomal dominant polycystic kidney disease. *N Engl J Med*. 1993;329(5):332-342.

Ravine D, Gibson RN, Walker RG, Sheffield LJ, Kincaid-Smith P, Danks DM. Evaluation of ultrasonographic diagnostic criteria for autosomal dominant polycystic kidney disease 1. *Lancet*. 1994;343(8901):824-827.

Wilson PD. Polycystic kidney disease. *N Engl J Med*. 2004;350(2):151-164.

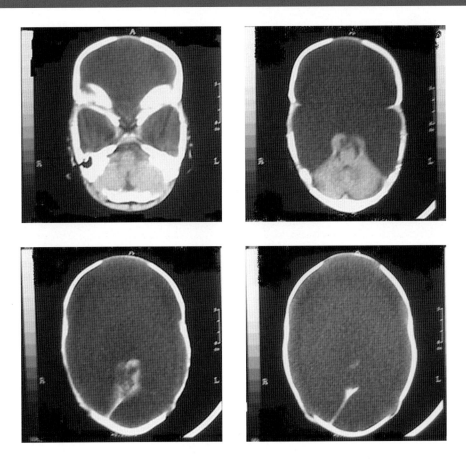

1. What is the diagnosis?

2. What are the risk factors of this entity?

3. Which vascular territory is not affected by this condition?

4. Enumerate few diagnoses in the differential.

5. What are the imaging findings?

Case ranking/difficulty:

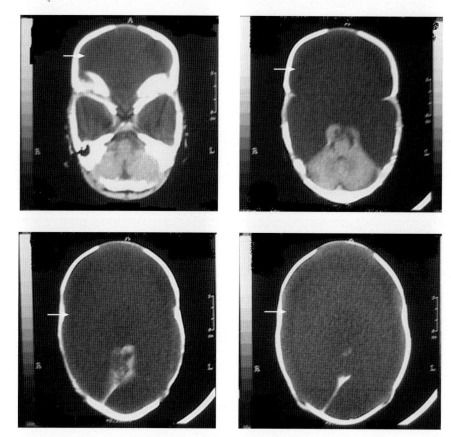

Axial enhanced CT of the brain demonstrates a complete absence of normal cortical mantle in the anterior and the middle cerebral artery territories (*arrow*), which helps in ruling out hydrocephalus. No fused thalami detected. There is a normal posterior fossa, including cerebellum. Brain stem can be atrophic; however, cerebellum is often normal.

Answers

1. The diagnosis is hydranencephaly.

2. Risk factors may include vascular compromise, toxic exposure such as tobacco, young maternal age, intrauterine infection, and twin-to-twin transfusion.

3. The posterior cerebral artery territory is not affected.

4. Porencephaly, Alobar holoprosencephaly, and hydrocephalus are parts of the differential diagnosis.

5. Imaging findings are absence of cerebral cortex in the anterior cerebral and middle cerebral artery territories and intact brain structures in the posterior cerebral artery territory.

Pearls

• Hydranencephaly is a rare congenital nervous system disorder characterized by absence of all or nearly all cerebral hemispheres with preservation of posterior fossa structures (occipital lobes, inferior temporal lobes, thalami, brainstem, and cerebellum), structures that are supplied by the posterior cerebral circulation.

• Cause is unknown, but insult of the anterior cerebral artery and middle cerebral artery territory is believed to be the case.

• Brain structures supplied by the posterior cerebral artery circulation remain intact.

• Images reveal no cerebral cortex in the anterior cerebral territory and in the middle cerebral artery territory.

Suggested Readings

Donnelly, Lane F. *Fundamentals of Pediatric Radiology.* Philadelphia, PA: Saunders/Elsevier; 2001.

Fenichel, GM. *Clinical Pediatric Neurology: A Signs and Symptoms Approach.* 6th ed. Philadelphia, PA: Saunders/Elsevier; 2009.

Quek, Y-W, et al. Hydranencephaly associated with interruption of bilateral internal carotid arteries. *Pediatr Neonatol.* 2008;49(2):43-47.

3-day-old premature newborn, with rapidly increasing head circumference

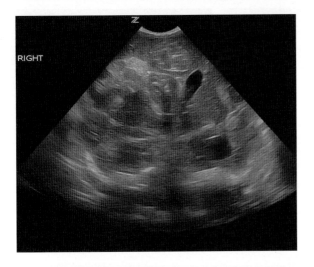

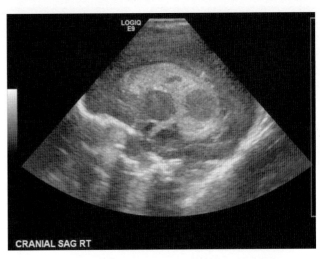

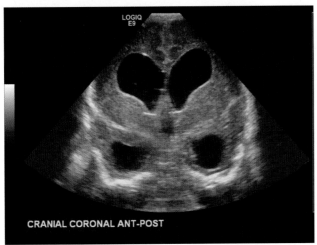

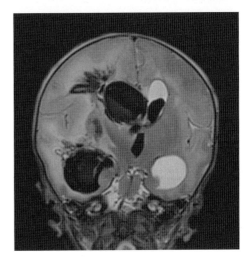

1. What are the findings?

2. What are the sequelae of this entity?

3. What are the risk factors for this entity?

4. What are the various grades of this entity?

5. What is the modality commonly used for this diagnosis?

Case ranking/difficulty: 🌰

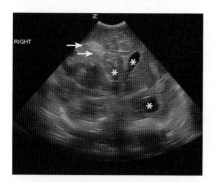

Coronal sonogram of the head of a preterm newborn reveals intraventricular hemorrhage in the right lateral ventricle, extending into brain parenchyma (*arrows*) consistent with grade IV hemorrhage. Ventricles are dilated (*asterisks*).

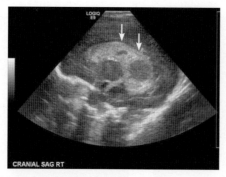

Sagittal sonogram of the head of a premature infant demonstrates intraventricular hemorrhage extending into brain parenchyma consistent with grade IV hemorrhage (*arrows*).

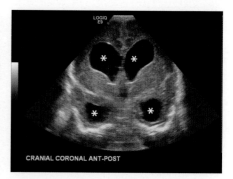

Coronal sonogram of the head of a premature infant demonstrates dilated ventricles (*asterisks*). This is a delayed complication of germinal matrix bleed.

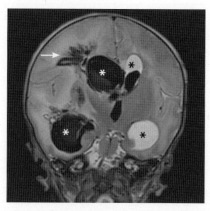

Coronal view of T2-weight MRI of the brain of a preterm newborn reveals acute bleed in the right lateral ventricle (*white asterisks*) and in the brain parenchyma (*arrow*). The hemorrhage is hypointense, due to deoxyhemoglobin. The ventricles are dilated with hyperintense CSF (*black asterisks*).

Answers

1. There is echogenicity in the lateral ventricles, anterior to the caudothalamic groove. Dilated lateral ventricles noted. The echogenicity extends to the brain parenchyma, consistent with grade IV hemorrhage. The MRI reveals hypointensity in the right ventricle and in the brain parenchyma due to deoxyhemoglobin, representing acute grade IV hemorrhage.

2. Sequelae include hydrocephalus, periventricular leukomalacia (PVL), and porencephaly. Usually intraventricular hemorrhage (IVH) grade I, II, and even III do not result in periventricular leukomalacia. Grade IV is more prone to the development of PVL and consequently porencephaly.

3. Premature infants with gestational age less than 32-week at birth and weighing less than 1500 grams are at higher risk for germinal matrix hemorrhage. Congenital heart disease, surgeries and severe respiratory distress increase the risk. It is usually seen in the first week of life.

4. Grade I - Confined to germinal matrix.
   Grade II - Extends into the ventricle but no ventricular dilatation.
   Grade III - Extends into the ventricles with ventricular dilatation.
   Grade IV - Bleeding due to venous/hemorrhagic infarction in the drainage area of the thalamostriate veins after compression /thrombosis.

5. Portable ultrasound is most commonly used to diagnose this entity. CT scan is not preferred as it involves ionizing radiation. MRI can diagnose this better than ultrasound, but transport of these sick babies to MRI scanner is not easy.

Pearls

- Germinal matrix is extensively located along the ventricular wall.
- It contains migrating neurons and vessel precursors.
- On sonography acute hemorrhage appears echogenic. Retracting blood clots are hypoechoic.

Suggested Readings

Burstein J, Papile LA, Burstein R. Intraventricular hemorrhage and hydrocephalus in premature newborns: a prospective study with CT. *AJR Am J Roentgenol.* 1979;132(4):631-635.

Volpe JJ. Intracranial hemorrhage: germinal matrix-Intraventricular hemorrhage of the preterm infant. In: *Neurology of the Newborn.* 5th ed. Philadelphia, PA: Saunders/Elsevier; 2008;517-588.

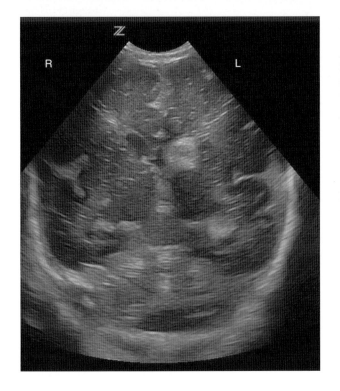 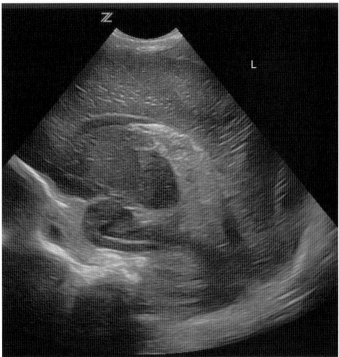

1. What are the findings?

2. What is the diagnosis?

3. Where does intracranial bleeding occur most frequently in the premature neonate?

4. What are the possible complications?

5. What is the natural course of the lesion?

Case ranking/difficulty:

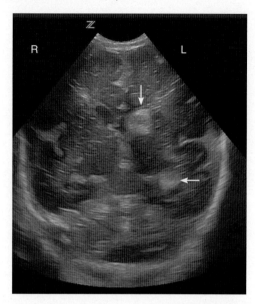

Coronal view with hyperechogenicity and dilatation of the left choroid plexus filling in the left side ventricle, including the left temporal horn (*white arrows*). There is no ventricular dilatation.

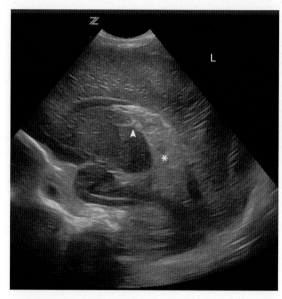

On the sagittal images, the bleeding is clearly centered within the choroid plexus (*white asterisk*) and not at the level of the caudo-thalamic groove (*white arrowhead*).

Answers

1. The left choroid plexus is dilated and hyperechogenic compared to the right side. Dilatation typically involves also the plexus at the level of the temporal horn. There is no parenchymal involvement. There is no hydrocephalus.

2. The hyperechogenicity of the choroid plexus represents acute hemorrhage and the bleeding is not centered at the level of the caudo-thalamic groove but within the plexus itself.

3. Germinal matrix residues occur at the level of the caudo-thalamic notch. They are composed of primitive vessels which demonstrate on histology weaker vessel walls compared to usual vessel wall architecture, making them more prone to rupture.

4. Secondary bleeding into the ventricular system after choroid plexus hemorrhage may occur in up to 25 to 30% of cases. As with all intraventricular hemorrhage, obstruction of cerebrospinal fluid normal outflow through the aqueduct may lead to obstructive hydrocephalus. Especially bilateral choroid plexus bleedings may produce relevant blood loss and hematocrit drop, leading to hemorrhagic shock symptoms.

5. In the absence of rebleeding, the hematoma will progressively become hypoechogenic and central cavitation and/or cystic degeneration will occur. After complete hematoma resorption, the plexus will resume its normal shape, but residual calcifications may be seen.

Pearls

- Up to 25% of intracranial hemorrages in the neonatal period occur at the plexus choroideus.
- May involve both plexus.
- Complications are intraventricular bleeding, hydrocephalus and hemorrhagic shock symptoms.

Suggested Readings

Naeini RM, Yoo JH, Hunter JV. Spectrum of choroid plexus lesions in children. *AJR Am J Roentgenol.* 2009;192(1):32-40.

Reeder JD, Kaude JV, Setzer ES. Choroid plexus hemorrhage in premature neonates: recognition by sonography. *AJNR Am J Neuroradiol.* 1982;3(6):619-622.

Neonatal convulsions

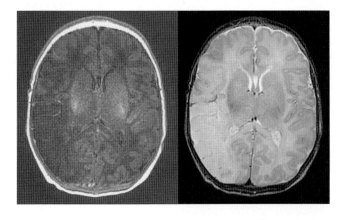

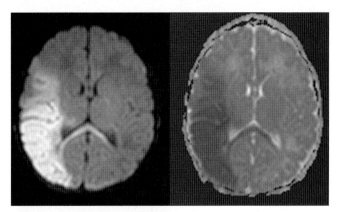

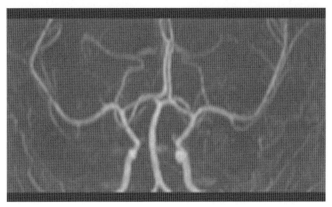

1. What is your diagnosis?

2. Which acute clinical sign is mostly encountered in these neonates?

3. What are the characteristical findings on MR angiography of a neonatal infarction?

4. Why does the splenium of the corpus callosum show diffusion restriction?

5. What are the two most common etiologies of this entity?

Case ranking/difficulty:

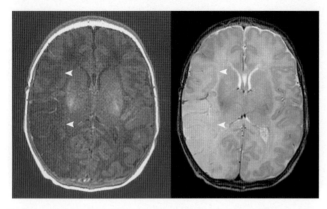

T2-hyperintensity and T1-hypointensitiy with cortical blurring and edema in the region of the right middle cerebral artery (*white arrowheads*).

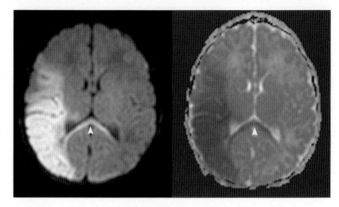

Diffusion restriction with DWI hyperintensity and ADC reduction in the region of the right middle cerebral artery, also involving the splenium of the corpus callosum (*white arrowheads*).

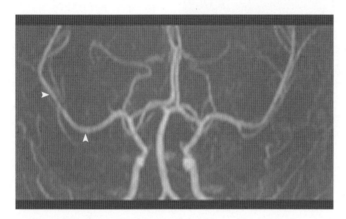

Normal appearance of the all the branches of the cerebral arteries, especially at the level of the right middle cerebral artery (*white arrowheads*).

Answers

1. Neonatal infarctions occur typically in the distribution of the middle cerebral artery, and the left side is the most common location. In this patient, there is a sparing of the basal ganglia, hence a peripheral middle cerebral artery occlusion must be postulated.

2. Most neonates present with seizures in the first few days after birth, sometimes coupled with unilateral motor weakness.

3. Neonatal infarctions typically undergo delayed MR imaging due to the fact that there is no acute clinical sign (in contrast to the adult counterpart). Due to the time delay, fragmentation of most of the thromboemboli will have taken place. Therefore, in almost all cases, MR angiography will display normal vessel anatomy, not even showing residual vascular irregularity at the primary obstruction site.

4. Wallerian degeneration and secondary ADC restriction have been described in tracts with sufficiently large white matter bundles especially at the level of the corticospinal tract (eg, cerebral peduncle, brainstem also), and also in the corpus callosum or the optic radiations.

5. Coagulopathy and congenital heart defects are the most common causes of neonatal infarctions, representing more than 2/3 of all cases. An open foramen ovale is a normal finding in neonates and can only be considered a possible cause in older children.

Pearls

- Neonatal infarctions mostly occur in the distribution of the left middle cerebral artery.
- Typical sign: "missing cortex" in all sequences.
- Wallerian degeneration and secondary diffusion restriction often occur in large projectional white matter tracts.

Suggested Readings

Rutherford MA, Ramenghi LA, Cowan FM, eds. Neonatal stroke. *Arch Dis Child Fetal Neonatal*. 2012;97(5): F377-F384.

Schulzke S, Weber P, Luetschg J, Fahnenstich H. Incidence and diagnosis of unilateral arterial cerebral infarction in newborn infants. *J Perinat Med*. 2005;33(2):170-175.

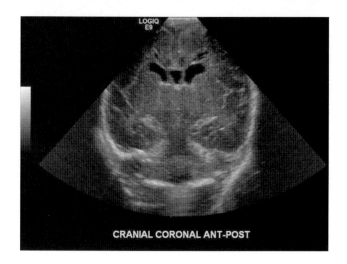

CRANIAL CORONAL ANT-POST

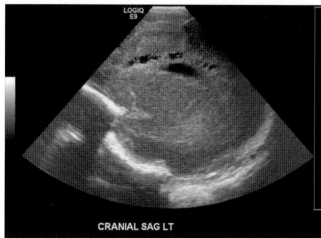

CRANIAL SAG LT

1. In which part of the brain the abnormality occurs?

2. What are the early sonographic findings of this entity?

3. What are the risk factors for the development of this entity?

4. Please enumerate at least two late sonographic findings of this entity.

5. What are the clinical complications of this entity?

Case ranking/difficulty:

Category: Head

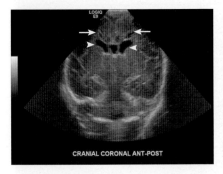

Coronal sonogram of the brain shows multiple tiny cysts (*arrows*) in the periventricular white matter bilaterally. The *arrowheads* point to the lateral ventricles.

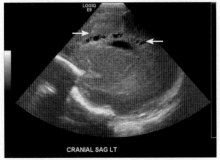

Sagittal sonogram of the brain shows multiple tiny cysts (*arrows*) in the left periventricular white matter.

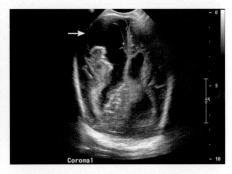

Coronal sonogram of the brain shows development of porencephaly that communicates with the right ventricle (*arrow*). This is seen as a late complication of periventricular leukomalacia.

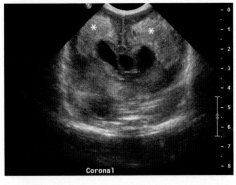

Coronal sonogram of the brain shows increased echogenicity of the periventricular white matter (*asteriks*). This is seen in the early stages of periventricular leukomalacia.

Pearls

- Periventricular leukomalacia (PVL) is the most common ischemic brain injury in premature infants.
- Necrosis results from ischemic changes in the white matter adjacent to the lateral ventricles.
- Sonogram of the brain is the easiest modality to diagnose PVL.
- Initially sonogram demonstrates increased echogenicity of the periventricular white matter.
- Later few small cysts appear that represent foci of brain parenchymal loss.
- These cysts may coalesce to form a larger cyst called porencephaly. This cyst is filled with cerebrospinal fluid and represents a focal loss of brain parenchyma.

Answers

1. Periventricular leukomalacia occurs in the periventricular white matter.

2. Early sonographic findings of this entity are echogenic periventricular white matter.

3. Risk factors for the development of periventricular leukomalacia include prematurity, germinal matrix hemorrhage, and hypoxic ischemic insult.

4. Porencephaly and hydrocephalus are late complications of periventricular leukomalacia.

5. Complications of periventricular leukomalacia include hydrocephalus, developmental delay, and cerebral palsy.

Suggested Readings

De Vries LS, Van Haastert IL, Rademaker KJ, Koopman C, Groenendaal F. Ultrasound abnormalities preceding cerebral palsy in high-risk preterm infants. *J Pediatr.* 2004;144(6):815-820.

Paul DA, Pearlman SA, Finkelstein MS, Stefano JL. Cranial sonography in very-low-birth-weight infants: do all infants need to be screened? *Clin Pediatr (Phila).* 1999;38(9):503-509.

Tzarouchi LC, Astrakas LG, Zikou A, et al. Periventricular leukomalacia in preterm children: assessment of grey and white matter and cerebrospinal fluid changes by MRI. *Pediatr Radiol.* 2009;39(12):1327-1332.

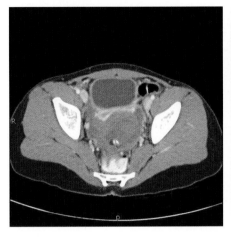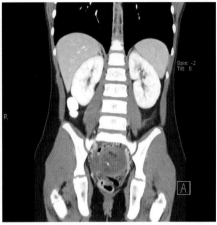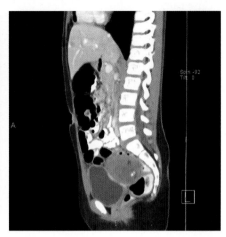

1. What are the findings?

2. What are the elements of the germ layer that this entity contains?

3. What are the most common complications of this entity?

4. What is the most important factor that correlates with the torsion of the structure that is shown in this case?

5. What are the treatment options?

Case ranking/difficulty:

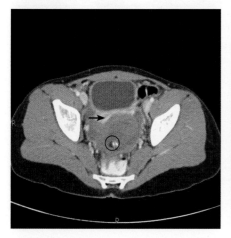

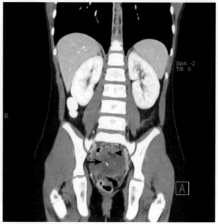

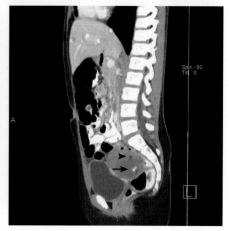

Axial contrast CT of the pelvis reveals pelvic mass arising from the right ovary (*arrow*) calcifications and fat seen inside the mass (*circle*).

Coronal CT demonstrates a pelvic mass with calcifications (*arrow*) and fat (*arrowhead*).

Sagittal CT demonstrates a pelvic mass with calcifications (*arrow*) and fat (*arrowhead*).

Answers

1. There is a pelvic mass that appears solid and contains fat and calcifications. There is no evidence of blood.

2. The mass contains all the three elements of the germ layer: Ectoderm, mesoderm, and entoderm.

3. The most common complication of mature teratoma arising from the ovary is ovarian torsion.

4. Torsion is by far the most significant cause of morbidity, occurring in 3 to 11% of cases. Increasing tumor size correlates with increased risk of torsion.

5. Complete surgical removal is necessary to avoid and prevent ovarian torsion.

Pearls

- Mature teratoma has the three germ layer components: Ectoderm, mesoderm, and entoderm.
- In young women, mature teratoma usually arises from an ovary.
- May contain hair, teeth and bone.
- It is a benign neoplasm.
- Contains fat and calcifications which are easily seen in cross-sectional imaging.
- Surgical excision is necessary to avoid the risk of ovarian torsion.

Suggested Readings

Damarey B, Farine M, Vinatier D, et al. Mature and immature ovarian teratomas: US, CT and MR imaging features. *J Radiol*. 2010;91(1 Pt 1):27-36.

Park SB, Kim JK, Kim KR, Cho KS. Imaging findings of complications and unusual manifestations of ovarian teratomas. *Radiographics*. 2008;28(4):969-983.

Rouanet JP, Maubon A, Juhan V, Meny R, Salanon AP, Daclin PY. Imaging of benign ovarian tumors. *J Radiol*. 2000;81(12 Suppl):1823-1830.

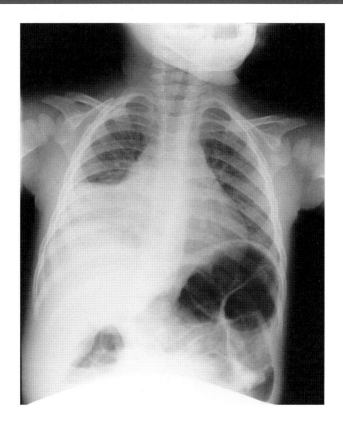

1. What is the leading cause of death in patients with sickle cell disease?

2. What is the genetic etiology of sickle cell disease?

3. What is the pathophysiology of the case in a sickle cell patient?

4. What is the definition of acute chest syndrome?

5. What are the treatment options?

Case ranking/difficulty:

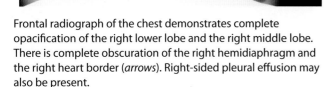

Frontal radiograph of the chest demonstrates complete opacification of the right lower lobe and the right middle lobe. There is complete obscuration of the right hemidiaphragm and the right heart border (*arrows*). Right-sided pleural effusion may also be present.

Answers

1. Acute chest syndrome is the leading cause of death and hospitalization among patients with sickle cell disease.

2. The genetic etiology of this disease is substitution of the amino acid valine with glutamic acid in the sixth position of the B-chain of the hemoglobin tetramer. The amino acid substitution causes the red blood cell to sickle and elongate upon deoxygenation.

3. The amino acid substitution causes the red blood cell to sickle and elongate upon deoxygenation. This leads to microvascular obstruction, tissue ischemia, and infarction.

4. Acute chest syndrome is defined as a new infiltrate on chest radiograph in a patient with sickle cell disease in conjunction with one other new symptom: chest pain, cough, wheezing, tachypnea, and/or fever.

5. The management of acute chest syndrome encompasses a multimodal approach. The potential for infection should be addressed with broad-spectrum antibiotics including mycoplasma coverage. Any degree of dehydration should be addressed by replacing the fluid deficit giving maintenance fluid plus insensible loses. The tachypnea, hypoxia, and anemia should be addressed by bronchodilators, oxygen therapy, and early transfusion. Some patients may require respiratory support with non-invasive mechanical ventilation or intubation.

Pearls

- Acute chest syndrome is defined as a new infiltrate on chest radiograph in a patient with sickle cell disease in conjunction with one other new symptom: chest pain, cough, wheezing, tachypnea, and/or fever.
- The red blood cells sickle and elongate upon deoxygenation. This leads to microvascular obstruction, tissue ischemia, and infarction.

Suggested Readings

Bernard AW, Yasin Z, Venkat A. Acute chest syndrome of sickle cell disease. *Hospital Physician*. 2007;44:15-23.

Charache S, Scott JC, Charache P. Acute chest syndrome in adults with sickle cell anemia. Microbiology, treatment, and prevention. *Arch Intern Med*. 1979;139:67-69.

Platt OS. The acute chest syndrome of sickle cell disease. *N Eng J Med*. 2000;342:1904-1907.

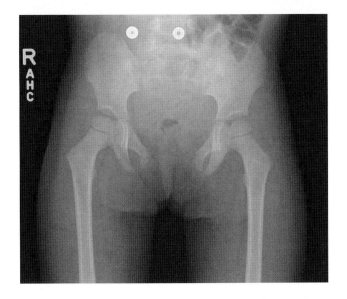 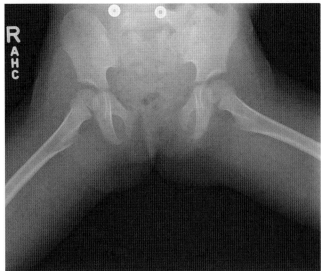

1. What are the findings?

2. What are the causes of this entity?

3. What are the clinical conditions associated with the congenital form of this entity?

4. What are the features associated with cleidocranial dysostosis?

5. What is the pathophysiology of the widening of the symphysis pubis in cleidocranial dysostosis?

Case ranking/difficulty:

Category: Genitourinary

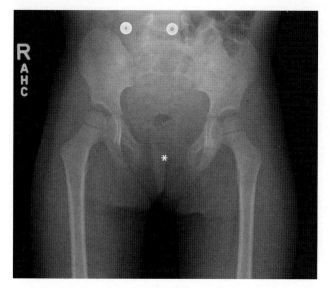 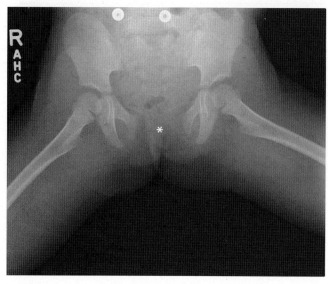

Frontal view of the pelvis reveals widening of the symphysis pubis (*asterisk*).

Answers

1. Frontal views of the pelvis show diastasis of the symphysis pubis.

2. Widening of the pubic symphysis may be congenital or an acquired condition secondary to trauma, pregnancy and delivery, infection, or osteolytic neoplasm.

3. Congenital widening of the symphysis pubis may be associated with exstrophy of the bladder, cloacal exstrophy, epispadias, anorectal anomalies, cleidocranial dysostosis, and hydrocolpos.

4. Features associated with cleidocranial dysostosis are diastasis of the symphysis pubis, wormian bones, and aplasia or hypoplasia of the clavicle.

5. Diastasis of the symphysis pubis in cleidocranial dysostosis is due to delayed maturation of the pubic symphysis cartilage.

Pearls

- Diastasis of the symphysis pubic bones may be an important clue to the presence of congenital genitourinary anomalies.
- Normal width of the symphysis pubis depends on the age and gender. Women and children have wider symphysis pubis. The symphysis pubis measures up to 10 mm in children, 6 mm in young adults, and 3 mm in late adult life.
- Common causes of widened symphysis in adults are osteitis pubis, pregnancy, or trauma.
- Causes of widened symphysis pubis in a child include bladder exstrophy, epispadias, hypospadias, imperforate anus, prune belly syndrome, and cleidocranial dysostosis.
- In cleidocranial dysostosis, the widening of the pubic symphysis seen on radiograph is due to delayed mineralization of the cartilage of the pubic bones rather than due to a true separation of the pubic bones.

Suggested Readings

Caffey J, Madell SH. Ossification of pubic bones at birth. *Radiology*. 1956;67(3):346-350.

Muecke ED, Currarino G. Congenital widening of the pubic symphysis. *Am J Roentgenol Radium Ther Nucl Med*. 1968;103(1):179-185.

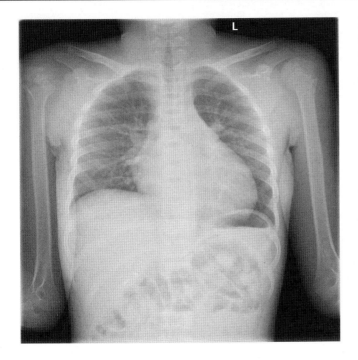
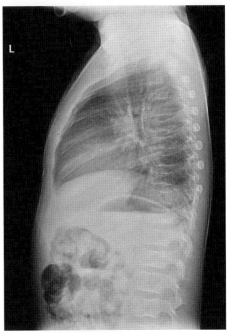

1. What are the spinal findings?

2. What are the findings outside the spine?

3. What is the pathophysiology of the findings?

4. What are the other organs that may be affected in association with this entity?

5. What are the treatment options?

Case ranking/difficulty:

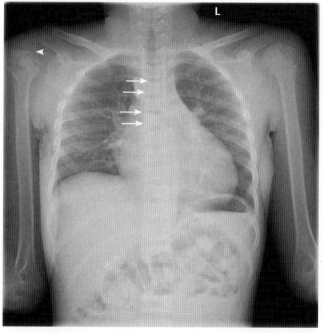

Frontal view of the chest reveals clear lungs. The right humeral head is sclerotic and irregular (*arrowhead*) due to avascular necrosis. The vertebral bodies demonstrate concavities of the end plates (*arrows*). This corresponds to bony changes of a sickle cell patient.

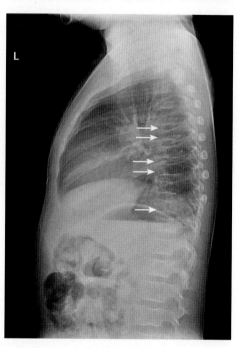

Lateral view of the chest reveals clear lungs. The vertebral bodies demonstrate concavities of the end plates (*arrows*). This corresponds to bony changes of a sickle cell patient.

Answers

1. Spinal changes in sickle cell disease as shown in the images are concavities of the end plates of the vertebral bodies, pattern of a fish shape. There is decrease in the height of the vertebral bodies with osteopenia.

2. There are sclerosis and irregularities of the right humeral head.

3. There is abnormal erythropoiesis, and the radiographic findings are primarily related to poor blood flow, either from frank infarction or from sludging of red blood cells.

4. Other organs that may be associated with sickle cell disease are central nervous system (with cerebrovascular complications of hemiparesis), spleen (with progressive shrinkage leading to autosplenectomy), lung (with massive, slowly clearing pulmonary densities), and kidneys (with renal papillary necrosis).

5. There is no definite treatment. Treatment is essentially supportive. Hydration needs to be maintained. Infections need to be controlled. Blood transfusion is necessary for severe anemia.

Pearls

- Spine changes in sickle-cell anemia show "fish-shaped" vertebral bodies secondary to osteoporotic collapse.
- Radiographic findings are primarily related to poor blood flow, either from frank infarction or from sludging of red blood cells.
- Abnormalities are seen in the bones (dactylitis, aseptic necrosis of the femoral and humeral heads), central nervous system (with cerebrovascular complications of hemiparesis), spleen (with progressive shrinkage leading to autosplenectomy), lung (with massive, slowly clearing pulmonary densities), and kidneys (with renal papillary necrosis).

Suggested Readings

Cooley TB, Witwer ER, Lee P. Anemia in children with splenomegaly and peculiar changes in bones: report of cases. *Am J Dis Child*. 1927;34(3):347-363.

Reynolds J. A re-evaluation of the "fish vertebra" sign in sickle cell hemoglobinopathy. *Am J Roentgenol Radium Ther Nucl Med*. 1966;97(3):693-707.

Reynolds J. *The Roentgenological Features of Sickle Cell Disease and Related Hemoglobinopathies*. Springfield, Ill: Charles C Thomas; 1965.

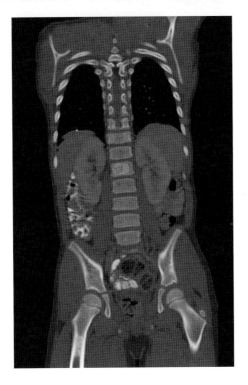
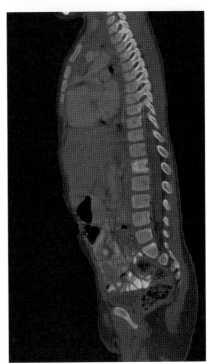

1. What are the findings?

2. What anomalies can be associated with this entity?

3. What are MRI findings of such a case?

4. The appearance of spinal hemangioma in plain radiograph is sclerotic vertebral body. What is the pathophysiology for this appearance?

5. What are the treatment options?

Case ranking/difficulty:

Category: Spine

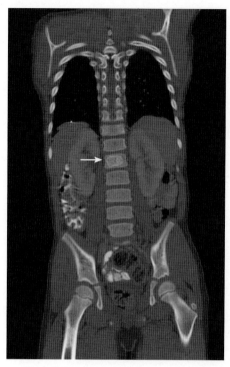

Coronal CT in a bone window demonstrates dense structure in the vertebral body of L1 (*arrow*). The structure has two tiny foci of low attenuation in its center representing fat, and consistent with osseous hemangioma.

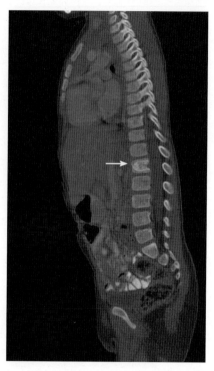

Sagittal CT in a bone window demonstrates dense structure in the vertebral body of L1 (*arrow*). The structure has two tiny foci of low attenuation in its center representing fat and consistent with osseous hemangioma.

Answers

1. There is a dense structure limited to L1 vertebral body. Tiny foci of low attenuation noted inside this structure representing fat.

2. There is association with spinal abnormalities in hemangiomas overlying the lumbosacral spine. The most common malformation is a tethered cord, often accompanied by an occult lipomyelomeningocele. Rarely, genitourinary abnormalities may be seen. Cutaneous anomalies may be associated.

3. MRI features largely depend on the proportion of fat and vascularity of the lesions. With T1-weighted MRI, particularly in vertebral hemangiomas, areas of high fat content appear as areas of high signal intensity. On T2-weighted images, high signal intensity typically corresponds to the vascularity of hemangiomas.

4. Most vertebral hemangiomas are small and cannot be seen on plain radiographs. The characteristic radiographic appearance is of a sclerotic or ivory vertebra with coarse, thickened vertical trabeculae giving a corduroy, accordion, or honeycomb appearance. This appearance is due to resorption of horizontal trabeculae, caused by vascular channels and consequent reinforcement of vertical trabeculae.

5. Treatment depends on location. If asymptomatic, it should be left alone. Involution is the natural course of infantile spinal hemangioma. Laser treatment is an option if patient is symptomatic.

Pearls

- A spinal hemangioma is a primary, benign tumor most common in the thoracic and lumbar spine.
- It is most common in patients aged between 30 to 50 years. It can be seen sometimes in the pediatric population.
- Lumbar infantile hemangioma may be associated with spinal anomalies.

Suggested Readings

Resnik D, Kyriakos M, Greenway GD. Tumors and tumor-like lesions of bone. In: *Diagnosis of Bone and Joint Disorders*. 4th ed. Philadelphia: WB Saunders; 2002: 3979-3985.

Ross JS, Masaryk TJ, Modic MT, Carter JR, Mapstone T, Dengel FH. Vertebral haemangiomas: MR imaging. *Radiology*. 1987;165(1):165-169.

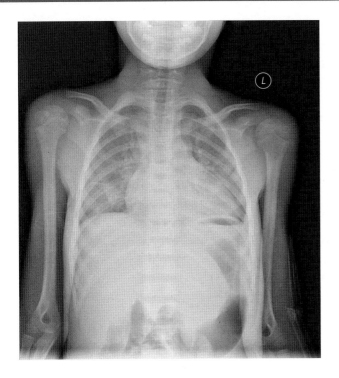 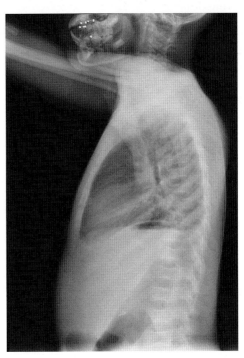

1. What are the findings?

2. What kind of spinal deformities may be seen in sickle cell patients?

3. What are the pathological processes leading to this entity?

4. At what age, this entity commonly starts to occur in sickle cell patients?

5. What is the differential diagnosis?

Case ranking/difficulty:

Category: Spine

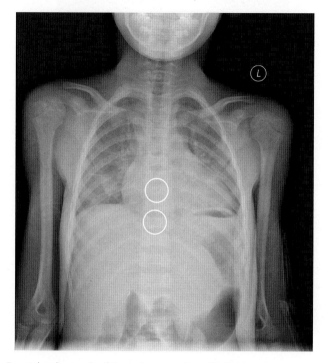

Frontal radiograph of the spine reveals multiple biconcave vertebral bodies (*circles*) representing collapse of the vertebral bodies due to osteonecrosis.

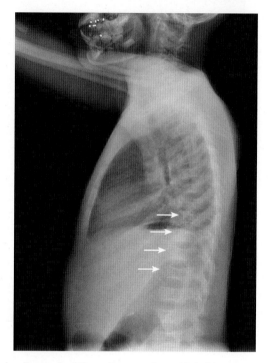

Lateral radiograph of the spine reveals multiple biconcave vertebral bodies (*arrows*) representing collapse of the vertebral bodies due to osteonecrosis.

Answers

1. There are multiple biconcave vertebral bodies representing collapse due to osteonecrosis in sickle cell patients.

2. The spinal deformities that may be seen in sickle cell patients include avascular necrosis with collapse, infectious spondylitis, course trabeculation, anterior vertebral notching, and trapezoid (biconcave) vertebral bodies.

3. The pathological processes leading to deformity of the vertebral bodies in sickle cell patients are sickling of red blood cells and marrow hyperplasia which lead to infection, ischemia, and necrosis.

4. Spinal involvement in sickle cell disease is not uncommon. It is related to the severity and duration of the disease and occurs more commonly during and after the second decade.

5. Collapse of the vertebral bodies may be seen with osteoporosis, Langerhans cell histiocytosis, multiple vertebral infections, and in multiple fractures due to trauma.

Pearls

- Bony changes in sickle cell disease are due to marrow hyperplasia and sickling of the red blood cells.
- This leads to infection, ischemia, and necrosis.
- Consequently there is collapse of the vertebral bodies leading to the H-shape or biconcave appearance shown in radiographs of the spine.

Suggested Readings

Diggs LW. Bone and joint lesions in sickle-cell disease. *Clin Orthop Relat Res*. 1967;52:119-143.

Henkin WA. Collapse of the vertebral bodies in sickle cell anemia. *Am J Roentgenol Radium Ther*. 1949;62(3): 395-401.

Mandell GA, Kricun ME. Exaggerated anterior vertebral notching. *Radiology*. 1979;131(2):367-369.

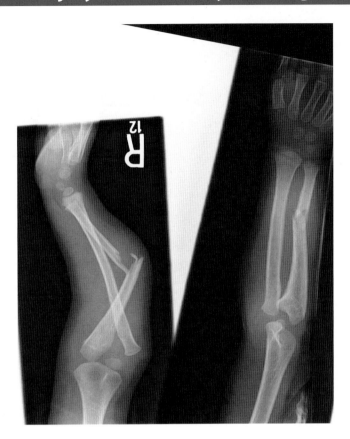

1. What are the findings?

2. What is the Bado type classification of the shown case?

3. What is the mechanism of the injury?

4. What are the complications of this case?

5. How is the reduction of the radial head dislocation achieved in the pediatric population?

Case ranking/difficulty: 🐾 🐾

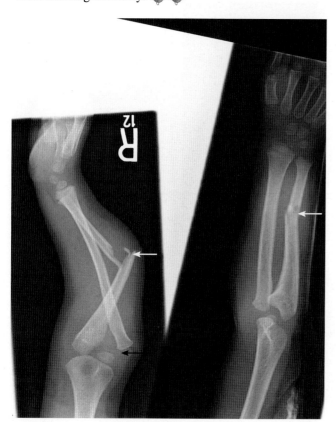

Frontal (right) and lateral (left) radiographs of the right forearm demonstrate fracture of the midshaft of the right ulna (*white arrows*) with apex dorsal angulation. In the lateral view, the radial head does not intersect with the capitulum (*black arrow*).

Answers

1. There is a fracture of the mid shaft of the ulna with apex dorsal angulation. The radial head does not intersect with the capitulum, consistent with dislocation. This is Monteggia fracture-dislocation.

2. This is type II Monteggia fracture-dislocation. There is posterior dislocation of the radial head.

3. Monteggia fractures are primarily associated with falls on an outstretched hand with forced pronation.

4. The ulnar-trochlear joint is not affected in Monteggia fracture-dislocation. The interosseous membrane proximal to the fracture is disrupted which may lead to radial nerve injury. Injuries to the median and the ulnar nerves have also been reported.

5. In the pediatric population, mostly it is closed reduction with supination of the forearm, traction, and direct pressure on the radial head.

Pearls

- The Monteggia fracture is a fracture of the ulna with the dislocation of the head of radius.
- There are four types of the fracture according to the Bado classification.
- The mechanism is primarily associated with falls on an outstretched hand with forced pronation.

Suggested Readings

Bado JL. The Monteggia lesion. *Clin Orthop Relat Res.* 1967;50:71-86.

John SD, Wherry K, Swischuk LE, Phillips WA. Improving detection of pediatric elbow fractures by understanding their mechanics. *Radiographics.* 1996;16(6):1443-1460; quiz 1463-1464.

Kay RM, Skaggs DL. The pediatric Monteggia fracture. *Am J Orthop.* 1998;27(9):606-609.

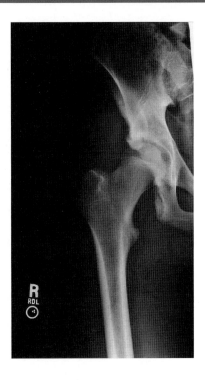 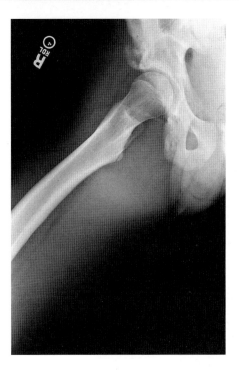

1. What are the findings?

2. Which muscle inserts in the anterior superior iliac spine?

3. Which muscle inserts in the anterior inferior iliac spine?

4. Where in the pelvis does the hamstring muscle insert?

5. Where does the iliacus muscle insert?

Case ranking/difficulty:

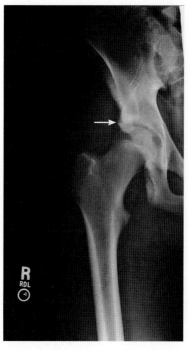

Frontal radiograph of the right hip reveals bony irregularity detached from the right anterior inferior iliac spine (*arrow*).

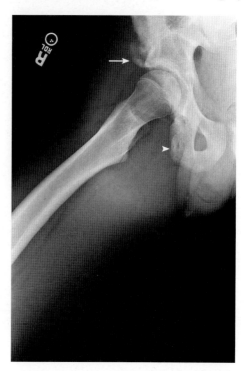

Abduction radiograph of the right hip reveals bony irregularity detached from the right anterior inferior iliac spine (*arrow*), representing avulsion fracture. There is also bony irregularity adjacent to the ischial tuberosity (*arrowhead*), which may represent old avulsion fracture.

Answers

1. There is avulsion fracture of the anterior inferior iliac spine. Irregularities are noted adjacent to the right ischial tuberosity, which may represent old avulsion fracture.

2. Sartorius inserts in the anterior superior iliac spine.

3. Rectus femoris inserts in the anterior inferior iliac spine.

4. The Hamstring muscle inserts in the ischial tuberosity.

5. The iliacus muscle inserts in the lesser trochanter of the femur.

Suggested Readings

Anderson MW, Kaplan PA, Dussault RG. Adductor insertion avulsion syndrome (thigh splints): spectrum of MR imaging features. *AJR Am J Roentgenol.* 2001;177(3):673-675.

Bui-Mansfield LT, Chew FS, Lenchik L, Kline MJ, Boles CA. Nontraumatic avulsions of the pelvis. *AJR Am J Roentgenol.* 2002;178(2):423-427.

Stevens MA, El-Khoury GY, Kathol MH, Brandser EA, Chow S. Imaging features of avulsion injuries. *Radiographics.* 1999;19(3):655-672.

Pearls

- Avulsion fracture is a fracture that results in a fragment that is pulled from the parent bone by contraction of a tendon or a ligament.
- Usually appears in the apophyses of the pelvis.
- Occurs most commonly during puberty.
- Most common apophysis to avulse is the ischial tuberosity.

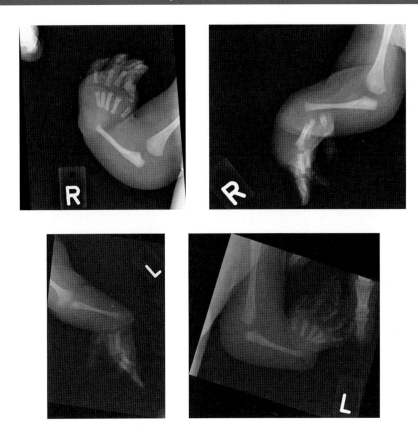

1. What is wrong with the patient's forearms?

2. What is the differential diagnosis?

3. The patient was found to have thrombocytopenia. What is the diagnosis?

4. Assuming that the patient has aplastic anemia, what would have been the diagnosis?

5. Assuming that the patient has atrial septal defect, what would have been the diagnosis?

Case ranking/difficulty: **Category:** Syndromes

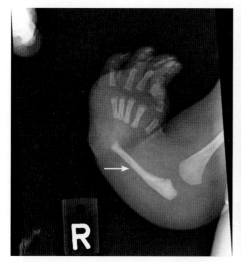

Frontal radiograph of the right forearm reveals absence of radius. The forearm has only one bone–the ulna (*arrow*).

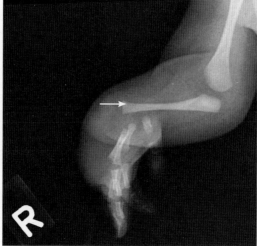

Lateral radiograph of the right forearm reveals absence of radius. The forearm has only one bone– the ulna (*arrow*).

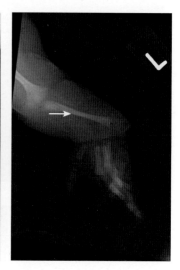

Frontal radiograph of the left forearm reveals absence of radius. The forearm has only one bone–the ulna (*arrow*).

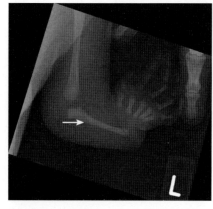

Lateral radiograph of the left forearm reveals absence of radius. The forearm has only one bone–the ulna (*arrow*).

Pearls

- TAR syndrome (thrombocytopenia with absent radius) is characterized by thrombocytopenia and absence of the radii.
- Associated anomalies may include additional skeletal defects of other bones, congenital heart disease, and renal anomalies.
- Treatment is supportive. Avoid trauma and if necessary, platelet concentrate transfusion.

Suggested Readings

Costelloe CM, De Mouy EH, Neitzschman HR. Radiology case of the month. Congenital limb and bleeding disorder. Thrombocytopenia absent radius syndrome (TAR). *J La State Med Soc*. 2000;152(11):551-552.

Giuffrè L, Cammarata M, Corsello G, Vitaliti SM. Two new cases of thrombocytopenia absent radius (TAR) syndrome: clinical, genetic and nosologic features. *Klin Padiatr*. 1989;200(1):10-14.

Answers

1. The radii are absent bilaterally.

2. Differential diagnosis includes Fanconi anemia, Holt-Oram syndrome, and thrombocytopenia-absent radius (TAR). These entities have absence of radii.

3. The diagnosis is TAR.

4. The diagnosis would have been Fanconi anemia.

5. The diagnosis would have been Holt-Oram syndrome.

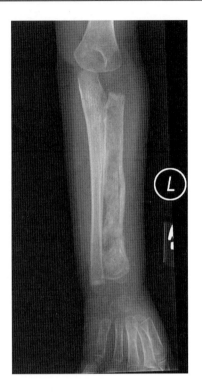 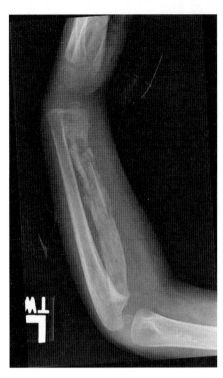

1. What are the findings?

2. What is the diagnosis?

3. What is the most common causative agent
   of the case in the general population?

4. What is the most common causative agent
   of the case in sickle cell patients?

5. What is involucrum?

Case ranking/difficulty: 🐾 🐾

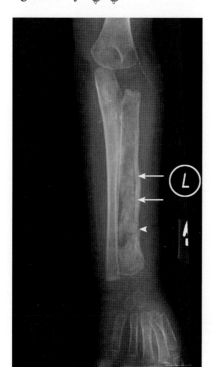

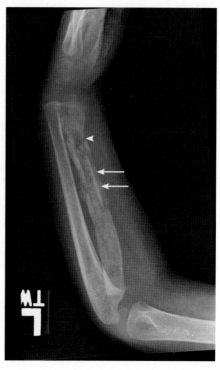

Frontal radiograph of the left forearm demonstrates diffuse heterogeneous left radius with areas of cortical disruption and periosteal reaction. Fracture is noted (*arrowhead*) involving the distal diametaphyseal left radius with near normal anatomic alignment of the fracture fragments. The *arrows* point to the involucrum.

Lateral radiograph of the left forearm demonstrates diffuse heterogeneous left radius with areas of cortical disruption and periosteal reaction. Fracture is noted (*arrowhead*) involving the distal diametaphyseal left radius with near normal anatomic alignment of the fracture fragments. The *arrows* point to the involucrum.

Answers

1. There is diffusely heterogeneous left radius. Fracture of the distal diametaphyseal left radius is seen. New periosteal reaction noted representing involucrum.

2. The pattern seen in the images with a history of sickle cell disease is most consistent with chronic osteomyelitis.

3. The most common causative agent of osteomyelitis in the general population is *Staphylococcus aureus*.

4. The most common causative agent of osteomyelitis in sickle cell patients is due to *Salmonella* species.

5. Involucrum is a periosteal reaction that acts to circumscribe the sequestrum.

- The inflammatory process inside the bone during the chronic phase of osteomyelitis produces intramedullary pressure. The inflammatory exudate stripes the periosteum and produces isolated, avascular, and infected piece of bone called sequestrum.
- The striped periosteum acts to circumscribe the sequestrum and to produce a thick sheet of new bone called involucrum.

Suggested Readings

Akakpo-Numado GK, Gnassingbe K, Boume MA, Songne B, Tekou H. Current bacterial causes of osteomyelitis in children with sickle cell disease. *Sante*. 2009;18(2):67-70.

Givner LB, Luddy RE, Schwartz AD. Etiology of osteomyelitis in patients with major sickle hemoglobinopathies. *J Pediatr*. 1981;99:411-413.

Mallough A, Talab Y. Bone and joint infections in patients with sickle cell disease. *J Pediatr Orthop*. 1985;5:158-162.

Pearls

- A chronic osteomyelitis results from an inflammatory process that continues over time, leading to osseous deformity.

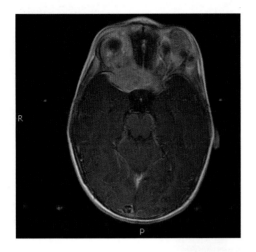
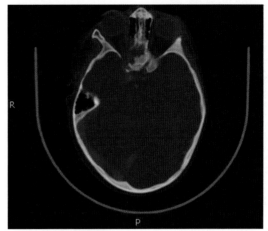
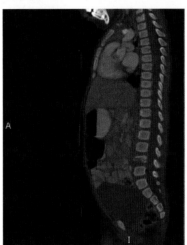

1. Describe the findings in the axial CT and the MRI.

2. Describe the findings in the sagittal CT of the lumbar spine.

3. What are the entities that may be included in the differential diagnosis?

4. How this case may present clinically?

5. What are the treatment options?

Case ranking/difficulty:

Category: Generalized diseases

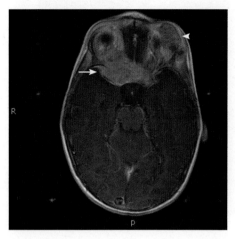

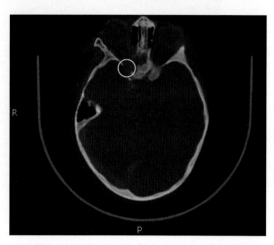

Axial T1 MRI with contrast reveals destructive lesion at the right orbital posterior ethmoid roof invading the lesser sphenoid wing and medial orbital wall extending to the orbital apex, and involving the right optic canal with erosion of the optic strut (*arrow*). A second destructive lesion with irregular margins is noted at the superolateral left orbital wall destroying the zygomatic process of the frontal bone (*arrowhead*).

Axial CT in bone window reveals destruction of the right orbital and posterior ethmoid roof and the lesser sphenoid wing (*circle*).

5. Treatment option includes chemotherapy, radiation therapy, and surgical excision of large tumors.

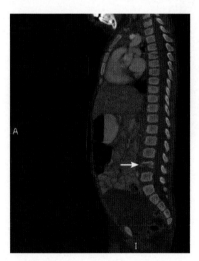

Sagittal CT in bone window reveals lytic lesion of L4 with decrease in the height of the vertebral body (*arrow*).

Answers

1. There are destructive enhancing heterogeneous lesions involving both orbits.

2. There is decreased height of L4 with lytic lesion in the vertebral body.

3. Differential diagnosis may include lymphoma, leukemia, mastocytosis, myeloma, and neuroblastoma.

4. Langerhans cell histiocytosis (LCH) may present with fever, lethargy, bone pain weight loss, and specific symptoms pertaining to the involved organ.

Pearls

- LCH is part of a group of clinical syndromes called histiocytosis, which are characterized by an abnormal proliferation of histiocytes.
- The disease has several names, including Hand-Schüller-Christian disease, Letterer-Siwe for disseminated disease, eosinophlic granuloma for a local disease, and histiocytosis X.
- LCH may lead to a non-specific inflammatory response, which includes fever, lethargy, and weight loss.
- LCH may affect multiple organs.
- Lytic lesions are seen in the bones.
- Vertebral plana is classic radiographic findings.
- Skull is the most frequent bone affected with destructive intracranial lesions and bevelled edge appearance seen on tangential view.
- Hepatosplenomegaly may be present.

Suggested Readings

Komp DM. Historical perspectives of Langerhans cell histiocytosis. *Hematol Oncol Clin North Am*. 1987;1(1):9-21.

Minkov M, Prosch H, Steiner M, et al. Langerhans cell histiocytosis in neonates. *Pediatr Blood Cancer*. 2005;45(6):802-807.

Windebank KP, Nanduri V. Langerhans Cell Histiocytosis. *Arch Dis Child*. 2009;94(1):904-908.

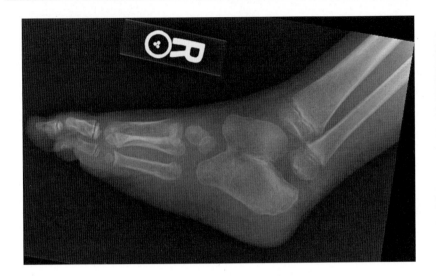
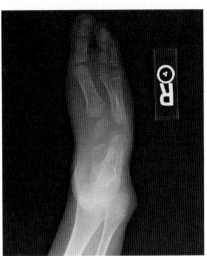

1. What is the diagnosis?

2. What is the normal range of the talocalcaneal angle in the lateral view of neonates?

3. What is the talocalcaneal angle in the lateral view of the shown case?

4. Describe the findings in the frontal view.

5. What may be included in the treatment options?

Case ranking/difficulty: 🍂🍂

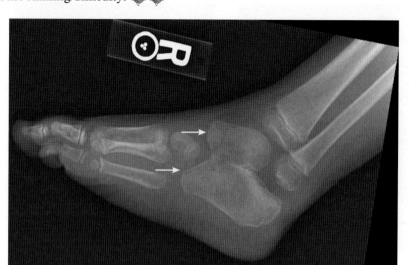

Lateral radiograph of the foot shows that the talus and the calcaneus are almost parallel to each other (*arrows*). Three metatarsals noted.

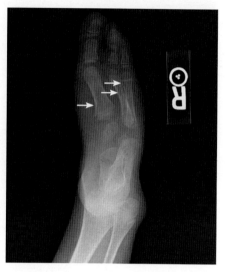

Frontal radiograph of the foot demonstrates metatarsus adductus. Three metatarsals noted (*arrows*).

Answers

1. The diagnosis is talipes equinovarus (more commonly known as club foot). There are a few missing metatarsals.

2. The normal range of the talocalcaneal angle in neonates is 25 to 55 degrees.

3. In a lateral radiograph of club foot, there is talocalcaneal parallelism.

4. In frontal radiograph of club foot, there is metatarsus adductus.

5. Treatment may include casting, splinting, and orthopedic surgical correction.

- In normal frontal view of the foot the long axis of the calcaneum is in continuity with the fifth metatarsal and the long axis of the talus is in continuity with the first metatarsal. In club foot, the first metatarsal is medial to this line–metatarsus adductus.
- The patient in the shown images was born with only three metatarsals. This is another congenital abnormality unrelated to the club foot.

Suggested Readings

Beaty JH. Congenital anomalies of the lower extremity. In: Canale ST, Beaty JH, eds. *Campbell's Operative Orthopaedics*. 11th ed. Philadelphia, PA: Mosby Elsevier; 2007:chap 26.

Hosalkar HS, Spiegel DA, Davidson RS. The foot and toes. In: Kliegman RM, Behrman RE, Jenson HB, Stanton BF, eds. *Nelson Textbook of Pediatrics*. 18th ed. Philadelphia, PA: Saunders Elsevier; 2007:chap 673.

Wynne-Davies R. Genetic and environmental factors in the etiology of talipes equinovarus. *Clin Orthop Relat Res*. 1972;84:9-13.

Pearls

- Clubfoot is a congenital deformity of the foot.
- The most common type of club foot is known as "talipes equino varus" in which the foot points down and deviates inwards.
- In normal lateral radiograph of neonates, the angle between the calcaneum and the talus ranges between 25 to 55 degrees. In club foot, the calcaneum and the talus tend to be parallel to each other.

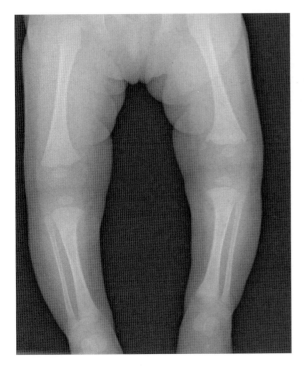
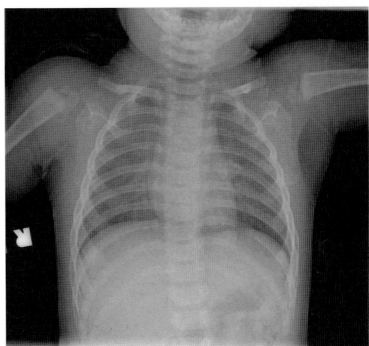

1. What is the most common location of injury in child abuse?

2. What is a bucket-handle fracture?

3. What fractures have moderate specificity for child abuse?

4. What fractures are highly specific for child abuse in an infant?

5. What is the role of nuclear medicine bone scan?

Case ranking/difficulty:

Category: Syndromes

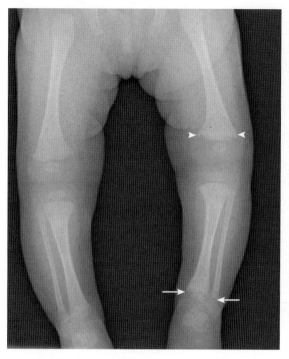

Frontal radiograph of the lower extremities shows corner fractures of the distal left femoral metaphysis (*arrowheads*). Bucket-handle fractures are seen in the distal metaphyses of the left tibia and fibula (*arrows*).

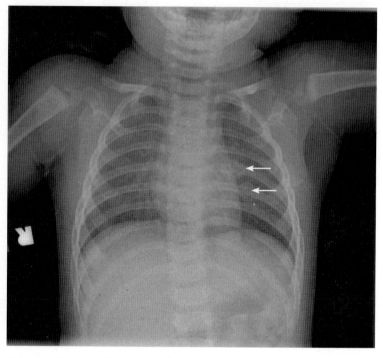

Frontal radiograph of the chest shows healing fractures of the left 6th and 7th posterior ribs (*arrows*).

Answers

1. Cutaneous/soft tissue injury is the most common injury due to child abuse followed by fractures.

2. A metaphyseal corner fracture when viewed obliquely appears as crescentic rim of bone separated from the metaphysis that looks like a bucket handle. It has high specificity for child abuse when seen in an infant.

3. Linear skull fracture has low specificity whereas complex skull fracture has moderate specificity for child abuse. Multiple bilateral fractures, fractures of varying ages, vertebral body fracture, finger fracture, and epiphyseal separation injury also have moderate specificity.

4. Rib, sternum, scapula and metaphyseal fractures in an infant have high specificity for child abuse.

5. Nuclear medicine bone scan is very helpful in detection of rib fractures. Radiographs are better than nuclear medicine bone scan for detection of skull fracture and metaphyseal fractures.

Pearls

- Diagnosis of child maltreatment syndrome/non-accidental trauma/child abuse requires a team approach between pediatrician, radiologist, and social service personnel.
- Metaphyseal corner fracture, bucket-handle fracture, fractures of rib, sternum, scapula, and spinous process in an infant are highly specific for child abuse.
- Radiographic skeletal survey is an important tool for this diagnosis.

Suggested Readings

Donnelly LF, Jones BV, O'hara SM, et al. Diagnostic imaging. *Pediatrics*. Salt Lake City, Utah, USA: Amirsys; 2005.

Kleinman PL, Kleinman PK, Savageau JA. Suspected infant abuse: radiographic skeletal survey practices in pediatric health care facilities. *Radiology*. 2004;233(2):477-485.

Mogbo KI, Slovis TL, Canady AI, Allasio DJ, Arfken CL. Appropriate imaging in children with skull fractures and suspicion of abuse. *Radiology*. 1998;208(2):521-524.

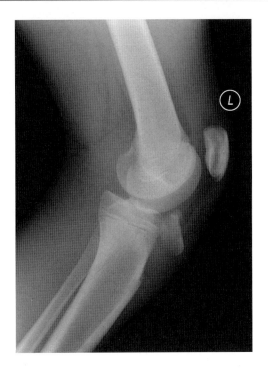
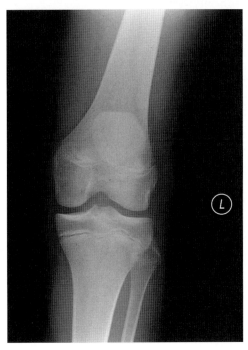

1. What are the findings?

2. What is the normal ratio between the patellar length and the length of the patellar tendon?

3. What is the best radiographic view to measure the ratio discussed in question 2?

4. Enumerate few of the etiologies causing patella alta.

5. Enumerate few of the etiologies causing patella baja.

Case ranking/difficulty:

Category: Lower extremities

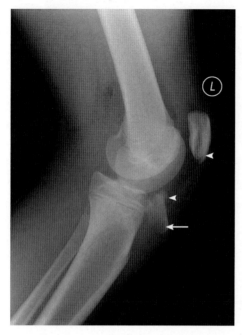

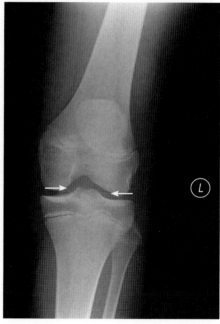

Lateral radiograph of the left knee reveals avulsion fracture of the anterior proximal tibial metaphysis (*arrow*). The avulsed fragment includes the tibial tubercle (*outlined arrowhead*). High riding patella is noted (*simple arrowhead*).

Frontal radiograph of the left knee demonstrates hazy density in the joint space, above the tibial spines (*arrows*) which represent a part of the avulsed fragment. Most of the avulsed fragment is obscured by the proximal tibial density.

Answers

1. There is avulsion of the anterior proximal tibial metaphysis. There is edema in the region of the patellar tendon. There is high-riding patella (patella alta) due to rupture of the patellar tendon.

2. The normal ratio between the patellar length (greatest diagonal length) and the patellar tendon length (from the lower pole of patella to its insertion on top of tibial tubercle) is between 0.8 and 1.2). Increase in the ratio is seen in patellar baja. Decrease in ratio is seen in patella alta.

3. The best view to measure the ratio between the patellar length and the distance from the lower pole of patella to the tibial tubercle is a lateral view of the knee with the knee flexed at 30 degrees.

4. Patellar tendon rupture and elongation will cause patella alta. Rupture of the quadricepital tendon causes patella baja. In children with cerebral palsy, there is spacticity of the quadricepital tendon that will pull the patella causing patella alta. Chondromalacia of the patella is associated with high riding patella.

5. Achondroplastic dwarf, quadriceps tendon rupture, flaccid neuromuscular disease such as polio, and status post operative patella (following tibial tubercle transfer or ACL reconstruction) are all causes for patellar baja. Patellar tendon rupture is a cause for patella alta.

Pearls

- Fracture of the anterior tibial tubercle may cause rupture of the patellar tendon which normally inserts in the lower patellar pole and in the anterior tibial tubercle.
- This leads to patella alta (high-riding patella) due to loss of the lower patellar support mechanism.
- Differential diagnosis of patella alta includes fracture of the anterior tibial tubercle (as seen in the case) with rupture or elongation of the patellar tendon. Patella alta can be seen in children with cerebral palsy due to spasticity of the quadricipital tendon, and in chondromalacia of the patella.

Suggested Readings

Insall J, Goldberg V, Salvati E. Recurrent dislocation and the high-ridings patella. *Clin Orthop Relat Res*. 1972;88:67-69.

Insall J, Salvati E. Patella position in the normal knee joint. *Radiology*. 1971;101:101-104.

Kannus PA. Long patellar tendon: radiographic sign of patellofemoral pain syndrome a prospective study. *Radiology*. 1992;185:859-863.

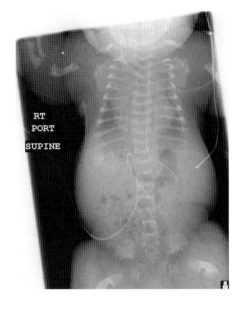 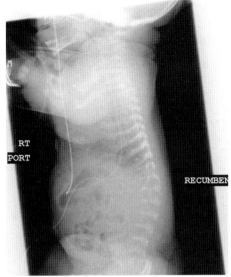 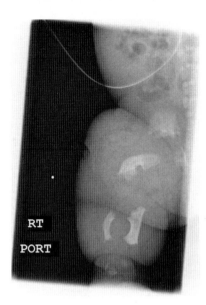

1. What are central nervous system abnormalities of the case?

2. What type of bony dysplasia is shown?

3. What are the spinal changes in this entity?

4. How will you describe the ribs?

5. The pattern of the femur resembles.

Case ranking/difficulty:

Category: Syndromes

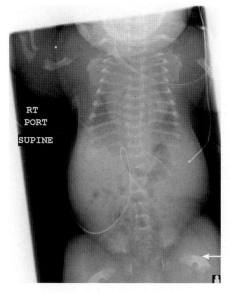

Frontal radiograph of the entire body of a newborn demonstrates short ribs, and platyspondyly. Increased ratio of the intervertebral disk space to the vertebral bodies height. Deformity of the extremities with the "telephone receiver" shape femur (*arrow*).

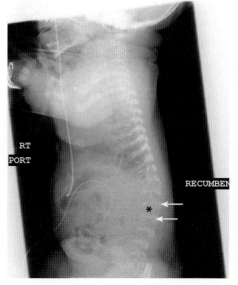

Lateral radiograph of the entire body of a newborn demonstrates short ribs, platyspondyly. There is increased ratio of the intervertebral disk space (*asterisk*) to the vertebral bodies height (*arrows*).

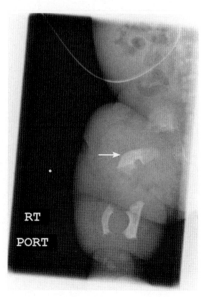

Frontal radiograph of the right femur demonstrates deformity of the lower extremity with the shape of the femur resembles the telephone receiver (*arrow*).

Answers

1. Thanatophoric dysplasia may have central nervous system abnormalities including temporal lobe malformations, hydrocephaly, brainstem hypoplasia, neuronal migration abnormalities.

2. Thanatophoric dysplasia is a rhizomelic dysplasia. The proximal portion of the extremities is shortened.

3. Spinal changes are platyspondyly, U-shaped vertebral bodies, and increased ratio between the intervertebral disk space and vertebral body height.

4. The ribs are shortened.

5. The femurs are bowed and resemble a telephone receiver.

- The femurs are bowed with the shape of telephone receiver. There are central nervous system abnormalities including temporal lobe malformations, hydrocephaly, brainstem hypoplasia, neuronal migration abnormalities.
- Treatment is palliative. In case of respiratory failure, intubation and placement in a ventilator is necessary.

Suggested Readings

Baker KM, Olson DS, Harding CO, Pauli RM. Long-term survival in typical thanatophoric dysplasia type 1. *Am J Med Genet.* 1997;70(4):427-436.

Garjian KV, Pretorius DH, Budorick NE, et al. Fetal skeletal dysplasia: three-dimensional US–initial experience. *Radiology.* 2000;214(3):717-723.

Kolble N, Sobetzko D, Ersch J. Diagnosis of skeletal dysplasia by multidisciplinary assessment: a report of two cases of thanatophoric dysplasia. *Ultrasound Obstet Gynecol.* 2002;19(1):92-98.

Pearls

- Thanatophoric dysplasia is the most common form of skeletal dysplasia that is lethal in the neonatal period.
- Radiographs show: rhizomelic shortening of the long bones, irregular metaphyses of the long bones, platyspondyly, U-shaped vertebral bodies, short ribs and small foramen magnum with brain stem compression.

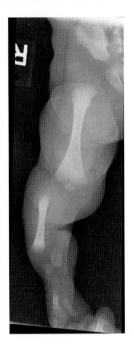 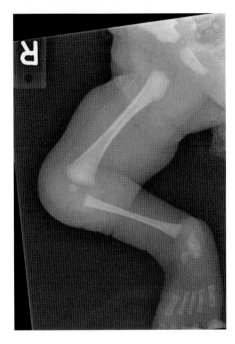 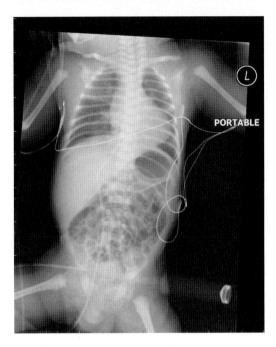

1. What is the most likely diagnosis?

2. What is shown in the lower extremity radiographs?

3. What does VACTERL stand for?

4. What is the frequency of VACTERL association?

5. In order to make the diagnosis of VACTERL association, how many anomaly sites should be present?

Case ranking/difficulty: 🐾 🐾

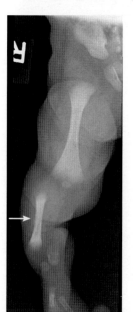

Frontal radiograph of the right leg demonstrates absence of the fibula. Only the tibia is present (*arrow*).

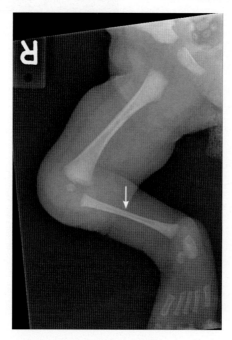

Lateral radiograph of the right leg demonstrates absence of the fibula. Only the tibia is present (*arrow*).

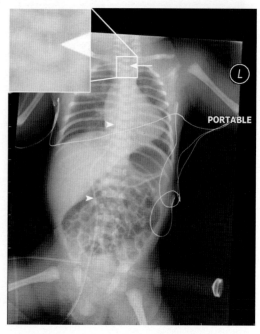

Frontal radiograph of the chest demonstrates an enteric tube (*arrow*) located in the upper esophagus. An umbilical venous catheter noted (*arrowheads*). The lungs are clear. Abdomen demonstrates normal bowel gas pattern.

Answers

1. The distal tip of the enteric tube is in the proximal esophagus. As clinically, the tube could not advance further, it is very suspicious for esophageal atresia.

2. The fibula is missing in the lower extremity radiographs.

3. The acronym VACTERL describes a combination of anomalies in few of the areas: Vertebrae, Anus, Cardiac, Trachea, Esophagus, Renal and/or Radius, and Limbs.

4. The frequency of VACTERL association is 16:100,000.

5. To make the diagnosis of VACTERL association, not all seven sites (according to the acronym VACTERL) need to be present.

Pearls

- VATER syndrome or VACTERL association is a combination of birth defects that affect many organs.
- Not all areas are involved in the anomalies.
- This case demonstrates two areas of anomalies: esophageal atresia and absence of fibula.
- There is gas in the bowel, meaning that there is distal tracheoesophageal fistula, which is the most common form (82%).

Suggested Readings

Barry JE, Auldist AW. The VATER association; one end of a spectrum of anomalies. *Am J Dis Child*. 1974;128(6): 769-771.

Czeizel A, Ludányi I. An aetiological study of the VACTERL-association. *Eur J Pediatr*. 1985;144:331-337.

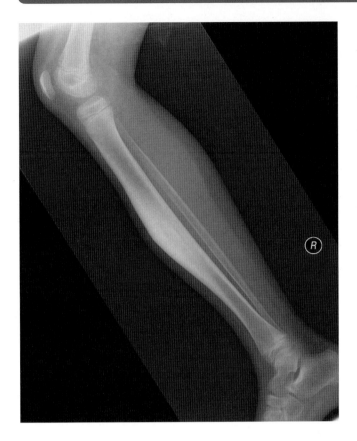
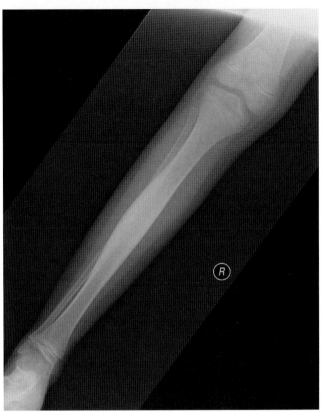

1. What are the radiographic findings?

2. What is the differential diagnosis?

3. What is the most likely diagnosis if the pain is worse at night, and relieved by aspirin?

4. What are the treatment options?

5. What leads to recurrence of this entity?

Case ranking/difficulty: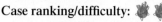

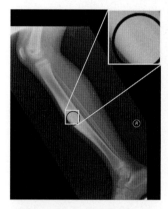

Lateral radiograph of the leg demonstrates thickening of the periosteum of the mid tibia. A small round lucency noted inside the thickened periosteum representing the nidus (*circle*).

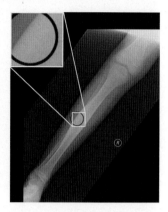

Frontal radiograph of the leg demonstrates thickening of the periosteum of the mid tibia. A small round lucency noted inside the thickened periosteum representing the nidus (*circle*).

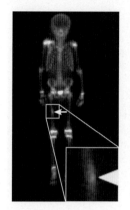

Anterior view of bone scintigraphy performed with Tc-99m-MDP in another patient shows increased activity in the mid-right femur representing osteoid osteoma. The nidus takes up the radiotracer (*arrow*). There is also increased activity in the right scapula. The patient had osteomyelitis of the right scapula.

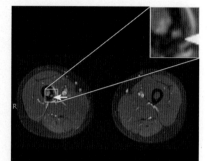

Axial MRI-T1 post contrast in the same patient of image 3 shows elevation of the periosteum of the mid-right femur with enhancement of the nidus (*arrow*).

Answers

1. There is thickening of the cortex in mid tibia with sclerosis surrounding a lytic nidus that is less than 1.5 cm in diameter.

2. Differential diagnosis includes Brodie abscess, osteoblastoma, osteomyelitis, healing fracture, and stress fracture.

3. Osteoid osteoma.

4. Aspirin, non-steroidal anti-inflammatory drugs and surgical ablation and CT guided radiofrequency thermal ablation of the nidus are the available treatment options. Sometimes, osteoid osteoma may regress spontaneously after months to years. Preferred treatment is CT guided percutaneous radio frequency thermal ablation.

5. Incomplete surgical resection or incomplete radio frequency thermal ablation of the nidus leads to recurrence of the lesion.

Pearls

- Osteoid osteoma is a benign bone-producing neoplasm of the skeletal system.
- Typical presentation is in the second decade of life with focal bony pain that is worse at night and is relieved by aspirin.
- Most (up to 70%) osteoid osteoma involves cortex of the diaphysis of long bones with femur and tibia comprising majority of the cases. Posterior elements of the spine are involved in 10% of the cases.

- The central lytic nidus is the neoplasm that is surrounded by reactive sclerosis. The nidus is usually smaller than 1.5 cm in diameter. The center of the nidus may have tiny sclerotic center.
- The lesion may be intracapsular at the femoral neck leading to arthritis. Radiograph is the initial examination of choice. CT scan is used for precise localization of the nidus and is used for guiding percutaneous radio frequency thermal ablation.
- Nidus is hyperintense on T2-weighted MRI with hypointense surrounding sclerosis.
- Nuclear medicine bone scan shows increased radiotracer uptake in the lesion.
- Sometimes, osteoid osteoma may regress spontaneously after months to years. Incomplete surgical resection/ablation of the nidus leads to recurrence of the lesion. Preferred treatment is CT guided percutaneous radio frequency thermal ablation.

Suggested Readings

Shukla S, Clarke AW, Saifuddin A. Imaging features of foot osteoid osteoma. *Skeletal Radiol.* 2010;39(7):683-689.

Stoller DW, Tirman PF, Bredella MA, Branstetter R, Blease S, Beltran S. Diagnostic Imaging. In: *Orthopaedics.* Salt Lake City, Utah, USA: Amirsys; 2003.

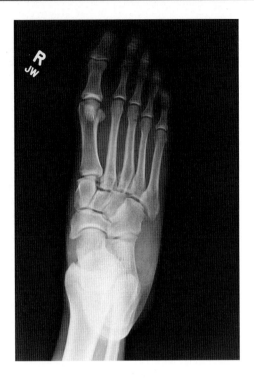 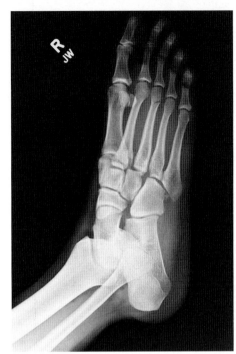

1. What are the findings?

2. In normal frontal radiograph of the foot, the lateral aspect of the first metatarsal should normally align with . . . .

3. In normal frontal radiograph of the foot, the medial aspect of the second metatarsal should normally align with . . . .

4. In normal oblique radiograph of the foot, the lateral aspect of the second metatarsal should normally align with . . . .

5. In normal oblique radiograph of the foot, the medial aspect of the third metatarsal should normally align with . . . .

Case ranking/difficulty:

Category: Lower extremities

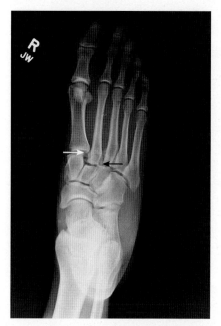

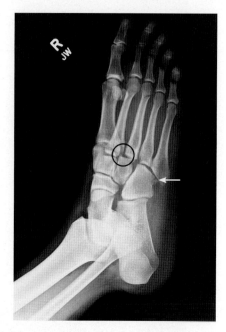

Frontal radiograph of the right foot shows that the lateral aspect of the first metatarsal bone does not align with the lateral aspect of the medial cuneiform (*white arrow*). The medial aspect of the third metatarsal does not align with the medial aspect of the lateral cuneiform (*black arrow*). There is a fracture of the lateral cuneiform with non-displaced fracture of the distal aspect of the third metatarsal.

Oblique radiograph of the right foot shows that the medial aspect of the third metatarsal does not align with the medial aspect of the lateral cuneiform. The lateral aspect of the second metatarsal does not align with the lateral aspect of the middle cuneiform (*circle*). There is a fracture of the lateral cuneiform with non-displaced fracture of the distal aspect of the third metatarsal. Fracture of the cuboid seen (*arrow*).

Answers

1. The alignment between the tarsal bones and the metatarsals is abnormal. The medial aspect of the third metatarsal does not align with the medial aspect of the lateral cuneiform. The lateral aspect of the first metatarsal does not align with the lateral aspect of the medial cuneiform and the medial aspect of the second metatarsal does not align with the medial aspect of the middle cuneiform. This is consistent with Lisfranc fracture-dislocation. There is a fracture of the lateral cuneiform and non-displaced fracture of the distal aspect of the third metatarsal.

2. In normal frontal radiograph of the foot, the lateral aspect of the first metatarsal should normally align with the lateral aspect of the medial cuneiform.

3. In normal frontal radiograph of the foot, the medial aspect of the second metatarsal should normally align with the medial aspect of the middle cuneiform.

4. In normal oblique radiograph of the foot, the lateral aspect of the second metatarsal should normally align with the lateral aspect of the middle cuneiform.

5. In normal oblique radiograph of the foot, the medial aspect of the third metatarsal should normally align with the medial aspect of the lateral cuneiform.

Pearls

- The most common injury to the Lisfranc joint occurs at the joint involving the first and second metatarsals and the medial cuneiform.
- In evaluating anteroposterior and oblique radiographs of the foot, it is essential to evaluate disruption of the normal anatomic alignment.
- Trauma is the most common etiology in children and young adults.
- In elderly, the most common etiology is diabetic foot and neurogenic joint.

Suggested Readings

Chaney DM. The Lisfranc joint. *Clin Podiatr Med Surg.* 2010;27(4):547-560.

Gupta RT, Wadhwa RP, Learch TJ, Herwick SM. Lisfranc injury: imaging findings for this important but often-missed diagnosis. *Curr Probl Diagn Radiol.* 2008;37(3):115-126.

Scolaro J, Ahn J, Mehta S. Lisfranc fracture dislocations. *Clin Orthop Relat Res.* 2011;469(7):2078-2080.

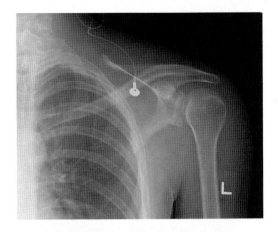
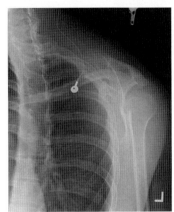
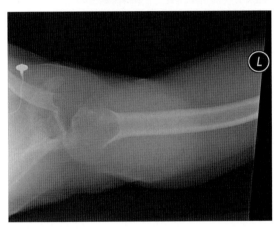
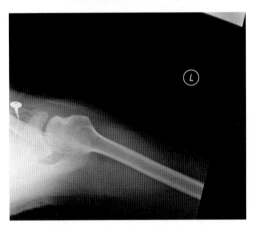

1. What is the diagnosis?

2. What is the location of the trough sign?

3. What is the rim sign in the shown entity?

4. What are the complications of the shown entity?

5. What is the "lightbulb sign" in the shown entity?

Case ranking/difficulty:

Category: Upper extremities

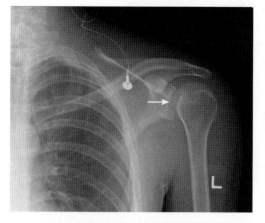

Frontal radiograph of the left shoulder demonstrates slight widening of the left shoulder joint space (*arrow*). This finding is very subtle and can be overlooked.

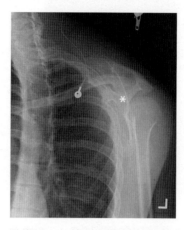

Radiograph of the left shoulder in trans-scapular Y-view reveals that the left shoulder is not centered in the center of the "Y" (*asterisk*). The left humerus head is displaced posteriorly.

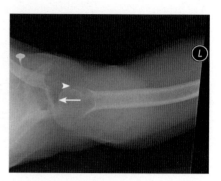

Axillary radiograph of the left shoulder reveals posterior dislocation. Reverse Hill-Sachs fracture or the trough sign noted (*arrow*). The *arrowhead* points to the normal bicepital groove.

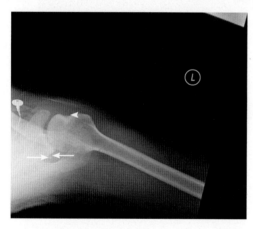

Axillary radiograph following reduction of the left shoulder reveals that the left humeral head is back in the normal position. Reverse Bankart fracture seen (*arrows*). The *arrowhead* points to the reverse Hill-Sachs fracture.

Answers

1. The diagnosis is posterior shoulder dislocation with reverse Hill-Sachs impaction fracture, and reverse Bankart lesion.

2. The trough sign is the reverse Hill-Sachs deformity, consisting with impaction fracture of the anteromedial humeral head.

3. Rim sign in posterior shoulder dislocation refers to the distance between medial border of humeral head and anterior glenoid rim >6 mm.

4. Complications include osteonecrosis of the humeral head, acute redislocation, recurrent posterior shoulder

instability, joint stiffness and functional incapacity, and post-traumatic osteoarthritis.

5. The lightbulb sign is the humeral head that is fixed in internal rotation, no matter how the forearm is turned.

Pearls

- Posterior shoulder dislocation is the second most common shoulder dislocation.
- It occurs during seizures or electrocution.
- Occasionally, severe direct blow may cause posterior dislocation.
- Plain radiographs in frontal view reveals widening of the joint space.
- On radiographs, diagnosis is confirmed with the trans-scapular Y view and/or the axillary views.
- Reverse Hill-Sachs impaction fracture occurs in the anteriomedial aspect of the femoral head.
- Reverse Bankart lesion is a fracture of the posterior glenoid rim.
- Complications are shoulder instability and recurrent dislocations.

Suggested Readings

Cisternino SJ, Rogers LF, Stufflebam BC, Kruglik GD. The trough line: a radiographic sign of posterior shoulder dislocation. *AJR Am J Roentgenol.* 1978;130(5):951-954.

Schmickal T, Kleine L, Doleschal S, Schuh A. Shoulder dislocation: diagnosis and treatment. *MMW Fortschr Med.* 2010;152(51-52):31-33.

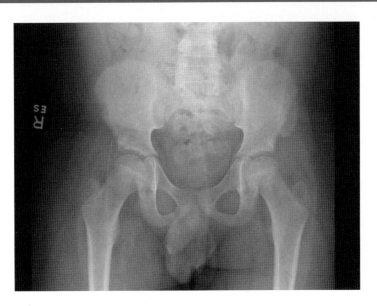

1. What is the etiology of the shown case?

2. What is the most common location of such a case?

3. What is Prussian's disease?

4. What is the pathophysiology of the case?

5. What are the treatment options?

Case ranking/difficulty: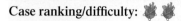

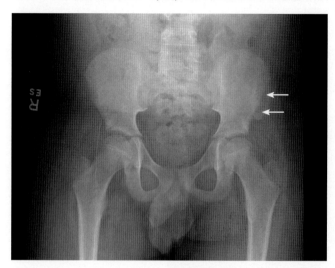

Frontal view of the pelvis demonstrates ossification around the left anterior superior iliac spine (*arrows*).

Pearls

- Myositis ossificans is an inflammatory response to local tissue trauma.
- The heterotopic bone that is formed contain more than the normal bone amount of osteoblasts.
- The most common anatomic sites involved are the quadriceps in the lower extremities and the brachialis muscles in the upper extremities.
- The most common type of myositis ossificans is the non-hereditary type that consists of ossifications surrounding injured muscles.
- The inherited type is very rare and is called myositis ossificans progressiva or fibrodysplasia ossificans progressiva that can occur without previous injury.
- Ossification is easily depicted by plain radiographs and in CT.
- Treatment is mostly conservative.

Answers

1. The etiology of myositis ossificans (heterotopic bone formation) is traumatic with ossification that occurs at the site of injured muscles.

2. Most (ie, 80%) ossifications arise in the thigh or arm, and are caused by a premature return to activity after an injury. Other sites include intercostal spaces, erector spinae, pectoralis muscles, glutei, and the chest.

3. "Prussian's disease" is myositis ossificans located in the adductor muscles.

4. The underlying process is thought to be an inflammatory process in response to local tissue trauma. Bone morphogenic protein is believed to be important in regulating the development of heterotopic ossification.

5. Treatment is initially conservative, as some patients' calcifications will spontaneously be reabsorbed, and others will have minimal symptoms. In occasional cases, surgical debridement of the abnormal tissue is required, although success of such therapy is limited. Treatment includes rest, immobilization, anti-inflammatory drugs, and physiotherapy.

Suggested Readings

Bowerman JW, McDonnell EJ. Radiology of athletic injuries: football. *Radiology*. 1975;117(1):33-36.

Hanna SL, Magill HL, Brooks MT, Burton EM, Boulden TF, Seidel FG. Cases of the day. Pediatric. Myositis ossificans circumscripta. *Radiographics*. 1990;10(5):945-949.

Olsen KM, Chew FS. Tumoral calcinosis: pearls, polemics, and alternative possibilities. *Radiographics*. 2008;26(3):871-885.

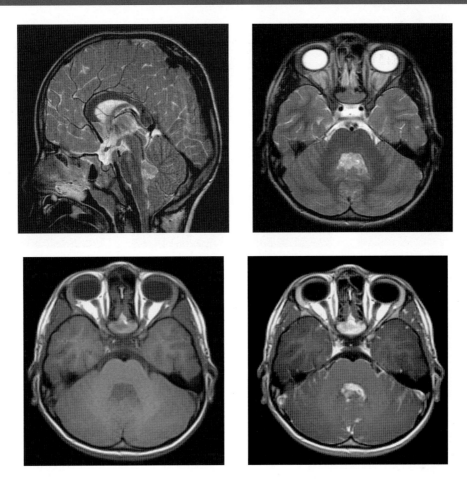

1. What is the differential diagnosis?

2. The symptoms of the case are due to . . . .

3. What are the MRI findings?

4. What are the diseases that may be associated with this case?

5. What are the treatment options?

Case ranking/difficulty: **Category:** Head

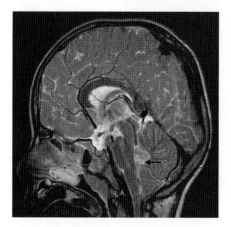

Sagittal T2-weighted image reveals hyperintense mass in the center of the fourth ventricle (*arrow*).

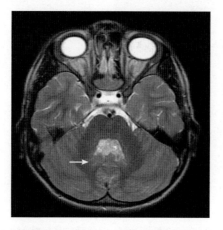

Axial T2-weighted image reveals hyperintense mass in the center of the fourth ventricle (*arrow*).

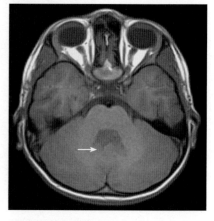

Axial T1-weighted image reveals hypointense mass in the center of the fourth ventricle (*arrow*).

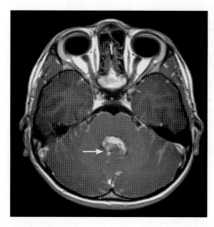

Axial T1-weighted image post contrast reveals heterogeneously enhancing mass in the center of the fourth ventricle (*arrow*). There is leptomeningeal enhancement in the region of the tentorium representing superficial leptomeningeal metastases (sugar coating).

Pearls

- Medulloblastoma is a highly malignant primary brain tumor that originates from the inferior medullary velum, which is a thin layer of white matter that forms the roof of the fourth ventricle.
- Medulloblastoma is the most common PNET originating in the brain.
- All PNET tumors of the brain are invasive and rapidly growing tumors that, unlike most brain tumors, spread through the cerebrospinal fluid and frequently metastasize to different locations in the brain and spine.
- The tumor is distinctive on T1- and T2-weighted MRI with heterogeneous enhancement and typical location adjacent to and extension into the fourth ventricle.

Answers

1. Differential diagnosis includes ependymoma, astrocytoma, medulloblastoma, meningioma, and atypical teratoid rhabdoid tumor.

2. Symptoms are mainly due to secondary increased intracranial pressure due to blockage of the fourth ventricle and are usually present for one to five months before diagnosis is made.

3. There is low signal in T1, high signal in T2, and heterogeneous pattern of enhancement.

4. Medulloblastomas are associated with Gorlin syndrome as well as with Turcot syndrome.

5. Treatment includes surgical resection, chemotherapy, and radiation therapy.

Suggested Readings

Allen JC, Epstein F. Medulloblastoma and other primary malignant neuroectodermal tumors of the CNS. The effect of patients' age and extent of disease on prognosis. *J Neurosurg*. 1982;57(4):446-451.

Koral K, Gargan L, Bowers DC, et al. Imaging characteristics of atypical teratoid-rhabdoid tumor in children compared with medulloblastoma. *AJR Am J Roentgenol*. 2008;190(3):809-814.

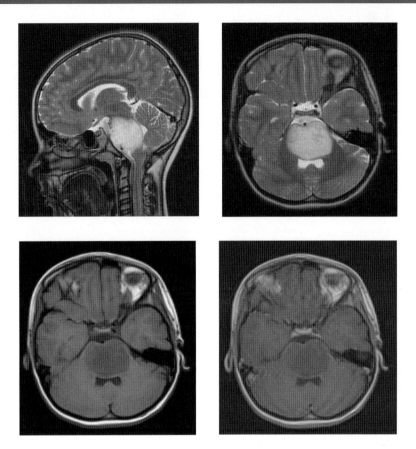

1. What is the differential diagnosis?

2. What is the disease that has increased incidence of this entity?

3. What is the location of such entity that hydrocephalus is a common presentation?

4. How do patients with cervicomedullary lesions present?

5. What are the common presenting symptoms of this case?

Case ranking/difficulty: 🦠 🦠

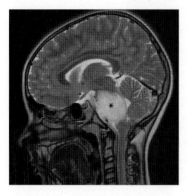

Sagittal MRI T2-weighted image reveals a heterogeneous hyperintense mass in the pons (*asterisk*) abutting and compressing the fourth ventricle. The mass is infiltrating between the tracts, inside the pons, seen as linear strands within the tumor. There is an exophytic growth of the tumor with encasement of the basilar artery.

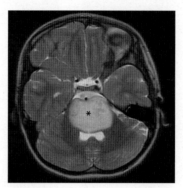

Axial MRI T2-weighted image reveals a heterogeneous hyperintense mass in the pons (*asterisk*) abutting and compressing the fourth ventricle. The mass is infiltrating between the tracts, inside the pons, seen as linear strands within the tumor. There is an exophytic growth of the tumor with encasement of the basilar artery.

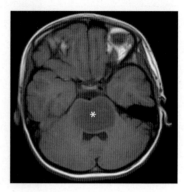

Axial MRI T1-weighted image reveals a hypointense mass in the pons (*asterisk*) abutting and compressing the fourth ventricle.

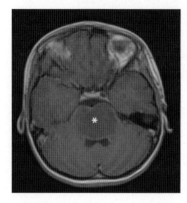

Axial MRI T1-weighted image post contrast reveals a hypointense mass in the pons (*asterisk*) abutting and compressing the fourth ventricle. The mass does not demonstrate significant enhancement.

Answers

1. Differential diagnosis includes brainstem glioma, meningioma, and metastatic disease to the brain. Ependymoma and medulloblastoma are not in the differential diagnosis, as they arise from the wall of the fourth ventricle and are primarily intraventricular.

2. Although no familial tendency is prominent overall, an increased incidence of pontine glioma has been observed consistently in patients with neurofibromatosis type 1.

3. Hydrocephalus is a common presentation, especially for tumors in periaqueductal or fourth ventricle outflow locations, because these regions have less tolerance of growth and higher risk of obstructive hydrocephalus.

4. Cervicomedullary lesions usually present with dysphagia, unsteadiness, nasal speech, vomiting, and weakness.

5. Common presenting symptoms include double vision, weakness, unsteady gait, difficulty in swallowing, dysarthria, headache, drowsiness, nausea, and vomiting. Rarely, behavioral changes or seizures may be seen in children. Older children may have deterioration of handwriting and speech.

Pearls

- Brainstem gliomas are highly aggressive brain tumors.
- Intrinsic pons glioma has a residual life expectancy of less than a year after diagnosis in over 90% of cases, except those associated with neurofibromatosis type I.
- Anatomic location determines the pathophysiological manifestation of the tumor.
- Common presenting symptoms include double vision, weakness, unsteady gait, difficulty in swallowing, dysarthria, headache, drowsiness, nausea, and vomiting.
- The typical MRI appearance of a brainstem glioma is an expansile, infiltrative process with low-to-normal signal intensity on T1-weighted images and heterogeneous high-signal intensity on T2-weighted images, with or without contrast enhancement.

Suggested Readings

Bilaniuk LT, Zimmerman RA, Littman P, et al. Computed tomography of brain stem gliomas in children. *Radiology*. 1980;134(1):89-95.

Scotti LN. Pontine arteries in brainstem glioma. *Radiology*. 1976;118(3):627-632.

Ueoka DI, Nogueira J, Campos JC, Maranhão Filho P, Ferman S, Lima MA. Brainstem gliomas–retrospective analysis of 86 patients. *J Neurol Sci*. 2009;281(1-2):20-23.

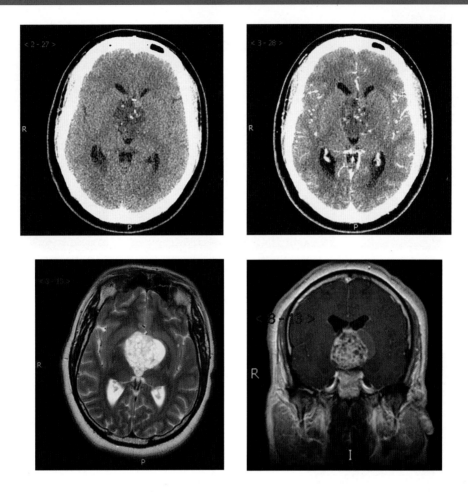

1. What is the differential diagnosis?

2. What are the two histologic types of the shown entity?

3. How can the two types of the shown entity be differentiated in neuro imaging?

4. What histologic type of the entity is demonstrated in the provided images?

5. What are the most common presenting symptoms?

Case ranking/difficulty:

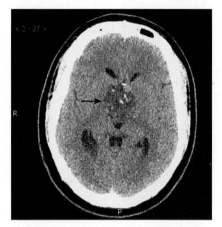

Non-contrast axial head CT reveals a suprasellar mass. The mass has slightly low attenuation in relation to the brain parenchyma (*arrow*). Calcification noted.

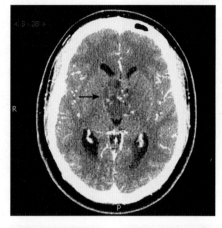

Contrast axial head CT reveals a suprasellar mass. The mass has slightly low attenuation in relation to the brain parenchyma (*arrow*). Minimal heterogeneous enhancement noted. Calcification noted.

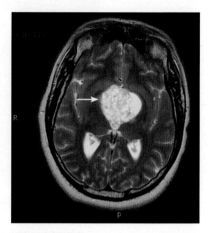

MRI-T2 of the head reveals a suprasellar mass. The mass has very high signal, same as the CSF (*arrow*). Punctuate areas of low signal noted inside the mass which may represent calcification.

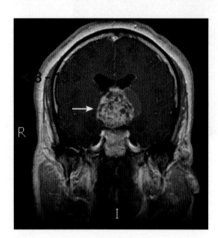

MRI-T1 of the head reveals a suprasellar mass. The mass has heterogeneous high signal (*arrow*). Punctuate areas of low signal noted inside the mass which may represent calcification.

Answers

1. The differential diagnosis may include meningioma, craniopharyngioma, neurosarcoidosis, cavernous sinus syndrome, and metastatic brain disease.

2. There are two histologic types of craniopharyngioma: adamantinomatous craniopharyngioma and papillary craniopharyngioma.

3. In the adamantinomatous type, calcifications are visible on neuro imaging and are helpful in diagnosis. The papillary type rarely calcifies.

4. The type shown has calcifications. Histologically, it was proven to be adamantinomatous craniopharyngioma.

5. Symptoms frequently develop insidiously and mostly become obvious only after the tumor attains a diameter of about 3 cm. The most common presenting symptoms are headache, endocrine dysfunction, and visual disturbances.

Pearls

- Craniopharyngioma is a tumor that arises from nests of odontogenic epithelium within the suprasellar/diencephalic region.
- The tumor contains deposits of calcium, which are evident on an x-ray.
- Craniopharyngioma is a rare, usually suprasellar neoplasm, which may be cystic, that develops from rests of epithelium derived from Rathke's pouch.
- The most common presenting symptoms are headache, endocrine dysfunction, and visual disturbances.

Suggested Readings

Bonneville F, Cattin F, Marsot-Dupuch K, Dormont D, Bonneville JF, Chiras J. T1 signal hyperintensity in the sellar region: spectrum of findings. *Radiographics*. 2006;26(1):93-113.

Bunin GR, Surawicz TS, Witman PA, Preston-Martin S, Davis F, Bruner JM. The descriptive epidemiology of craniopharyngioma. *J Neurosurg*. 1998;89(4):547-551.

Vinchon M, Dhellemmes P. Craniopharyngiomas in children: recurrence, reoperation and outcome. *Childs Nerv Syst*. 2008;24(2):211-217.

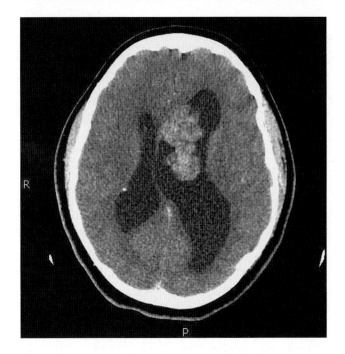
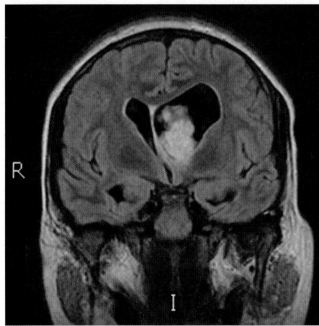

1. What are the findings?

2. What is the most likely diagnosis?

3. What can be found in the renal ultrasound of patients with tuberous sclerosis?

4. What can be found in cardiac MRI of patients with tuberous sclerosis?

5. Where in the nervous system are tubers seen?

Case ranking/difficulty:

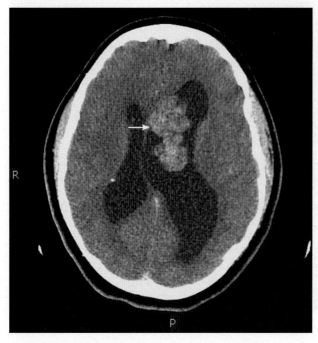

Axial contrast CT of the head reveals a large enhancing mass arising from the left lateral ventricle (*arrow*).

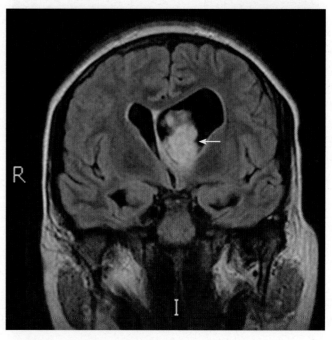

Coronal MRI FLAIR of the head reveals a large mass arising from the left lateral ventricle (*arrow*).

Answers

1. Findings consist of enhancing tumor arising from the wall of the left lateral ventricle.

2. In a patient with tuberous sclerosis, the most likely diagnosis is giant cell astrocytoma.

3. Patients with tuberous sclerosis tend to develop renal angiomyolipomas.

4. Patients with tuberous sclerosis tend to develop rhabdomyoma in the heart.

5. Tubers are noted most commonly in the cerebrum, without clear predilection for any particular lobe. They occur in the cerebellum as well, where they may be apparent only on microscopic examination. Rarely, they have been noted in the brain stem and spinal cord.

Pearls

- Giant cell astrocytoma is a common occurrence in patients with tuberous sclerosis.
- The neurological clinical findings in tuberous sclerosis are the result of growth of tubers, subependymal nodules, and giant cell astrocytoma.

- Subependymal nodules can degenerate into subependymal giant astrocytomas in 5% to 10% of cases.
- Giant cell astrocytoma occurs exclusively at the foramen of Monro. It can grow and lead to ventricular obstruction and hydrocephalus.
- Giant cell astrocytoma may be calcified.
- Intense enhancement seen following contrast administration.

Suggested Readings

Chen XZ, Dai JP. Tuberous sclerosis complex complicated with extraventricular cystic giant cell astrocytoma: case report. *Chin Med J*. 2007;120(9):854-856.

Franz DN, Leonard J, Tudor C, et al. Rapamycin causes regression of astrocytomas in tuberous sclerosis complex. *Ann Neurol*. 2006;59(3):490-498.

Jelinek J, Smirniotopoulos JG, Parisi JE, Kanzer M. Lateral ventricular neoplasms of the brain: differential diagnosis based on clinical, CT, and MR findings. *AJR Am J Roentgenol*. 1990;155(2):365-372.

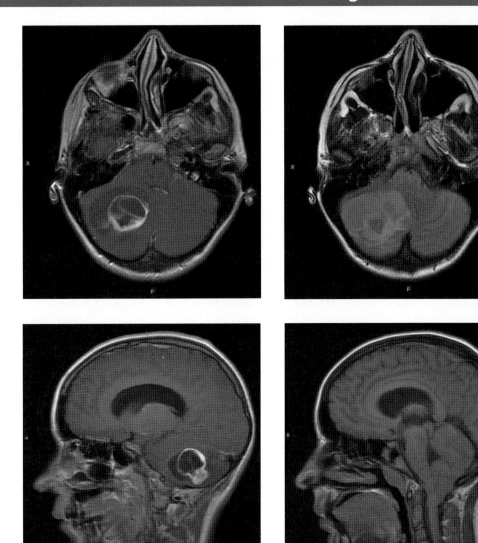

1. What are the locations where this entity can be found?

2. What is the most common anatomic location of this entity?

3. What are the imaging characteristics of this entity?

4. What are the presenting clinical symptoms of this entity?

5. What would MR spectroscopy show?

Case ranking/difficulty:

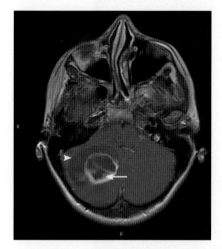

Axial MRI T1 image with contrast demonstrates a mass in the right lobe of the cerebellum. The mass appears to be cystic with solid component in the posterior and the inferior aspect of the mass (*arrow*). There is edema around the mass (*arrowhead*) and compression of the fourth ventricle.

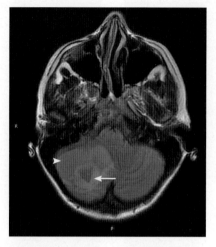

Axial MRI T2 image demonstrates a mass in the right lobe of the cerebellum. The mass appears to be cystic with solid component in the posterior and the inferior aspect of the mass (*arrow*). There is edema around the mass (*arrowhead*) and compression of the fourth ventricle.

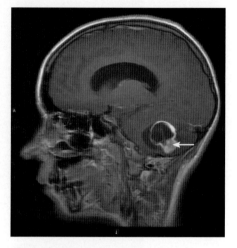

Sagittal MRI T1 image with contrast demonstrates a mass in the right lobe of the cerebellum. The mass appears to be cystic with solid component in the posterior and the inferior aspect of the mass. There is an enhancing mural nodule (*arrow*).

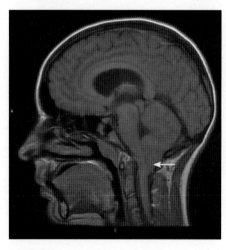

Sagittal MRI T1 image without contrast in the midline demonstrates tonsilar herniation (*arrow*).

Answers

1. Pilocytic astrocytoma (PA) can be found in the cerebellum, optic pathway, brainstem, hypothalamus, cerebral hemispheres, and the spinal cord.

2. The most common location of juvenile PA is the cerebellar hemisphere.

3. Imaging characteristics of juvenile PA is a well-marginated cystic mass with homogeneously enhancing mural nodule.

4. The presenting clinical symptoms are hydrocephalus, ataxia, and gait disturbance.

5. PAs are WHO grade I neoplasm that arise from astrocytes. They are usually well-circumscribed and have benign behavior. However, MR spectroscopy mimics aggressive appearing mass with elevated choline, decreased N-acetylaspartate (NAA), and elevated lactate.

Pearls

- PAs usually arise in the cerebellar hemispheres.
- PA can also be found along the optic pathway in patients with neurofibromatosis type I.
- PA can be all solid or solid mass with necrotic center. Calcification is uncommon, but can be seen in up to 20% of the PAs.
- Cerebellar PAs usually arise from cerebellar hemisphere and cause mass effect on 4th ventricle leading to obstructive hydrocephalus.
- Differential diagnosis of a posterior fossa mass in a child includes pilocytic astrocytoma, ependymoma, and medulloblastoma.

Suggested Readings

Donnelly LF, Jones BV, O'hara SM, et al. *Diagnostic Imaging: Pediatrics.* Salt Lake City, Utah, USA: Amirsys; 2005.

McLean MA, Sun A, Bradstreet TE, et al. Repeatability of edited lactate and other metabolites in astrocytoma at 3T. *J Magn Reson Imaging.* 2012;36(2):468-475.

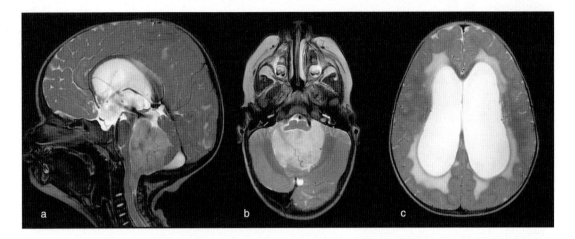

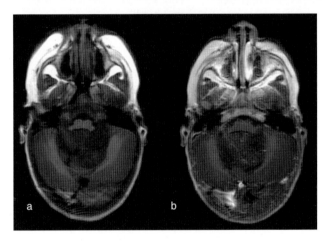
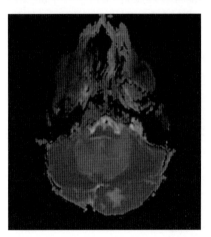

1. What is the differential diagnosis?

2. What are the most common symptoms
   at presentation?

3. What are the most common characteristics
   of this entity?

4. What are the therapeutic options?

5. What complementary examinations must
   be made?

Case ranking/difficulty: **Category:** Head

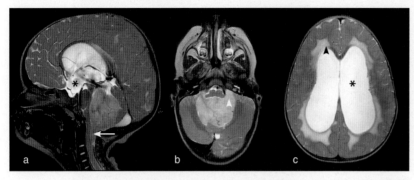

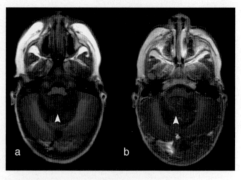

Sagittal (a) and axial (b, c) T2WI demonstrate T2-hyperintense posterior fossa tumor occupying the fourth ventricle with infiltration of the foramen of Luschka (*white arrowhead* on the left side) and foramen magnum (*white arrow*). CSF obstruction and hydrocephalus are present (*black asterisks* in (a) third ventricle and (c) side ventricles). Parenchymal CSF resorption is hindered due to elevated intraventricular pressure and "ventricular capping" developed (*black arrowhead* in 'c').

T1WI without (a) and with gadolinium (b). The tumor is mainly T1-hypointense and shows only minimal contrast enhancement (*white arowheads*).

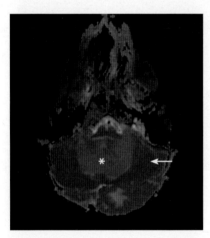

The majority of the tumor demonstrates higher diffusion values (*white asterisk*) than cerebellar hemispheres (*white arrow*) due to the less compact nature of the tumor and larger cytoplasmic areas of tumor cells.

Answers

1. A tumor originating from the fourth ventricle is most often either a medulloblastoma or an ependymoma. Rhabdoid tumor may sometimes mimick this presentation but tends to occur earlier in childhood and present with larger cysts.

2. Tumors invading the fourth ventricle may adhere and irritate the posterior wall of the brainstem in which the reticular formation and the vomiting center are located (in conjunction with the area postrema). Ataxia is a common non-specific sign, but its worsening must trigger neuroimaging to exclude posterior fossa tumor. Headaches are common in case of hydrocephalus.

3. Compared to medulloblastoma, ependymoma is a less compact tumor composed of larger cells with larger cytoplasmic component and smaller nuclei, hence the higher ADC values. Typical for ependymomas are encasement and infiltration/molding of the surrounding structures, whereas medullobastoma usually do not invade the foramen of Luschka.

4. The most important goal is to attempt complete tumoral resection, as this is directly related to survival. If more than 1 mL of tumor tissue is left, radiotherapy has been shown to ameliorate overall survival rate. Chemotherapy is not an option in ependymoma.

5. Spinal canal must be checked for drop metastasis. These are commonly found in the lower spinal recess. A postoperative MR scan is imperative to evaluate the amount of residual tumor in case of incomplete resection. Both examinations have a direct impact upon radiotherapy scheme.

Pearls

- Ependymoma is a tumor originating from ependymal cells mainly from the floor of the fourth ventricle.
- Tumoral infiltration of the foramen is a classical finding.
- Spinal metastasis must be sought after.

Suggested Reading

Schneider JF, Confort-Gouny S, Viola A, et al. Multiparametric differentiation of posterior fossa tumors in children using diffusion-weighted imaging and short echo-time 1H-MR spectroscopy. *J Magn Reson Imaging.* 2007;26(6):1390-1398.

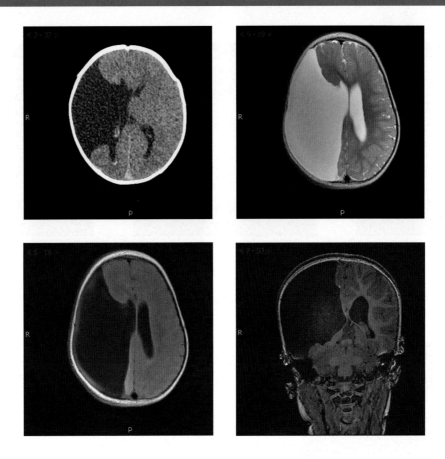

1. What are the findings?

2. What is the differential diagnosis?

3. What are the clinical manifestations?

4. What are the findings in type I of this entity?

5. What are the treatment options?

Schizencephaly

Case ranking/difficulty: 🌰 🌰

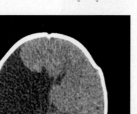 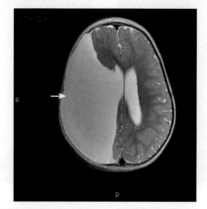 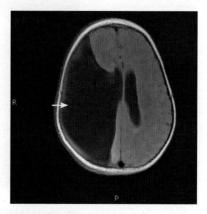

Axial CT of the brain shows cerebrospinal fluid-filled cleft, lined by a thin line of gray matter, extending through the right hemisphere from the ependyma centrally to the pia peripherally (*arrow*).

Axial MRI-T2 of the brain shows cerebrospinal fluid-filled cleft, lined by a thin line of gray matter, extending through the right hemisphere from the ependyma centrally to the pia peripherally (*arrow*).

Axial MRI-T1 of the brain shows cerebrospinal fluid-filled cleft, lined by a thin line of gray matter, extending through the right hemisphere from the ependyma centrally to the pia peripherally (*arrow*).

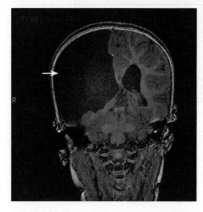

Coronal MRI-T1 of the brain shows cerebrospinal fluid-filled cleft, lined by a thin line of gray matter, extending through the right hemisphere from the ependyma centrally to the pia peripherally (*arrow*).

lips closing one end of an abnormal fluid cleft through the hemisphere.

5. Treatment for individuals with schizencephaly generally consists of physical therapy, occupational therapy, treatment for seizures, and, in cases that are complicated by hydrocephalus, a shunt.

Answers

1. Schizencephaly type II is seen with a CSF cleft that extends from the pial surface to the ventricle wall. The lips of the cleft are lined with gray matter. The disorder is unilateral.

2. Differential diagnosis includes CSF-containing abnormalities such as porencephalic cyst, hydranencephaly, arachnoid cyst, ventriculomegaly, and monoventricle in holoprosencephaly.

3. Clinical manifestations may include seizure disorders, developmental delay, poor language skills, and spastic hemiparesis.

4. Type I schizencephaly has a cord of gray matter tissue, either with no fluid cleft or with ventricular or cortical

Pearls

- Schizencephaly is a rare disorder, with an estimated frequency of 1.5:100,000 live births.
- This abnormality is caused by abnormal neural migration during the embryonic life.
- The disorder consists of a cleft in the brain. The lips of the cleft are lined by a thin layer of gray matter. The cleft extends from the ependyma to the pial surface of the brain.
- Two types of schizencephaly were described. Type I in which the lips of the cleft are fused, and type II in which the lips of the cleft are separated and the space between the lips is filled with cerebrospinal fluid.
- This disorder may be bilateral or unilateral.

Suggested Readings

Oh KY, Kennedy AM, Frias AE Jr, Byrne JL. Fetal schizencephaly: pre- and postnatal imaging with a review of the clinical manifestations. *Radiographics*. 2010;25(3):647-657.

Patel AC, Cohen HL, Hotson GC. US case of the day. Open-lip schizencephaly with an area of heterotopic gray matter and associated absence of the septa pellucida. *Radiographics*. 2002;17(1):236-239.

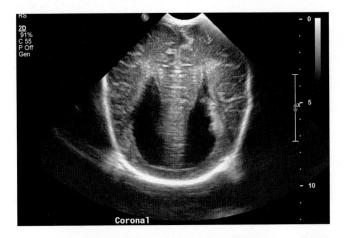
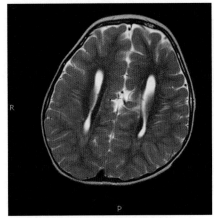
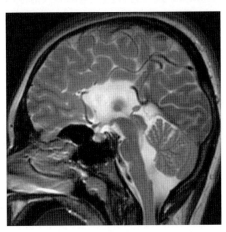
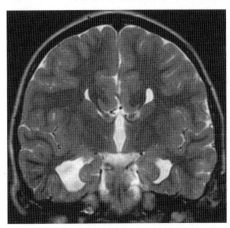

1. What are the findings?

2. What is the diagnosis?

3. What are the associated abnormalities?

4. What are Probst bundles?

5. What is colpocephaly?

Case ranking/difficulty:

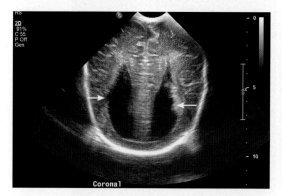
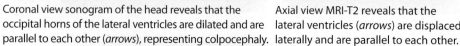
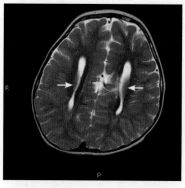
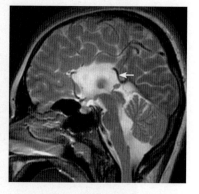

Coronal view sonogram of the head reveals that the occipital horns of the lateral ventricles are dilated and are parallel to each other (*arrows*), representing colpocephaly.

Axial view MRI-T2 reveals that the lateral ventricles (*arrows*) are displaced laterally and are parallel to each other.

Sagittal T2-weighted MRI of the brain reveals complete absence of the corpus callosum. The cingulate sulcus is absent, and the medial hemispheric sulci reach the third ventricle in a radial fashion (*arrow*).

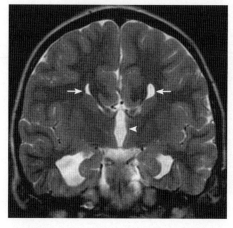

Coronal view MRI-T2 with contrast demonstrates that the lateral ventricles form a bull's-horn appearance (*arrows*) and are indented medially by the Probst bundle. There is high riding of the third ventricle (*arrowhead*).

Answers

1. There is colpocephaly. The lateral ventricles are parallel to each other and form a Viking helmet appearance. There is high riding of the third ventricle and the gyri radiate toward the third ventricle.

2. The diagnosis is agenesis of the corpus callosum.

3. Diseases that may be associated with agenesis of the corpus callosum are Arnold-Chiari malformation, Dandy-Walker syndrome, Aicardi syndrome, holoprosencephaly, and trisomy 18. Associated anomalies include migration anomalies, interhemispheric cyst, or pericallosal lipoma.

4. Probst bundles are white matter tracts that would have normally crossed in the corpus callosum run in anteroposterior direction medial to the lateral ventricles.

5. Colpocephaly is defined as disproportionate enlargement of the occipital horns of the lateral ventricles.

Pearls

- Corpus callosum is a commissural structure that connects the white matter of the two cerebral hemispheres.
- Partial agenesis/dysgenesis of corpus callosum usually shows presence of genu and absence of posterior parts or rostrum.
- Imaging features of agenesis of corpus callosum include:
  1. Gyri radiating toward the third ventricle
  2. Absence of cingulate gyrus
  3. Probst bundles
  4. High-riding third ventricle
  5. Colpocephaly – Enlarged occipital horns
  6. Parallel running lateral ventricles on axial view
  7. Lateral ventricles pointing superiorly resembling Viking
  8. Helmet or trident shape on coronal view
  9. Meandering anterior cerebral artery
- Isolated absence of corpus callosum has better prognosis than when it is associated with other anomalies.
- Less than 20% of agenesis of corpus callosum has chromosomal anomalies.
- Diffusion tractography on prenatal and postnatal MRI demonstrates non-crossing of fibers.

Suggested Readings

Byrd SE, Radkowski MA, Flannery A, McLone DG. The clinical and radiological evaluation of absence of the corpus callosum. *Eur J Radiol*. 1993;10(1):65-73.

Davidson HD, Abraham R, Steiner RE. Agenesis of the corpus callosum: magnetic resonance imaging. *Radiology*. 1985;155(2):371-373.

Warren ME, Cook JV. Agenesis of the corpus callosum. *Br J Radiol*. 1993;66(781):81-85.

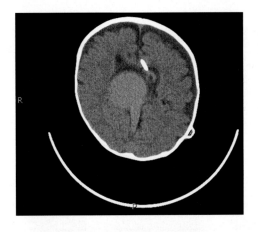
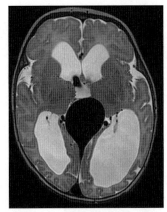
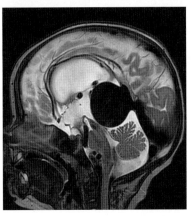
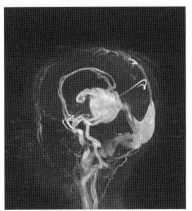

1. What are the findings?

2. What is the diagnosis?

3. What are the clinical signs that may be present in this entity?

4. What are the entities that may be included in the differential diagnosis?

5. What are the treatment options?

Case ranking/difficulty:

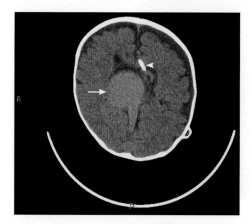

Axial non-contrast CT reveals density in the central region of the brain (*arrow*), representing the vein of Galen. The *arrowhead* represents the shunt tube.

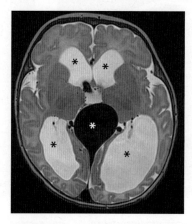

Axial MRI-T2 reveals flow void in the central region of the brain (*white asterisk*), representing the vein of Galen. There are dilated ventricles (*black asterisks*).

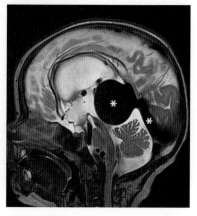

Sagittal MRI-T1 reveals flow void in the central region of the brain (*white asterisks*), representing the vein of Galen.

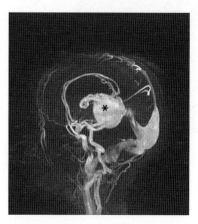

MRA in sagittal view reveals the vein of Galen malformation (*black asterisk*).

Answers

1. The MRI reveals flow void in the center of the brain. The non-contrast CT demonstrates density of blood attenuation in the same region. Ventricles are dilated.

2. The diagnosis is vein of Galen malformation. Hydrocephalus is associated.

3. Newborns may clinically present with high-output congestive heart failure, with developmental delay, hydrocephalus, and seizures.

4. Differential diagnosis may include arteriovenous malformation, cavernous sinus malformation, and hydrocephalus.

5. Treatment options may include selective catheterization and therapeutic embolization of feeding arteries, surgical ligation of the arterial feeders, embolic glue to occlude

the arteriovenous fistula on the arterial side, treatment of cardiac failure, and relieve hydrocephalus if present by a ventriculo-peritoneal shunt.

Pearls

- The vein of Galen is located under the cerebral hemispheres, and drains the anterior and central regions of the brain into the sinuses of the posterior cerebral fossa.
- Vein of Galen malformation results from the median prosencephalic vein, which is a precursor of the vein of Galen, and becomes aneurysmatic due to lack of regression.
- Aneurysmal malformations of the vein of Galen typically result in high-output congestive heart failure or may present with developmental delay, hydrocephalus, and seizures.
- The malformation is identified by CT or MRI.
- Treatment includes occlusion of the vein itself or feeding artery, treating the heart failure, and relieving the hydrocephalus if present.

Suggested Readings

Golombek SG, Ally S, Woolf PK. A newborn with cardiac failure secondary to a large vein of Galen malformation. *South Med J.* 2004;97(5):516-518.

Hoang S, Choudhri O, Edwards M, Guzman R. Vein of Galen malformation. *Neurosurg Focus.* 2009;27(5):E8.

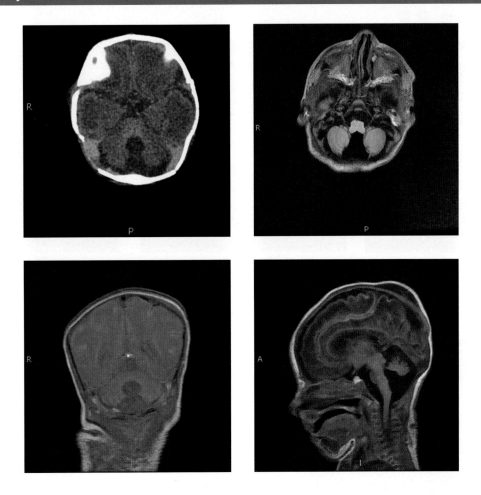

1. What is in the differential diagnosis of this entity?

2. What is the frequency of occurrence of this case?

3. What are the radiographic findings that may be seen in this entity?

4. What is the imaging modality of choice for the diagnosis?

5. What are the treatment options?

Case ranking/difficulty:

Category: Head

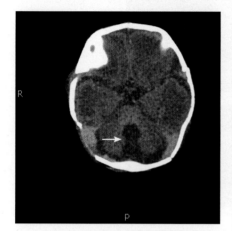

Axial CT demonstrates hypoplasia of the cerebellar hemispheres and communication between the fourth ventricle and the cisterna magna (*arrow*).

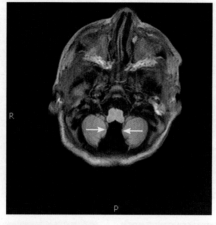

Axial MRI-T2 Flair demonstrates hypoplasia of the cerebellar hemispheres and communication between the fourth ventricle and the cisterna magna (*arrows*).

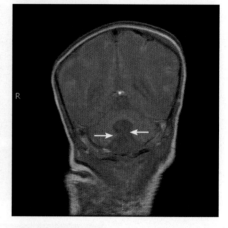

Coronal MRI-T2 Flair demonstrates hypoplasia of the cerebellar hemispheres and communication between the fourth ventricle and the cisterna magna (*arrows*).

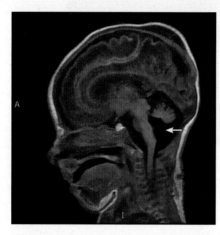

Sagittal MRI-T2 Flair demonstrates hypoplasia of the cerebellar hemispheres and partial lower agenesis of the vermis. There is a communication between the fourth ventricle and the cisterna magna (*arrow*).

Answers

1. Differential diagnosis includes mega cisterna magna and retrocerebellar arachnoid cyst.

2. The frequency of occurrence of Dandy-Walker malformation is 1:25,000.

3. Dandy-Walker variant consists of communication between the cisterna magna and the fourth ventricle with hypoplasia of the vermis. There is no enlargement of the posterior fossa. The findings of the Dandy-Walker complex may include hydrocephalus, agenesis of the corpus callosum, torcular-lambdoid inversion, and absence of the vermis.

4. MRI and CT in the sagittal plan are the best imaging modalities for the diagnosis of Dandy-Walker malformation.

5. There is no specific therapy for Dandy-Walker complex or variant. Treatment is geared to relieve the associated manifestations and symptoms.

Pearls

- The Dandy-Walker complex is a continuum of aberrant development of the posterior fossa.
- There may be association with multiple congenital anomalies, radiographic anomalies, and developmental delay.
- Dandy-Walker malformation is characterized by agenesis or hypoplasia of the cerebellar vermis.
- The cerebellar hemispheres are small and hypoplastic.
- There is a posterior fossa cyst that is in continuation with the fourth ventricle.
- Hydrocephalus may be present.

Suggested Readings

Barkovich AJ, Kjos BO, Norman D, Edwards MS. Revised classification of posterior fossa cysts and cystlike malformations based on the results of multiplanar MR imaging. *AJR Am J Roentgenol.* 1989;153(6):1289-1300.

Sasaki-Adams D, Elbabaa SK, Jewells V, Carter L, Campbell JW, Ritter AM. The Dandy-Walker variant: a case series of 24 pediatric patients and evaluation of associated anomalies, incidence of hydrocephalus, and developmental outcomes. *J Neurosurg Pediatr.* 2008;2(3):194-199.

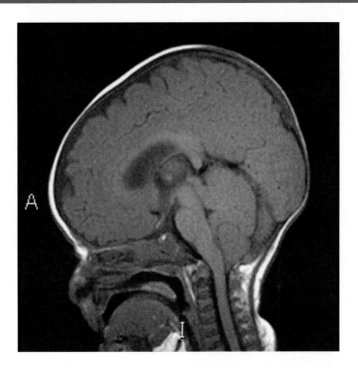

1. What are the findings?

2. What can be the associated osseous anomalies?

3. What is the most common associated anomaly of the spinal cord?

4. What is the finding that is associated with the type II, but not with the type I of this case?

5. What are the treatment options?

Case ranking/difficulty: **Category:** Head

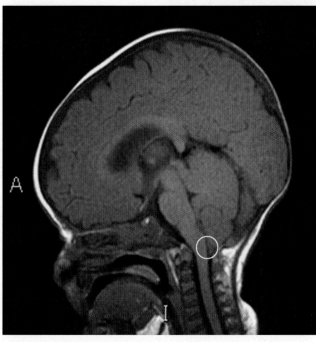

Sagittal MRI-T1 of the brain shows low-lying peg-shaped cerebellar tonsils below the level of the foramen magnum (*circle*).

Pearls

- Chiari I malformation is the most common type of all other Chiari malformations.
- The cerebellar tonsils herniate through the foramen magnum, a process that may lead to obstruction of cerebrospinal fluid outflow and a non-communicating hydrocephalus.
- Syringomyelia is present in 25% of patients with Chiari I malformation. The most common location is the cervical cord.
- Skeletal anomalies may be associated.
- MRI is the diagnostic modality of choice.

Suggested Readings

Ball WS, Crone KR. Chiari I malformation: from Dr Chiari to MR imaging. *Radiology*. 1995;195(3):602-604.

Milhorat TH, Chou MW, Trinidad EM, et al. Chiari I malformation redefined: clinical and radiographic findings for 364 symptomatic patients. *Neurosurgery*. 1999;44(5): 1005-1117.

Novegno F, Caldarelli M, Massa A, et al. The natural history of the Chiari Type I anomaly. *J Neurosurg Pediatr*. 2008; 2(3):179-187.

Answers

1. There is displacement of cerebellar tonsils below the level of the foramen magnum in a peg-like shape.

2. Associated osseous anomalies may include Klippel-Feil syndrome, platybasia, basilar invagination, incomplete ossification of C1 ring, retroflexed odontoid process, and scoliosis.

3. Syringohydromyelia is the most common associated anomaly of the spinal cord.

4. Myelomeningocele is associated with the type II Chiari malformation. It is not associated with the type I Chiari malformation.

5. Surgical treatment of choice is posterior fossa decompression. If hydrocephalus is present, then V-P shunt tubing may be necessary. If associated anomalies are present, each one should be respectively evaluated and if necessary, treated. Conservative and supportive treatment if condition is very mild.

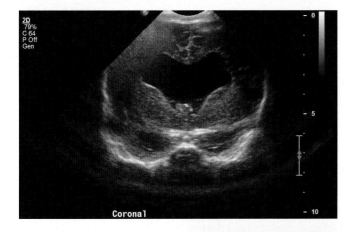

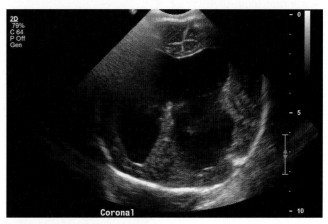

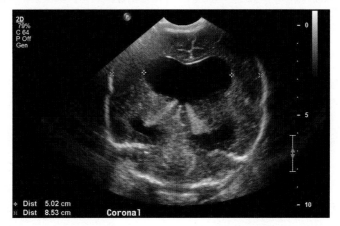

1. What is the diagnosis?

2. What are few of the clinical features of this entity?

3. What are the sonographic findings?

4. What are some of the imaging modalities that may demonstrate the findings?

5. What are the complications of this case?

Case ranking/difficulty:

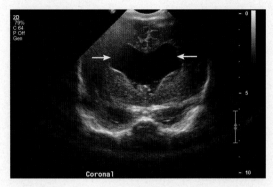

Coronal head sonogram of a newborn through the anterior fontanel demonstrates the frontal horns of the lateral ventricles (*arrows*). Note that the septum pellucidum is absent and there is communication between the lateral ventricles. Lateral ventricles are dilated. There is squared appearance of the frontal horns and the low-lying fornices are typical.

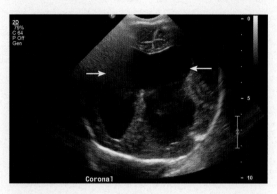

Coronal head sonogram of a newborn through the anterior fontanel demonstrates the mid brain and the lateral ventricles (*arrows*). Note that the septum pellucidum is absent and there is communication between the lateral ventricles. The lateral ventricles are dilated.

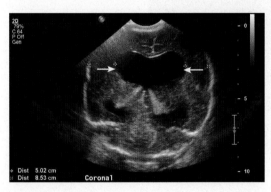

Coronal head sonogram of a newborn through the anterior fontanel demonstrates the occipital horns of the lateral ventricles (*arrows*). Note that the septum pellucidum is absent and there is communication between the lateral ventricles. Lateral ventricles are dilated.

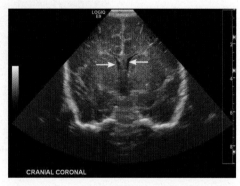

Normal coronal head sonogram of a newborn through the anterior fontanel shows that the two frontal horns of the lateral ventricles (*arrows*) are completely separated.

Answers

1. This is De Morsier disease or septo-optic dysplasia.

2. Ophthalmologic abnormalities, diverticulation abnormalities, hypopituitarism, and diabetes insipidus.

3. Fusion of the anterior horn of both lateral ventricles.

4. Imaging modalities that may demonstrate septo-optic dysplasia are CT, MRI, and ultrasound.

5. Complications of the shown entity may include seizures, blindness, developmental delay, and hypopituitarism.

Pearls

- Septo-optic dysplasia is a rare disorder characterized by optic nerve dysplasia, pituitary deficiencies, and absence of the septum pellucidum.

- Symptoms may include blindness in one or both eyes, pupil dilation in response to light, nystagmus, hypotonia, hormonal problems, and seizures.
- This entity is in the lowest spectrum of severity of the congenital structural forebrain malformations characterized by midline hemisphere fusion.
- Sonogram shows communication between the frontal horns of the 2 lateral ventricles.
- MRI demonstrates atrophy of the optic nerves.
- Typically in coronal images, there is squared appearance of the frontal horns and low-lying fornices.

Suggested Reading

Barkovich AJ, Fram EK, Norman D. Septo-optic dysplasia: MR imaging. *Radiology*. 1989;171:189-192.

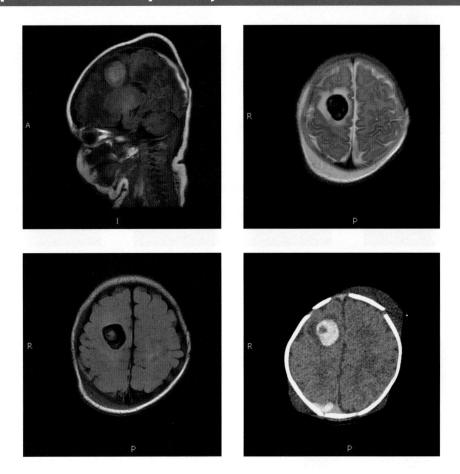

1. What is the diagnosis?

2. What is the age of the bleed based on the MRI images?

3. How is chronic hemorrhage seen in T1 and T2 MRI sequences?

4. Which chemical state of hemoglobin manifests as dark signal on MRI-T1 and dark signal on MRI-T2?

5. How does intracellular oxyhemoglobin manifest in MRI?

Case ranking/difficulty: **Category:** Head

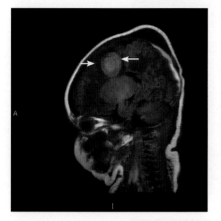

Sagittal MRI-T1 reveals a mass in the right frontal lobe that demonstrates increased signal (*arrows*). Edema surrounds the hemorrhage. Caput succedaneum noted.

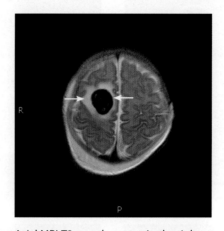

Axial MRI-T2 reveals a mass in the right frontal lobe that demonstrates dark signal (*arrows*). Edema surrounds the hemorrhage. Caput succedaneum noted.

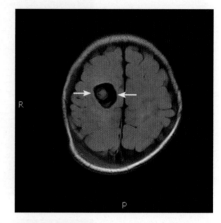

Axial MRI-FLAIR reveals a mass in the right frontal lobe that demonstrates dark signal (*arrows*). Edema surrounds the hemorrhage.

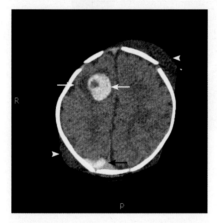

This non-contrast CT was performed 5 days before the MRI. There is hyperattenuating mass in the right frontal lobe (*white arrows*). This represents hyperacute hemorrhage. Edema surrounds the hemorrhage. Acute subdural hematoma noted in the right parieto-occipital lobe (*black arrow*). Caput succedaneum noted (*arrowheads*).

Pearls

- The most common cause of intracerebral hemorrhage in preterm newborns is hypoxic-ischemic injury.
- Age of the hemorrhage can be assessed in CT and more accurately in MRI.
- The signal intensity of a hemorrhage in MRI depends on the chemical state of iron in the hemoglobin molecule and on the integrity of the red blood cell membrane.
- On CT, acute hemorrhage is dense and hyperattenuating. The attenuation decreases with advanced age of bleeding.

Suggested Readings

Bradley WG Jr. MR appearance of hemorrhage in the brain. *Radiology.* 1993;189(1):15-26.

Gomori JM, Grossman RI, Goldberg HI, et al. Intracranial hematomas: imaging by high-field MR. *Radiology.* 1985;157(1):87-93.

Answers

1. The diagnosis is intracerebral hemorrhage.

2. The hemorrhagic mass in the MRI images is bright on T1 and dark on T2, representing early subacute hemorrhage (4 to 7 days).

3. Chronic hemorrhage is seen as dark on T1 and dark on T2.

4. Hemosiderin manifests as dark signal on MRI-T1 and dark signal on MRI-T2.

5. On MRI, intracellular oxyhemoglobin manifests as isointense on T1 and bright on T2.

Multiple café-au-lait spots. Figures on top, at the age of 2 years at diagnosis, figures on bottom, at the age of 7 years

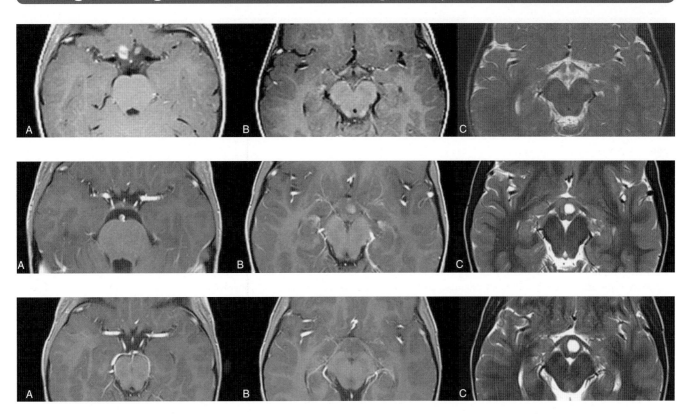

1. What is the diagnosis?

2. What is the other name of this entity?

3. Which cranial osseous structure may be involved?

4. Which are the peripheral tumors associated with this disease?

5. What are the possible explanations for macrocephaly in this disease?

Case ranking/difficulty: **Category:** Head

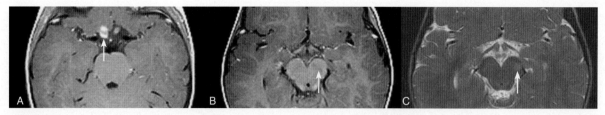

At 2 years, right optic nerve is enlarged and enhancing (a, *white arrow*). Enhancing and T2-hyperintense lesion within the left cerebral peduncle (b and c, *white arrows*).

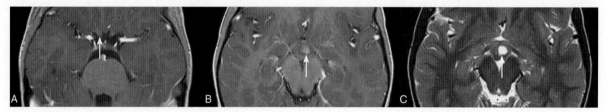

At 7 years, right optic nerve is minimally enlarged and non-enhancing (a, *white arrow*). T2-hyperintense cystic and enhancing lesion at the left fornix (b and c, *white arrows*).

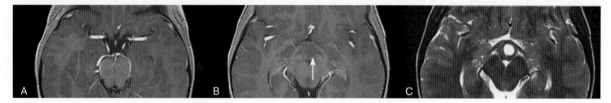

At 7½ years, enhancement disappeared in the left fornix lesion (b, *white arrow*).

Answers

1. Multiple T2-hyperintensities (hamartoma or dysmyelinated areas) and optic gliomas suggest neurofibromatosis Type I (NF-1).

2. NF-1 is also named von Recklinghausen disease.

3. Sphenoid wing deformity may be associated with NF-1. It may result from impaired development due to peripheral neurofibromas or a combination of structural dural weakness and CSF pulsation.

4. Neurofibrosarcoma are more frequent in children with NF1. There is also a higher incidence of chronic myeloid leukemia.

5. 30-50% of NF1 children have macrocephaly without hydrocephalus, due to a general increase of gray and white matter volume, in combination with altered white matter structure and reduced connectivity.

Pearls

- Neurofibromatosis type I is the most common neurocutaneous syndrome.

- NF1 is the most common single gene cause of learning disabilities.
- Cerebral lesions are mainly hamartoma, optic glioma, and parenchymal glioma.
- Lesions vary in time and may completely regress in the second decade.
- Optic glioma often shows contrast enhancement which is not suggestive of malignancy.
- Only parenchymal glioma rarely shows contrast enhancement, which if present, may suggest malignant degeneration.

Suggested Readings

Karlsgodt KH, Rosser T, Lutkenhoff ES, Cannon TD, Silva A, Bearden CE. Alterations in white matter microstructure in neurofibromatosis-1. *PLoS One.* 2012;7(10):e47854.

Sevick RJ, Barkovich AJ, Edwards MS, Koch T, Berg B, Lempert T. Evolution of white matter lesions in neurofibromatosis type 1: MR findings. *AJR Am J Roentgenol.* 1992;159(1):171-175.

Asymptomatic girl diagnosed after screening due to familial history. The girl developed an acute visual loss at the age of 9 years

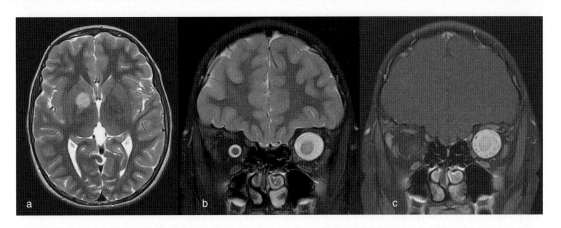

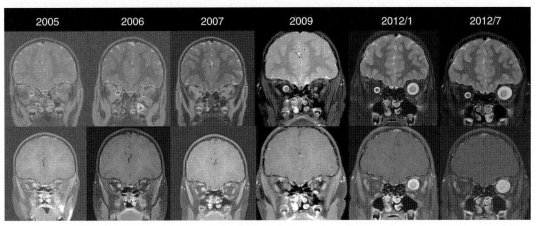

1. What is the reason for vision loss in this child?

2. What is the differential diagnosis?

3. Is surgery necessary?

4. What is an alternative treatment?

5. Does the lesions warrant follow-up?

Case ranking/difficulty: **Category:** Head

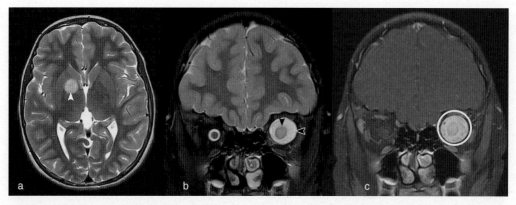

a: Axial T2WI; b: Coronal T2WI with fat saturation; c: Coronal T1WI + C with fat saturation. There is a T2-hyperintense space occupying lesions in the right globus pallidum and genu of the right internal capsule ('a', *white arrowhead*). There is a massive enlargement of the left retro-orbital optic nerve with a T2-hypointense compact core ('b', *black arrowhead*) and a T2-hyperintense mucinous peripheral rim ('b', *black outlined arrowhead*). Both layers demonstrate intensive contrast enhancement ('c', *white circle*).

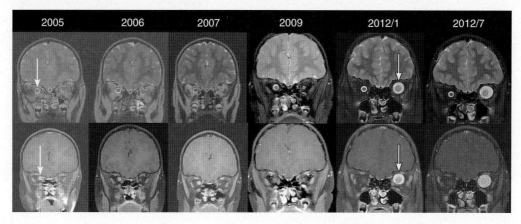

Time course of the optic nerve lesions. Upper row: T2WI with fat saturation; Lower row: T1WI + C with fat saturation. There is an initial moderate enlargement of the right optic nerve with contrast enhancement (*white arrows*) which first disappears in 2009 before the lesion minimally begins to shrink and the optic sheath enlarges in 2012. There is a sudden massive enlargement of the left optic nerve in 2012 with intensive contrast enhancement (*white outlined arrows*). There is a beginning subtle intratumoral peripheral cystic transformation in the second control in 2012.

Answers

1. Vision loss is often due to optic glioma.

2. Differential diagnosis is pilocytic astrocytoma.

3. Surgery is primarily not needed, due to spontaneous regression in the majority of cases.

4. Chemotherapy may be considered if case of progressive tumor volume and vision loss.

5. Yearly follow up of optic glioma is recommended.

Pearls

- Optic nerve enlargement with or without contrast enhancement is the hallmark of optic nerve glioma.
- It may involve both eyes and infiltrate the chiasma.

- Chemotherapy is considered in case of visual impairment and tumor progression.
- Surgery is considered to preserve contralateral vision in cases of prechiasmatic tumor progression.

Suggested Readings

Cassiman C, Legius E, Spileers W, Casteels I. Ophthalmological assessment of children with neurofibromatosis type 1. *Eur J Pediatr.* 2013 Oct;172(10):1327-1333. doi: 10.1007/s00431-013-2035-2. Epub 2013 May 25.

Spicer GJ, Kazim M, Glass LR, Harris GJ, Miller NR, Rootman J, Sullivan TJ. Accuracy of MRI in defining tumor-free margin in optic nerve glioma surgery. *Ophthal Plast Reconstr Surg.* 2013 Jul-Aug;29(4):277-280. doi: 10.1097/IOP.0b013e318291658e.

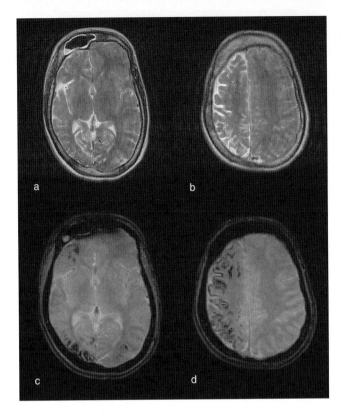

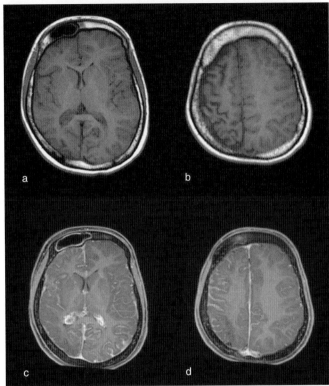

1. What are the findings?

2. What is the diagnosis?

3. Which other organ is almost invariably affected?

4. What are the clinical complications of this entity?

5. Which disease may share the same skin manifestations?

Case ranking/difficulty:

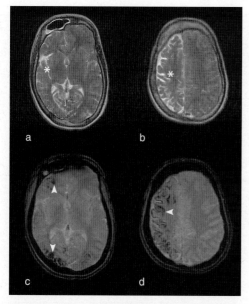

Extensive atrophy of the entire right cerebral hemisphere ('a', 'b', *white asterisks*), with preservation of the volume of the basal ganglia. On T2*GRE, widespread cortical superficial calcifications are seen on the right side ('c', 'd', *white arrowheads*).

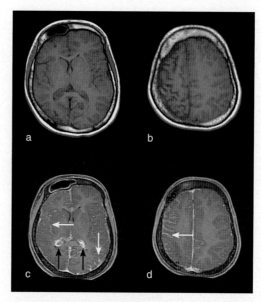

There is a diffuse bilateral leptomeningeal contrast enhancement ('c', 'd', *white arrows*), reflecting the dilated venous mesh of the angiomatosis. Furthermore, there is a characteristic engorgement of the plexus choroideus on both sides ('c', 'd', *black arrows*), signing disturbed deep venous drainage.

Answers

1. The presence of a pathological mesh of engorged venous vessels at the surface of the cortex, the leptomeningeal angiomatosis, is responsible for an imbalance in the perfusion of the cortical ribbon. This mainly leads to chronic ischemia, and results in atrophic changes of the affected hemisphere, including end-stage superficial calcifications.

2. The findings are characteristic for Sturge-Weber syndrome. As the skin is usually involved in the distribution of the trigeminal nerve (and most often the ocular branch), the alternative term of encephalotrigeminal angiomatosis is also used.

3. The angiomatosis involving the eye is a common finding in this disease. Vascular malformation may involve the conjunctive, the episclera, the choroid and retina. It leads to the development of glaucoma early in life.

4. Superficial leptomeningeal angiomatosis leads to chronic ischemia, calcifications and atrophy of the affected hemisphere, often resulting in spastic hemiparesis. It correlates with intractable seizures, developmental delay and mental retardation. Due to the early atrophic changes, hemihypertrophy of the contralateral body part may develop.

5. A nevus flammeus localized in the trigeminal ocular division is quite indicative of Sturge-Weber disease. But in other locations, Klippel-Trenaunay syndrome should

also be considered. In this entity however, body parts hypertrophy rather than hypotrophy is the rule.

Pearls

- There is an intensive contrast enhancement of the leptomeninges, revealing the extent of the angiomatosis.
- There is an engorgement of the plexus choroideus due to aberrant venous drainage of the deep and periventricular white matter.
- The angiomatosis produces a venous engorgement and steal phenomenon leading to acute and chronic ischemia of the affected cortex.
- There is a progressive atrophy of the affected hemisphere and extensive superficial dystrophic calcifications occur.

Suggested Readings

Di Rocco C, Tamburrini G. Sturge-Weber syndrome. *Childs Nerv Syst.* 2006;22(8):909-921.

Lin DD, Barker PB, Hatfield LA, Comi AM. Dynamic MR perfusion and proton MR spectroscopic imaging in Sturge-Weber syndrome: correlation with neurological symptoms. *J Magn Reson Imaging.* 2006;24(2):274-281.

Lo W, Marchuk DA, Ball KL, et al. Updates and future horizons on the understanding, diagnosis, and treatment of Sturge-Weber syndrome brain involvement. *Dev Med Child Neurol.* 2012;54(3):214-223.

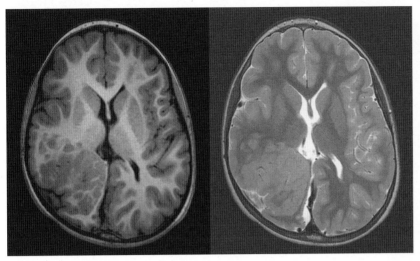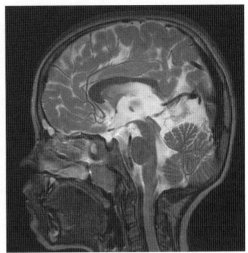

1. What are the findings?

2. What are the two findings suggesting white matter tract dysfunction?

3. From which structure do neurons originate?

4. What is the characteristic signal intensity of heterotopias compared to cortex?

5. What cells are responsible for neuronal migration?

Case ranking/difficulty:

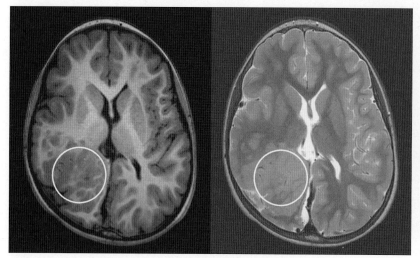

Mixed and multiple gray and white matter islands in the right temporal and occipital lobe, without normal layering (*white circle*). Atrophy of the right thalamus and malformation of the right occipital lobe (which is not visualized).

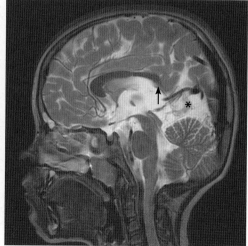

Malformation of the cerebellar tentorium with widening of the supravermian spaces (*black asterisk*). Atrophy of the splenium of the corpus callosum (*black arrow*).

Answers

1. There is an extensive cortical sulcation and gyrification anomaly, coupled to multiple gray matter islands with the white matter of the temporal occipital and parietal lobe. White matter tracts are consequently disrupted, and superficial cortical layer is thinned due to arrested migration of neurons which did not reach the cortical plate.

2. The extensive disruption of white matter tracts within the region involved by the giant heterotopia has resulted in atrophic changes in functionally connected structures, like the right thalamus and the entire right occipital lobe. Also, efferent white matter tracts, for instance, those connecting with the contralateral hemisphere are also atrophic, as seen in the splenium of the corpus callosum (connecting visual areas among others).

3. Neuronal and astroglial progenitor cells all originate from the germinal matrix (also called matrix primitive) located at the subependymal layer bordering both ventricular walls. There is also a primitive matrix around the fourth ventricle, responsible for the neuronal pool of the cerebellum.

4. Within heterotopias, myelination alteration as well as different cellular concentration and organization lead to FLAIR hyperintensity, while T1 and T2 remain comparable to the cortical layer.

5. Radial glial cells are central to the migration and differentiation processes. They show radial oriented extensions from the ventricular wall up to the pial surface. These cells serve not only as scaffold for the correct radial migration process but will eventually divide

in the subcortical region. They will then differentiate into cortical neurons and also into glia, not only during development but also after injury.

Pearls

- Heterotopias are accumulations of neurons which did not reach the cortex.
- Heterotopias are intrinsically epileptogenic foci.
- Heterotopias may retain functional connectivity with the corresponding cortex.
- Heterotopias are usually FLAIR hyperintense because of altered cellular content and myelination within the focus compared to normal cortex.

Suggested Readings

Colombo N, Citterio A, Galli C, et al. Neuroimaging of focal cortical dysplasia: neuropathological correlations. *Epileptic Disord.* 2003;5(Suppl 2):S67-S72.

Novegno F, Battaglia D, Chieffo D, et al. Giant subcortical heterotopia involving the temporo-parieto-occipital region: a challenging cause of drug-resistant epilepsy. *Epilepsy Res.* 2009;87(1):88-94.

Preul MC, Leblanc R, Cendes F, et al. Function and organization in dysgenic cortex. Case report. *J Neurosurg.* 1997;87(1):113-121.

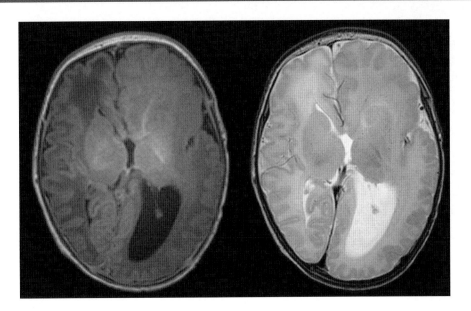

1. What are the findings?

2. What is the diagnosis?

3. Which syndromes may be associated with this entity?

4. What are the typical leading clinical signs of this entity?

5. What are the possible surgical options?

Case ranking/difficulty:

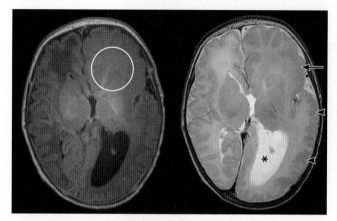

Left T1WI, right T2WI. Unilateral voluminous left cerebral hemisphere with enlargement of the left side ventricle (*black asterisk*). Fronto-opercular major thickening of the cortex with absence of gyrification and blurring of the cortico-subcortical border (pachygyria, *black outlined arrow*). Temporo-opercular and parieto-occipital minimal thickening of the cortex with multiple small superficial gyrification lacking secondary division (polymicrogyria, *black outlined arrowheads*). There is a considerable asymmetry in myelination state with a more advanced stage in the whole left hemisphere, especially in the deep white matter of the left frontal lobe (T1-hyperintensity, *white circle*), compared to the normal myelination (T1-hypointensity) of the contralateral side.

Answers

1. Unilateral hypertrophy of the left cerebral hemisphere is usually associated with malformative dilatation of the ipsilateral side ventricle and extensive areas of pachy-, and polimicrogyria. In this case, the contralateral side is normal.

2. In the absence of associated symptoms, the correct diagnosis is non-syndromic hemimegalencephaly.

3. There is an ipsilateral body and visceral hypertrophy in Proteus syndrome and in Klippel-Trenaunay-Weber syndrome, which may be associated with hemimegalencephaly (this association has not been reported in Beckwith-Wiedemann syndrome). In neurofibromatosis type I, hemimegalencephaly is extremely rare, and is associated with a milder clinical course (this association has not been reported in neurofibromatosis type II).

4. Macrocephaly is invariably present. Intracranial pressure is always normal in this entity. Enlargement of the side ventricle is of malformative nature and not due to increased intracranial pressure. Spasticity is classically unilateral. The degree of mental retardation is variable and related to seizure activity.

5. Cortical dysgenesis induces severe epilepsy which may be difficult to control. Intractable seizures induce profound mental retardation, and callosotomy as well as hemispherectomy (in cases of complete and severely dysgenetic hemisphere) must be considered to protect the normal contralateral hemisphere. In patients in whom epilepsy has been controlled, normal to subnormal developmental milestones can be achieved.

Pearls

- Hemimegalencephaly is an isolated or syndromic unilateral cerebral overgrowth.
- It is often associated with areas of polymicrogyria and pachygyria.
- There is malformative dilatation of at least parts of the ipsilateral side ventricle.
- Myelination delay or acceleration of the ipsilateral white matter is common.
- Cortical dysgenesis may also affect the contralateral hemisphere.

Suggested Readings

Alvarez RM, García-Díaz L, Márquez J, et al. Hemimegalencephaly: prenatal diagnosis and outcome. *Fetal Diagn Ther.* 2011;30(3):234-238.

Daghistani R, Widjaja E. Role of MRI in patient selection for surgical treatment of intractable epilepsy in infancy. *Brain Dev.* 2013;35(8):697-705.

Goldsberry G, Mitra D, MacDonald D, Patay Z. Accelerated myelination with motor system involvement in a neonate with immediate postnatal onset of seizures and hemimegalencephaly. *Epilepsy Behav.* 2011;22(2):391-394.

Slight hypotonic ataxia

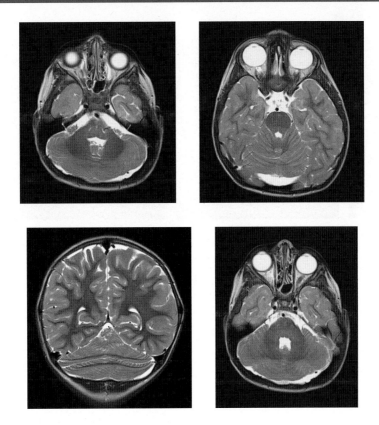

1. What are the findings?

2. Which complementary findings may be seen?

3. What is the origin of the fibers running through the superior cerebellar peduncle?

4. What is the name of the residual vermian tissue in figure on the extreme left?

5. What are the two syndromes which may be associated with this entity?

Case ranking/difficulty:

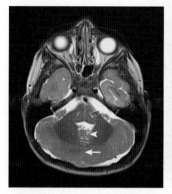

Dorsal fusion of the cerebellar hemispheres (*white arrow*) with absence of vermis. Residual dysplastic vermis structure can be seen at the roof of the fourth ventricle (*white arrowhead*).

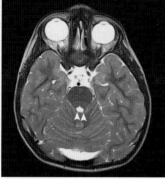

At the upper part of the cerebellum, the superior cerebellar peduncles form a V-shape pointing dorsally (*white arrowheads*). At this level no residual vermis is seen.

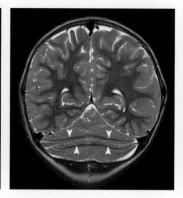

On coronal imaging, there is a bridging of white matter tracts from one hemisphere to the other crossing the midline (*white arrowheads*).

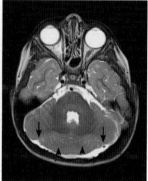

There is an abnormal third cerebellar lobe in the dorsal midline (*black arrowheads*) and two partial supplementary cerebellar fissures on each side (*black arrows*).

Answers

1. Fusion of the cerebellar hemispheres and the dentate nuclei, dysplastic or aplastic vermis, V-shaped superior cerebellar peduncles are present.

2. Due to the absence of the vermis, an abnormal third cerebellar lobe (lobus tertius) may form in the dorsal midline as in our patient. Tectum malformation may be present, which can induce aqueduct stenosis and hydrocephalus.

3. Efferent white matter tracts from the nuclei emboliformis, globosus and dentatus project through the superior cerebellar peduncle. These fibers may relay in the nucleus ruber or decussate and project to the ventrolateral and ventral anterior thalamus.

4. Centrally located remnants of the nodulus may be seen in the caudal midline.

5. Most frequent association is the Gomez-Lopez-Hernandez syndrome with a combination of parietal skin alopecia, trigeminal anaesthesia, and craniosynostosis.

Pearls

- Fusion of both cerebellar hemispheres.
- Absence or hypolasia of the vermis.
- White matter tracts cross the midline right-left best seen on coronal imaging.
- The superior cerebellar peduncles appear V-shaped due to fusion of the cerebellar efferent tracts.

Suggested Readings

Poretti A, Alber FD, Bürki S, Toelle SP, Boltshauser E. Cognitive outcome in children with rhombencephalosynapsis. *Eur J Paediatr Neurol*. 2009;13(1):28-33.

Toelle SP, Yalcinkaya C, Kocer N, et al. Rhombencephalosynapsis: clinical findings and neuroimaging in 9 children. *Neuropediatrics*. 2002;33(4):209-214.

Weaver J, Manjila S, Bahuleyan B, Bangert BA, Cohen AR. Rhombencephalosynapsis: embryopathology and management strategies of associated neurosurgical conditions with a review of the literature. *J Neurosurg Pediatr*. 2013;11(3):320-326.

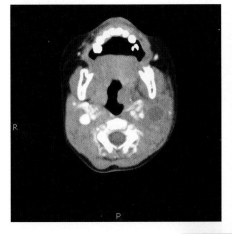
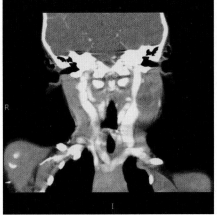
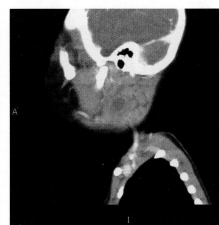

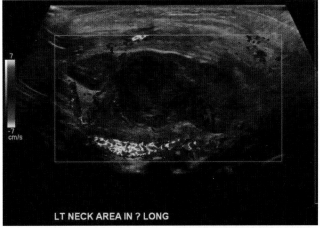

LT NECK AREA IN ? LONG

1. What is the differential diagnosis?

2. What type of this entity is most common?

3. What is the most common clinical presentation?

4. What is the most common anatomic location of this entity?

5. What are the treatment options?

Case ranking/difficulty:

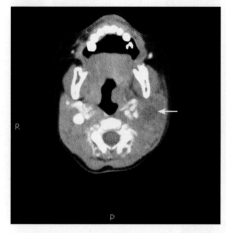

Axial CT of the neck with contrast demonstrates a cyst in the right side of the neck anterior to the sternocleidomastoid muscle (*arrow*).

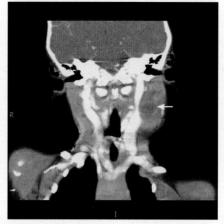

Coronal CT of the neck with contrast demonstrates a cyst in the right side of the neck anterior to the sternocleidomastoid muscle (*arrow*).

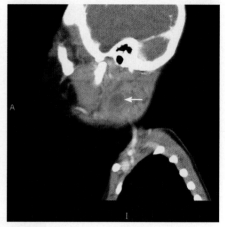

Sagittal CT of the neck with contrast demonstrates a cyst in the right side of the neck anterior to the sternocleidomastoid muscle (*arrow*).

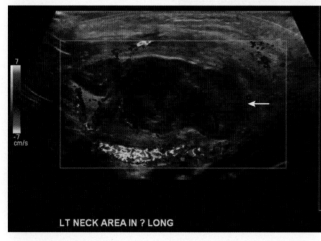

Longitudinal sonogram of the neck delineates the cystic nature of this lesion (*arrow*).

Answers

1. The differential diagnosis includes branchial cleft cyst, parapharyngeal mass, and cystic hygroma. Ranula is not in the differential diagnosis, as it is a sublingual cyst that results from obstruction sublingual salivary gland duct and is not anterior to the sternocleidomastoid muscle. Thyroglossal cyst also occurs in the midline and is not in the differential diagnosis.

2. The second branchial cleft cyst is the most common of all branchial cysts.

3. The most common clinical presentation of a second branchial cleft cyst is mass in the neck.

4. Second branchial cleft cysts are most frequently identified along the anterior border of the upper third of the sternocleidomastoid muscle and adjacent to the muscle.

5. Surgical excision is the treatment of choice. Antibiotics should be administered if the cyst becomes infected.

Pearls

- Branchial cleft cysts are the most common congenital cause of a neck mass.
- An estimated 2 to 3% of cases are bilateral.
- The second branchial cleft accounts for 95% of branchial anomalies.
- Cysts are most frequently identified along the anterior border of the upper third of the sternocleidomastoid muscle and adjacent to the muscle.
- Most branchial cleft cysts are asymptomatic, but they may become infected.
- Ultrasonography helps to delineate the cystic nature of these lesions.
- A contrast-enhanced CT scan shows a cystic and enhancing mass in the neck.

Suggested Readings

Bloch R. Images in emergency medicine. Branchial cleft cyst. *Ann Emerg Med*. 2006;47(3):291-308.

Koch BL. Cystic malformations of the neck in children. *Pediatr Radiol*. 2005;35(5):463-477.

Som PM, Sacher M, Stollman AL. Common tumors of the parapharyngeal space: refined imaging diagnosis. *Radiology*. 1988;169(1):81-85.

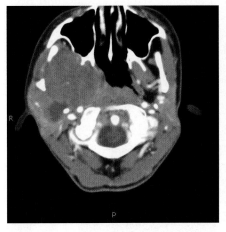 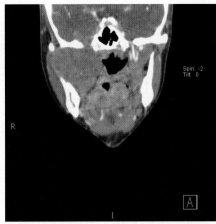 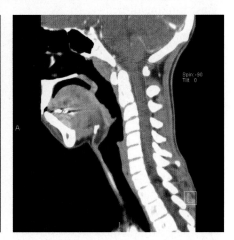

1. What are the findings?

2. What is the differential diagnosis?

3. What is the most common histologic type
    of this entity in the pediatric population?

4. Which histologic type carries the worst
    prognosis?

5. How is the final diagnosis made?

Category: Neck

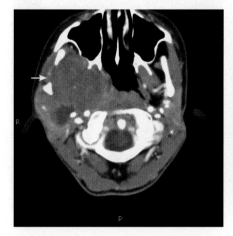

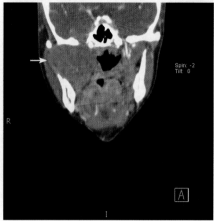

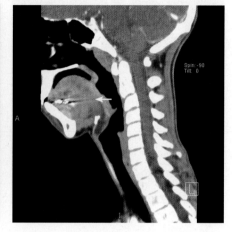

Contrast-enhanced axial CT of the neck demonstrates heterogeneous enhancing mass in the right masticator space (*arrow*) with foci of low attenuation representing necrosis and extending into the right masseter muscle, temporalis muscle, and medial and lateral pterygoid muscles.

Contrast-enhanced coronal CT of the neck demonstrates heterogeneous enhancing mass in the right masticator space (*arrow*) with foci of low attenuation representing necrosis and extending into the right masseter muscle, temporalis muscle, and medial and lateral pterygoid muscles.

Contrast-enhanced sagittal CT of the neck demonstrates heterogeneous enhancing mass in the right masticator space (*arrow*) with foci of low attenuation representing necrosis and extending into the right masseter muscle, temporalis muscle, and medial and lateral pterygoid muscles.

Answers

1. In the enhanced CT of the neck, there is heterogeneous enhancing mass in the right masticator space with foci of low attenuation representing necrosis. The mass extends into the right masseter muscle, temporalis muscle and medial and lateral pterygoid muscles.

2. Differential diagnosis may include lymphoma, synovial sarcoma, leukemia, primitive neuroectodermal tumor, and liposarcoma.

3. The most common rhabdomyosarcoma in the pediatric population is the embryonal type.

4. Alveolar rhabdomyosarcoma carries the worst prognosis.

5. Final diagnosis is histologic by tissue biopsy.

Pearls

- There are three known pathologic subtypes of rhabdomyosarcoma: embryonal, which is the most common, alveolar, and pleomorphic which occurs almost exclusively in adults.
- In children, there are 2 main subtypes of rhabdomyosarcoma: embryonal and alveolar.
- Rhabdomyosarcoma originates most commonly from the genitourinary system and the soft tissue of the neck, but can originate from anywhere.
- The diagnosis is made with cross-sectional imaging and is not different from any other tumors.
- Gold standard for the diagnosis is specimen biopsy.

Suggested Readings

Franco A, Lewis KN, Lee JR. Pediatric rhabdomyosarcoma at presentation: Can cross-sectional imaging findings predict pathologic tumor subtype? *Eur J Radiol.* 2011;80(3):e446-e450.

McCarville MB, Spunt SL, Pappo AS. Rhabdomyosarcoma in pediatric patients: the good, the bad, and the unusual. *AJR.* 2001;176:1563-1569.

Van Rijn RR, Wilde JCH, Bras J, Oldenburger F, McHugh KMC, Merks JHM. Imaging findings in noncraniofacial childhood rhabdomyosarcoma. *Pediatr Radiol.* 2008;38:617-634.

2-week-old male with hypothyroidism and increased thyroid-stimulating hormone

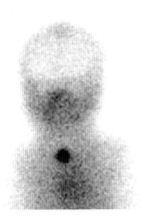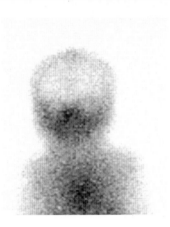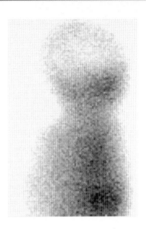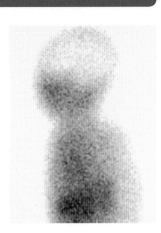

1. What are the findings?

2. What are the radiopharmaceuticals that are used for thyroid imaging?

3. What is the organidication process in the thyroid?

4. Why treatment of the shown case is urgent?

5. What are the treatment options?

Case ranking/difficulty:

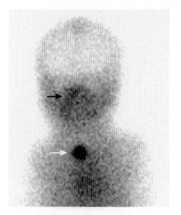

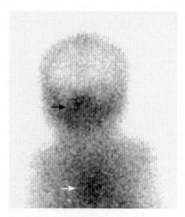

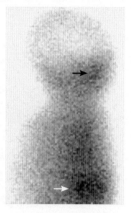

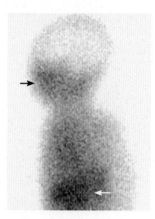

Thyroid scintigraphy. Anteroposterior view of the neck performed following in intravenous administration of 0.5 mCi of Tc-99m pertechnetate demonstrates absence of thyroid gland. *White arrow* points to a marker in the sternal notch. *Black arrow* demonstrates increased radiotracer activity in the nasopharynx.

Thyroid scintigraphy. Anteroposterior view of the neck performed following in intravenous administration of 0.5 mCi of Tc-99m pertechnetate demonstrates absence of thyroid gland. *Black arrow* demonstrates increased radiotracer activity in the nasopharynx. *White arrow* points to increased blood pool activity in the heart.

Thyroid scintigraphy. Right anterior oblique view of the neck performed following intravenous administration of 0.5 mCi of Tc-99m pertechnetate demonstrates the absence of thyroid gland. *Black arrow* demonstrates increased radiotracer activity in the nasopharynx. *White arrow* points to increased blood pool activity in the heart.

Thyroid scintigraphy. Left anterior oblique view of the neck performed following intravenous administration of 0.5 mCi of Tc-99m pertechnetate demonstrates absence of thyroid gland. *Black arrow* demonstrates increased radiotracer activity in the nasopharynx. *White arrow* points to increased blood pool activity in the heart.

Answers

1. The thyroid gland is not visualized.

2. The radiopharmaceuticals used for thyroid imaging are iodine (I-123 or I-131) and Tc-99m pertechnetate. Currently, Iodine-131 is not routinely used for imaging due to the high radiation burden.

3. Organification is the process of incorporation of the iodine in the thyroglobulin molecule to form the thyroid hormone. The process is facilitated by the enzyme peroxidase. Technetium is trapped by the thyroid gland, but not organified. Iodine is trapped and organified.

4. Without early hormone replacement therapy, developmental delay and irreversible mental retardation may occur.

5. In the absence of thyroid gland, life-long thyroid hormone replacement therapy is necessary.

Pearls

- Agenesis of the thyroid gland is a rare disorder with congenital absence of the thyroid gland.
- Treatment is urgent as there is increased risk for developmental delay and mental retardation.
- Diagnosis is made with nuclear imaging studies (radioactive iodine or free pertechnetate) that demonstrate complete nonvisualization of the gland.

Suggested Readings

Clerc J, Monpeyssen H, Chevalier A, et al. Scintigraphic imaging of paediatric thyroid dysfunction. *Horm Res.* 2008;70(1):1-13.

Rastogi MV, LaFranchi SH. Congenital hypothyroidism. *Orphanet J Rare Dis.* 2010;5(5):17.

5-year-old male with drooling and painful to talk

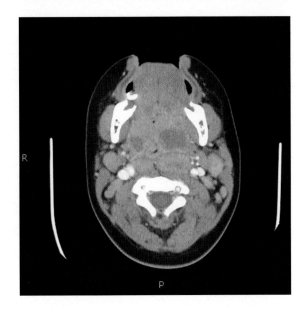 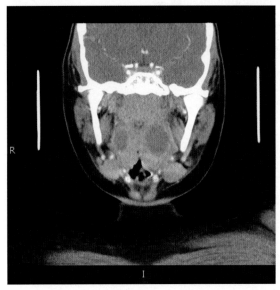

1. What are the findings?

2. What are the complications of this entity?

3. How does this entity occur?

4. What is the most common source of this entity
   in the pediatric population?

5. Why is treatment of this entity urgent?

Case ranking/difficulty:

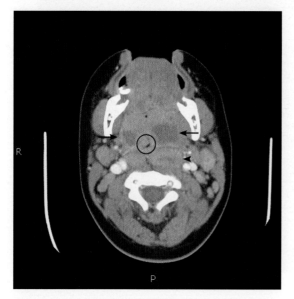

Axial-enhanced CT of the neck demonstrates the tonsils (*arrows*) with low attenuation in their center and enhancing wall representing an abscess. In addition, enlarged lymph node noted in the retropharyngeal area (*arrowhead*) with low attenuation in its center representing an abscess. Note is made of compression of the trachea (*circle*).

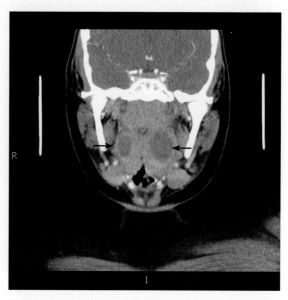

Coronal-enhanced CT of the neck demonstrates the tonsils (*arrows*) with low attenuation in their center and enhancing wall representing an abscess.

Answers

1. There is bilateral enlargement of the palatine tonsils with round areas of hypodensities and peripheral enhancement. There is narrowing/compromise of the oropharyngeal airway and prominent paripharyngeal lymphadenopathy left greater than right.

2. Complication of retropharyngeal abscess may include mass effect and airway compression, rupture of the abscess, aspiration of pus, and spread of the infection.

3. The retropharyngeal space can become infected in 2 ways: spread of infection from a contiguous area and/or direct inoculation from penetrating trauma.

4. Upper respiratory infection is the most common source. It may spread to retropharyngeal lymph nodes, which in turn may form an abscess.

5. Retropharyngeal abscesses are an immediate life-threatening emergency. It has a potential for airway compromise and obstruction.

Pearls

- Retropharyngeal abscess is immediate life-threatening emergency due to risk of airway compression.
- Most pediatric patients acquire the disease through spread from upper respiratory infection.
- Complications may include abscess rupture and aspiration of pus, airway compromise, mass effect, irritation, and erosion of the trachea.
- Computerized tomography of the neck is the imaging modality of choice for diagnosis.

Suggested Readings

Shefelbine SE, Mancuso AA, Gajewski BJ, Ojiri H, Stringer S, Sedwick JD. Pediatric retropharyngeal lymphadenitis: differentiation from retropharyngeal abscess and treatment implications. *Otolaryngol Head Neck Surg.* 2007;136(2):182-188.

Ungkanont K, Yellon RF, Weissman JL, et al. Head and neck space infections in infants and children. *Otolaryngol Head Neck Surg.* 1995;112(3):375-382.

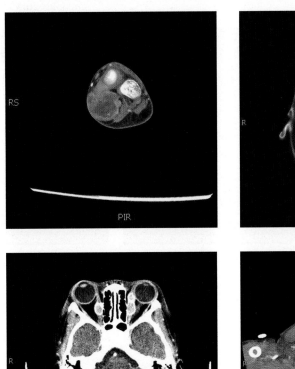

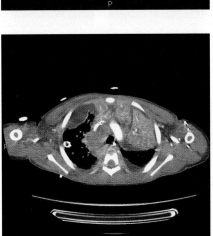

1. What is the diagnosis?

2. Which is the most common subtype of this entity in children?

3. What are the two most common locations that this disease originates?

4. Name the anatomic structure that is involved by the tumor as seen in the CT and MRI of the brain.

5. What are the treatment options?

Case ranking/difficulty: 🐢🐢

Category: Generalized diseases

Coronal CT of the foot reveals a mass in the soft tissue, medial aspect of the left foot (*arrow*).

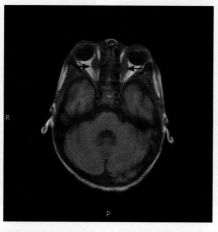

MRI-FLAIR, axial view of the head reveals a mass arising from the medial rectus muscle bilaterally (*arrows*).

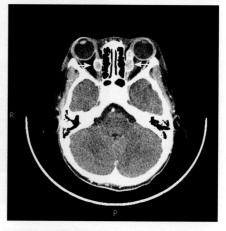

Axial CT of the head reveals enhancement of a mass arising from the medial rectus muscle bilaterally (*arrows*).

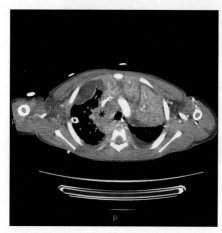

Axial CT of the chest reveals bilateral loculated pleural effusion, atelectatic changes, and large right hilar conglomerate of necrotic lymph nodes (*asterisk*).

Pearls

- The 2 histologic types of rhabdomyosarcoma in children are the embryonal and the alveolar types.
- Alveolar subtype carries worse prognosis than the embryonal type.
- Rhabdomyosarcoma originates most commonly from the genitourinary system and the soft tissue of the neck, but can originate from everywhere.
- Diagnosis is made with cross-sectional imaging and is not different from any other tumor.
- Gold standard for diagnosis is specimen biopsy.

Answers

1. The diagnosis is rhabdomyosarcoma.

2. Embryonal rhabdomyosarcoma is the most common subtype.

3. The 2 most common locations that rhabdomyosarcoma originates in the pediatric population are the genitourinary system and the soft tissue of the neck.

4. In the provided CT and MRI of the head, the medial rectus muscle is affected by the tumor bilaterally.

5. Treatment options include chemotherapy, radiation therapy, and surgery.

Suggested Readings

Franco A, Lewis KN, Lee JR. Pediatric rhabdomyosarcoma at presentation: Can cross-sectional imaging findings predict pathologic tumor subtype? *European Journal of Radiology*. 2011;80:e446-e450.

McCarville MB, Spunt SL, Pappo AS. Rhabdomyosarcoma in pediatric patients: the good, the bad, and the unusual. *AJR*. 2001;176:1563-1569.

Newton WA Jr, Gehan EA, Webber BL, et al. Classification of rhabdomyosarcoma and related sarcomas: Pathologic aspects and proposal for a new classification. *Cancer*. 1995;76:1073-1085.

8-year-old female with a pencil stuck in his left neck

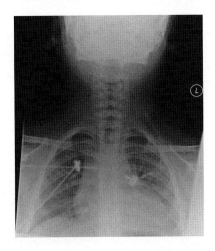
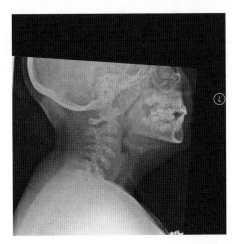
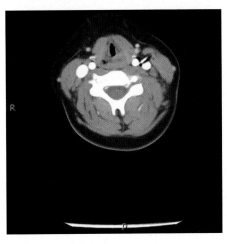
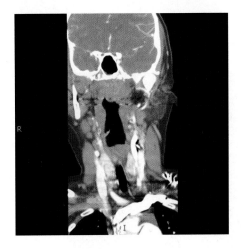

1. In the provided images, where is the tip of the pencil located?

2. In the provided images, which tissue has been damaged?

3. What should be the initial management of penetrating trauma in the neck?

4. What are the clinical signs of vascular injury in the neck?

5. What are the clinical signs of airway injury in the neck?

Case ranking/difficulty:

Category: Neck

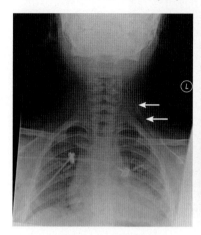

Frontal radiograph of the neck reveals a pencil stuck in the patient's neck (*arrows*).

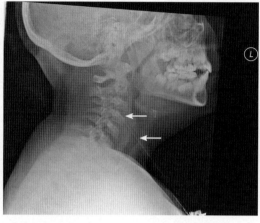

Lateral radiograph reveals a pencil stuck in the patient's neck (*arrows*), the tip overlying the cervical spine.

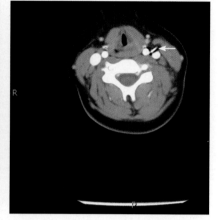

Axial-enhanced CT of the neck reveals a pencil that passes between the left common carotid artery and the left internal jugular vein (*arrow*). Vascular structure was not damaged.

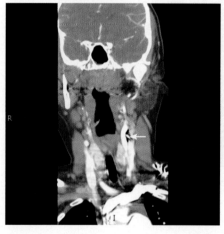

Coronal-enhanced CT of the neck reveals a pencil that passes between the left common carotid artery and the left internal jugular vein (*arrow*). Vascular structure was not damaged.

Answers

1. The tip of the pencil is between the left internal jugular vein and the left common carotid artery.

2. The pencil is noted to be between the left internal jugular vein and the left common carotid artery, but it did not penetrate the vessels. No tissue damage is seen.

3. The ABC rule applies. First airway patency needs to be maintained. Breathing should be normal. Circulation should be assessed and if necessary, fluids should be given to avoid hypotension and shock. The object trajectory should be assessed either by CT or if necessary, by immediate surgical exploration.

4. Clinical signs of vascular injury in the neck may include shock, expanding hematoma, profuse bleeding, hematemesis, and evolving stroke.

5. Clinical signs of airway injury in the neck may include subcutaneous emphysema, hoarseness, stridor, and respiratory distress.

Pearls

- Penetrating wounds of the neck are common in the civilian trauma population.
- Risk of significant injury to vital structures in the neck is dependent upon the penetrating object.
- Management should initially be focused on maintaining the vital signs (air ways, blood pressure).
- CT is an excellent tool to assess internal tissue damage.
- In other cases, surgical exploration may be necessary for assessment of the damage and treatment.
- If the penetrating object is still stuck in the neck, removal should be prudent to avoid further damage. Surgical intervention is safer.

Suggested Readings

Bhattacharya P, Mandal MC, Das S, Mukhopadhyay S, Basu SR. Airway management of two patients with penetrating neck trauma. *Indian J Anaesth.* 2009;53(3):348-351.

Hussain Zaidi SM, Ahmad R. Penetrating neck trauma: a case for conservative approach. *Am J Otolaryngol.* 2011;32(6):591-596.

Schroeder JW, Baskaran V, Aygun N. Imaging of traumatic arterial injuries in the neck with an emphasis on CTA. *Emerg Radiol.* 2010;17(2):109-122.

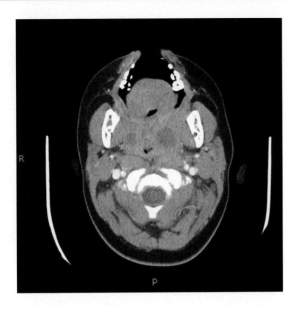
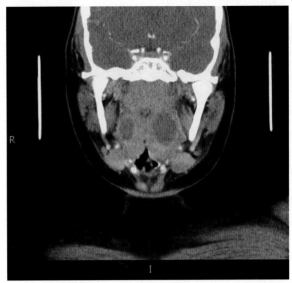

1. What are the findings?

2. What is the diagnosis?

3. What is the most common micro-organism causing this entity in children?

4. What are the complications of this entity?

5. What are the treatment options?

Case ranking/difficulty:

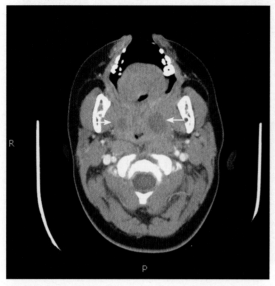

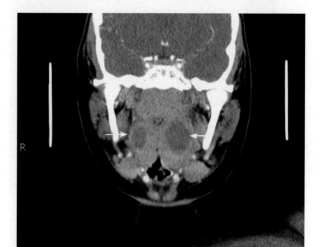

Axial-enhanced CT demonstrates marked bilateral enlargement of the palatine tonsils which contain rounded areas of hypodensity with mild peripheral enhancement (*arrows*). Findings are consistent with bilateral intratonsillar abscesses, left larger than right. There are enlarged lobular soft tissue densities in the retropharyngeal space, left larger than right suspected to represent significant retropharyngeal lymphadenopathy. The left-sided retropharyngeal lymph node is significantly larger than the right and contains central hypodensity consistent with suppuration.

Answers

1. There is enlargement of the palatine tonsils with rounded areas of hypodensity with mild peripheral enhancement and prominent retropharyngeal lymphadenopathy.

2. The diagnosis is intratonsillar abscess.

3. The most common bacteria which cause this disease include group A, B, C, and G hemolytic streptococci.

4. Complications of intratonsillar abscess may include septicemia, generalized cervical lymphadenitis, hemorrhagic adenitis, mass effect and compression of the pharynx and airways, and rheumatic fever.

5. Treatment options may include intravenous and oral antibiotics, needle or surgical drainage. Tonsillectomy may also be performed in rare cases.

Coronal-enhanced CT demonstrates marked bilateral enlargement of the palatine tonsils which contain rounded areas of hypodensity with mild peripheral enhancement (*arrows*). Findings are consistent with bilateral intratonsillar abscesses, left larger than right.

Pearls

- Intratonsillar abscess is a rare infection in children.
- Complications may include spread of infection with septicemia, mass effect and compression of the pharynx and larynx, and generalized cervical lymphadenitis.
- The symptoms and the treatment for this complication are the same as in the case of peritonsillar abscess.

Suggested Readings

Childs EW, Baugh RF, Diaz JA. Tonsillar abscess. *J Natl Med Assoc*. 1991;83(4):333-336.

Gan EC, Ng YH, Hwang SY, Lu PK. Intratonsillar abscess: a rare cause for a common clinical presentation. *Ear Nose Throat J*. 2008;87(12):E9.

Hsu CH, Lin YS, Lee JC. Intratonsillar abscess. *Otolaryngol Head Neck Surg*. 2008;139(6):861-862.

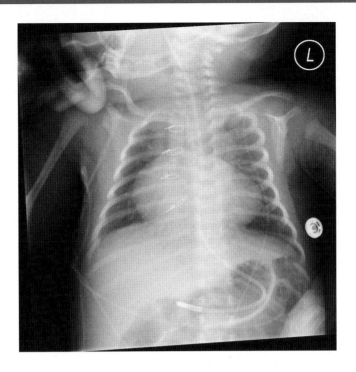

1. What is the finding?

2. What are the features of this entity?

3. What category does this entity belong to?

4. What is the treatment?

5. What are the sequelae of the treatment?

Case ranking/difficulty:

Category: Thorax

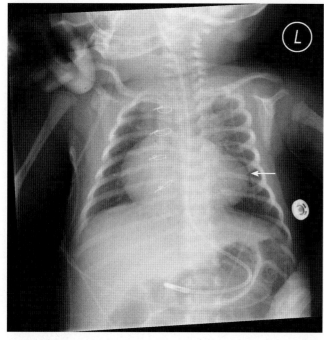

Frontal view of the chest demonstrates cardiomegaly. The left cardiac border shows uplifted apex (*arrow*). This has a boot-shaped pattern. Sternal sutures noted following Blalock-Taussig surgical intervention.

Answers

1. Boot-shaped heart is seen in Tetralogy of Fallot (TOF). It is due to uplifting of the cardiac apex because of right ventricular hypertrophy and concavity of the main pulmonary artery. The shadow of the pulmonary arterial trunk is almost invariably absent and there is decreased pulmonary vascularity.

2. The features of TOF are: right ventricular outflow tract obstruction, ventricular septal defect (VSD), right ventricular hypertrophy, and over-riding of the aorta over the VSD.

3. VSD allows mixing of oxygenated and deoxygenated blood from the left and right ventricles. Due to right ventricular outflow tract obstruction, this mixed blood flows preferentially to the aorta, thereby creating right to left shunt. Hence, the pulmonary vascularity is not increased in TOF, unlike in patients with isolated VSD. Patients are cyanotic and cyanosis relieves in squatting position.

4. Palliative procedure modified Blalock-Taussig shunt using a Gore-Tex graft. The corrective surgery involves repair of the ventricular septal defect and enlargement of the right ventricular outflow tract.

5. Pulmonary regurgitation is well tolerated initially. However, it leads to progressive dilatation of the right ventricle (RV) and RV outflow tract. RV dilatation causes tricuspid regurgitation, arrhythmia, and RV diastolic dysfunction. RV diastolic dysfunction may progress to irreversible RV systolic dysfunction requiring another surgery. Revision of RV outflow tract is performed using a valved conduit.

Pearls

- The four components of TOF are pulmonary infundibular stenosis, ventricular septal defect (VSD), overriding of the aorta above the VSD, and hypertrophy of the right ventricle.
- Cardiomegaly is mainly due to right ventricular hypertrophy that uplifts the cardiac apex producing the typical boot-shaped configuration (coeur en sabot) of the heart on frontal radiograph. Absent or small main pulmonary artery along with small thymus produces narrower upper part of this boot shape.
- Initially, a palliative procedure called modified Blalock-Taussig shunt is performed using a Gore-Tex graft between the subclavian artery and pulmonary artery to direct the blood to the lungs for more oxygenation.
- Corrective surgery is performed at a later stage. However, some surgeons prefer to perform corrective surgery. The corrective surgery involves repair of the ventricular septal defect and enlargement of the right ventricular outflow tract obstruction, which leads to pulmonary regurgitation.

Suggested Readings

Ferguson EC, Krishnamurthy R, Oldham SA. Classic imaging signs of congenital cardiovascular abnormalities. *Radiographics.* 2008;27(5):1323-1334.

Haider EA. The boot-shaped heart sign. *Radiology.* 2008;246(1):328-329.

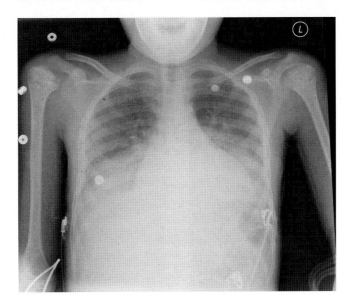

1. What are the findings?

2. What is the diagnosis?

3. What is the underlying defect?

4. What is the pathophysiology of the findings in the humeral heads?

5. What are other radiographic findings that may be seen in this entity (not explicitly shown in the provided image)?

Case ranking/difficulty: 🥉🥉

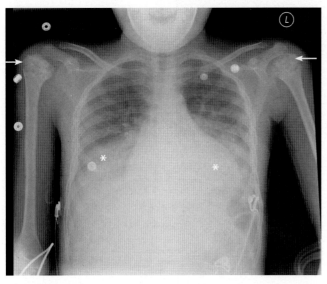

Frontal view of the chest demonstrates opacities of the right lower lobe and the left lower lobe (*asterisks*) representing consolidations. Sclerosis of the humeral head bilaterally noted, representing avascular necrosis (*arrows*).

Answers

1. Bilateral lower-lobe opacities, cardiomegaly, and bilateral humeral-head sclerosis and deformation.

2. Bilateral humeral-head sclerosis is most likely from avascular necrosis in an African-American child. The opacities in the lower lobe are probably from pneumonia causing acute chest syndrome. Combination of both findings should suggest sickle cell disease.

3. Replacement of the normally present glutamic acid at the sixth position of the beta chain of the hemoglobin by valine causes sickle cell anemia (SCA).

4. During deoxygenation, the abnormal hemoglobin undergoes polymerization causing irreversible change in the shape of the red blood cells (RBCs). RBCs become sickle shaped and are less deformable. Deformability of normal RBCs allow their passage through the microvasculature. This leads to microvascular obstruction leading to tissue ischemia and infarction. Microvascular obstruction is further increased by intimal hyperplasia seen in these patients. The RBCs in SCA patients have increased affinity for vascular endothelium promoting vascular obstruction.

5. Abdominal radiograph may show small or absent splenic shadow, calcified spleen, gall stones, surgical clips from cholecystectomy, and H-shaped vertebrae or Lincoln log vertebrae due to central end plate depressions.

Pearls

- Replacement of the normally present glutamic acid at the sixth position of the beta chain of the hemoglobin by valine causes sickle cell anemia (SCA).
- Avascular necrosis, osteomyelitis, acute chest syndrome, splenic infarct, splenic sequestration, stroke, papillary necrosis, and renal failure are frequently seen in SCA.
- Organisms causing pneumonia in SCA patients are streptococcus, hemophilus, staphylococcus, chlamydia, and salmonella. Pneumonia can lead to acute chest syndrome.
- Daily oral penicillin prophylaxis is given to SCA children from 3 months to 5 years of age.
- Abdominal radiograph may show small or absent splenic shadow, calcified spleen, gall stones, surgical clips from cholecystectomy, and H-shaped vertebrae or Lincoln log vertebrae due to central end plate depressions.

Suggested Readings

Crowley JJ, Sarnaik S. Imaging of sickle cell disease. *Pediatr Radiol.* 1999;29(9):646-661.

Khoury RA, Musallam KM, Mroueh S, Abboud MR. Pulmonary complications of sickle cell disease. *Hemoglobin.* 2011;35(5-6):625-635.

Lonergan GJ, Cline DB, Abbondanzo SL. Sickle cell anemia. *Radiographics.* 2001;21(4):971-994.

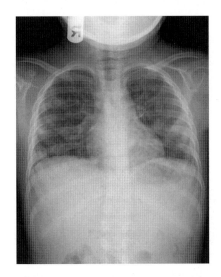
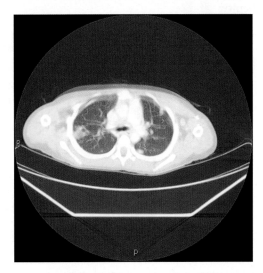
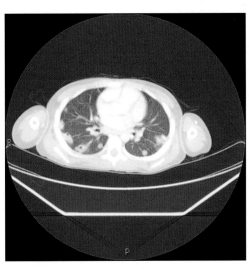
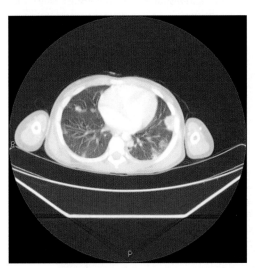

1. What are the findings?

2. What is the differential diagnosis?

3. How can methicillin-resistant *Staphylococcus aureus* (MRSA) be acquired?

4. Among hospital-acquired *Staphylococcus aureus* infections, what is the percentage of MRSA infection?

5. What are the treatment options?

Case ranking/difficulty: **Category:** Thorax

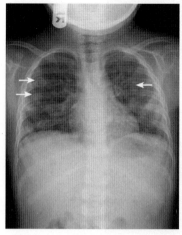

Frontal chest radiograph demonstrates multiple lung nodules (*arrows*).

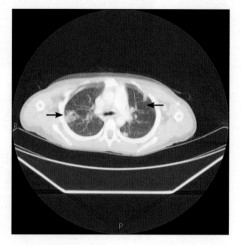
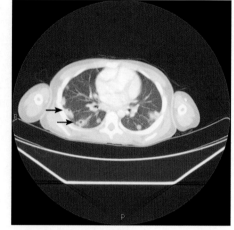

Non-contrast axial CT in lung window demonstrates multiple lung nodules, some of them are cavitary representing central necrosis (*arrows*).

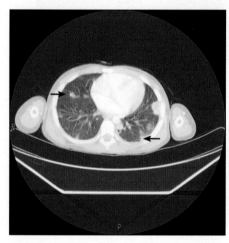

Non-contrast axial CT in lung window demonstrates multiple lung nodules, some of them are cavitary representing central necrosis (*arrows*).

Answers

1. There are multiple lung nodules in both lungs. Few of the nodules have lucent center representing necrosis. These are cavitary lesions, due to small abscesses in a patient with MRSA pneumonia.

2. Differential diagnosis may include septic emboli, Wegener's granulomatosis, tuberculosis, squamous or transitional cell metastatic disease, and rheumatoid nodules.

3. Methicillin-resistant *Staphylococcus aureus* (MRSA) can be either hospital-acquired or community-acquired. MRSA can be transmitted by direct (through skin and body fluids) and indirect contact (from towels, diapers, and toys) to uninfected people.

4. Fifty percent of hospital-acquired *Staphylococcus aureus* infections are caused by MRSA.

5. Oxygen and ventilation should be maintained. Hydration should be maintained. Treatment should be directed by the etiology and the causative agent.

Pearls

- In cavitary pneumonia, the lung parenchymal architecture is filled with cavitary nodules.
- Small cavitary lung lesions are seen in the plain radiograph and in CT. The cavitary lesions have central lucency representing necrosis or abscesses.
- The differential diagnosis includes necrotizing pneumonia, tuberculosis, vasculitis (Wegener's granulomatosis), sarcoidosis, fungal infection, and collagen vascular disease.

Suggested Readings

Donnelly LF, Klosterman LA. Cavitary necrosis complicating pneumonia in children: sequential findings on chest radiography. *Am J Roentgenol.* 1998;171(1):253-256.

Donnelly LF, Klosterman LA. The yield of CT of children who have complicated pneumonia and noncontributory chest radiography. *Am J Roentgenol.* 1998;170(6):1627-1631.

Morikawa K, Okada F, Ando Y, et al. Methicillin-resistant *Staphylococcus aureus* and methicillin-susceptible *S. aureus* pneumonia: comparison of clinical and thin-section CT findings. *Br J Radiol.* 2012;85(1014):e168-e175.

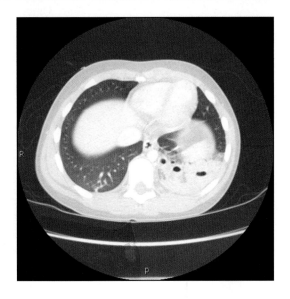 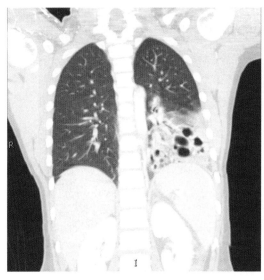

1. What is the diagnosis?

2. What are diseases that may be included in the differential diagnosis?

3. What are the risk factors?

4. Describe the imaging findings of this entity.

5. What are the clinical signs of this entity?

Case ranking/difficulty: **Category:** Thorax

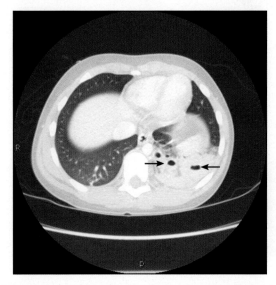

Axial CT in lung window at the level of the lower lobes reveals opacity of the left lower lobe with foci of air in it (*arrows*). The air is isolated without communication with the bronchi.

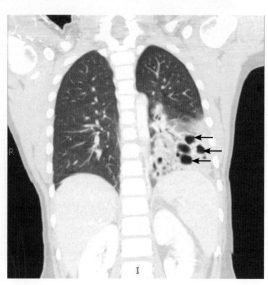

Coronal CT in lung window reveals opacity of the left lower lobe with foci of air in it (*arrows*). The air is isolated without communication with the bronchi.

Answers

1. The diagnosis is necrotizing pneumonia.

2. Diseases that may be included in the differential diagnosis are congenital pulmonary airway malformation, pulmonary sequestration, and Wegener's granulomatosis. Any cause of pulmonary cavitation is in the differential.

3. Risk factors include immunodeficiency, delayed treatment, alcoholism, and nosocomial infection.

4. Imaging findings include cavitation, densities with air inside. The air is isolated and does not communicate with the bronchi. Pleural effusion may be present.

5. Clinical signs include fever, chills, fatigue, and dyspnea. Complications may include development of acute respiratory distress syndrome (ARDS), sepsis, and shock.

Pearls

- Necrotizing pneumonia is a serious complication of community-acquired pneumonia.
- There is cavitation and liquefaction of the lung tissue.
- Clinical manifestations are fever, chills, and dyspnea.
- Complications associated with necrotizing pneumonia can include ARDS, sepsis, and shock.
- *Klebsiella pneumonia* is a micro-organism that can cause aggressive form of the disease.
- Methicillin-resistant *Staphylococcus aureus* (MRSA) is among the causative agents.
- Treatment is with antibiotics.

Suggested Readings

Barreira ER, Souza DC, Góes PF, Bousso A. Septic shock, necrotizing pneumonitis, and meningoencephalitis caused by *Mycoplasma pneumoniae* in a child: a case report. *Clin Pediatr (Phila)*. 2009;48(3):320-322.

Lichtenstein D, Peyrouset O. Is lung ultrasound superior to CT? The example of a CT occult necrotizing pneumonia. *Intensive Care Med*. 2006;32(2):334-335.

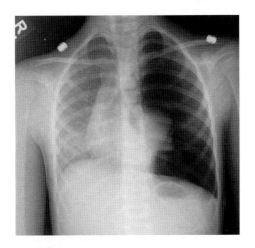
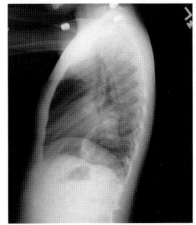
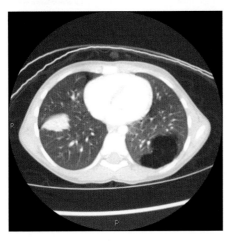
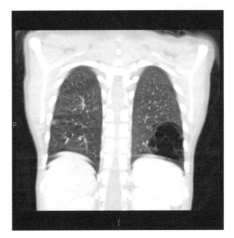

1. Describe the findings in the plain chest radiographs.

2. Describe the findings in the computerized tomography.

3. What is the size of type I in the classification of the shown entity?

4. What are the entities that may be included in the differential diagnosis?

5. According to the Stocker classification of the shown entity, which type is the most common?

Case ranking/difficulty: **Category:** Thorax

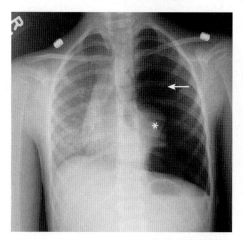

Frontal radiograph of the chest reveals left-sided pneumothorax (*arrow*). The left lung is collapsed (*asterisk*).

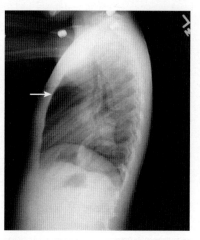

Lateral radiograph of the chest reveals left-sided pneumothorax (*arrow*).

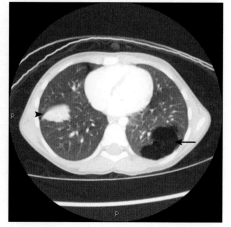

Axial view of chest CT in lung window reveals a septated air-filled cyst in the left lower lobe (*arrow*). Opacity is noted in the right lower lobe (*arrowhead*) representing consolidation. The CT was performed a week after resolution of the pneumothorax.

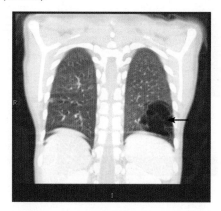

Coronal view of chest CT in lung window reveals a septated air-filled cyst in the left lower lobe (*arrow*). The CT was performed a week after resolution of the pneumothorax.

Answers

1. There is tension left-sided pneumothorax with collapse of the left lung. There is shift of the mediastinum to the right.

2. There is septated air-filled cyst in the left lower lobe seen in the axial and the coronal image. The axial image demonstrates consolidation of the right lower lobe.

3. Congenital pulmonary airway malformation is classified according to its size. Type I has large (>2 cm) multiloculated cysts.

4. The differential diagnosis for neonatal lung space-occupying lesions includes diaphragmatic hernia, pulmonary sequestration, bronchogenic cysts, bronchiectasis, cystic fibrosis, and congenital lobar emphysema.

5. The Stocker type I accounts for 50 to 70% of diagnosed cases. Type II lesions represent 18 to 40% of cases, and type III lesions represent 10% of diagnosed cases.

Pearls

- Congenital pulmonary airway malformation (CPAM) was previously known as congenital cystic adenomatoid malformation (CCAM).
- In CPAM, usually an entire lobe of lung is replaced by a non-working cystic piece of abnormal lung tissue.
- CPAMs are classified into three different types based largely on their gross appearance.
- Stocker classification type I has large (>2 cm) multiloculated cysts.
- Stocker classification type II has smaller, uniform cysts.
- Stocker classification type III is not grossly cystic, referred to as the "adenomatoid" type.
- Clinical presentation includes respiratory distress, recurrent infections, hemoptysis, or pneumothorax.
- Treatment is usually supportive and geared to treat the complications.

Suggested Readings

Kim WS, Lee KS, Kim IO, et al. Congenital cystic adenomatoid malformation of the lung: CT-pathologic correlation. *AJR Am J Roentgenol.* 1997;168(1):47-53.

Stocker JT, Madewell JE, Drake RM. Congenital cystic adenomatoid malformation of the lung. Classification and morphologic spectrum. *Hum Pathol.* 1977;8(2):155-171.

Wilson RD, Hedrick HL, Liechty KW, et al. Cystic adenomatoid malformation of the lung: review of genetics, prenatal diagnosis, and in utero treatment. *Am J Med Genet A.* 2006;140(2):151-155.

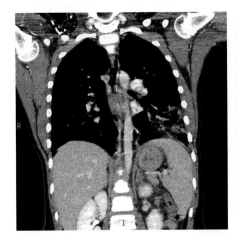 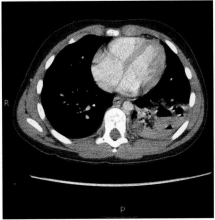 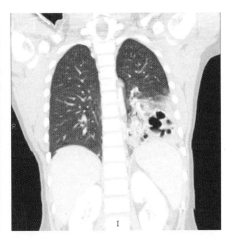

1. What is the differential diagnosis of this entity?

2. What is the most likely diagnosis?

3. The coronal CT (lung window) shows air cysts. What do they represent?

4. What is the most common anatomic location of this entity?

5. What are the characteristics of intralobar pulmonary sequestration?

Case ranking/difficulty:

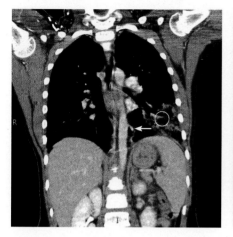

Coronal-contrast CT of the chest reveals heterogeneous opacities in the posterior left lower lobe (*circle*). Feeding arterial vessel noted (*arrow*).

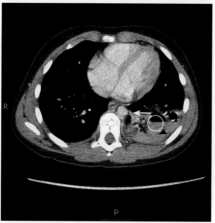

Axial-contrast CT of the chest reveals heterogeneous opacities in the posterior left lower lobe (*circle*). Feeding arterial vessel noted (*arrow*).

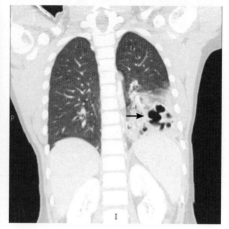

Coronal-contrast CT of the chest in lung window reveals air inside the heterogeneous structure (*arrow*). The air represents infection of the known pulmonary sequestration.

Answers

1. Differential diagnosis may include intralobar pulmonary sequestration, extralobar pulmonary sequestration, congenital pulmonary airway malformation (CPAM), necrotizing pneumonia, and left lower lobe abscess.

2. Most likely diagnosis is intralobar pulmonary sequestration, as the structure is ill-defined and feeding arterial vessel visualized. The coronal CT in lung window image reveals air inside the structure that represents a necrotizing infection. The sequestration is infected.

3. The air cysts represent necrotizing infection of an intralobar sequestration.

4. The most common location of pulmonary sequestration is left lower lobe.

5. Intralobar sequestration has a systemic feeding artery and pulmonary venous return. It shares the visceral pleura that covers the adjacent lung tissue.

Pearls

- Pulmonary sequestration is a cystic or solid mass composed of nonfunctioning primitive tissue that does not communicate with the tracheobronchial tree.
- Pulmonary sequestration has anomalous systemic blood supply. Its blood supply is from systemic circulation rather than the pulmonary circulation.
- The two forms of pulmonary sequestration are intralobar and extralobar.
- Intralobar sequestration shares the visceral pleura that covers the adjacent lung tissue. Venous drainage is commonly provided to the left atrium via the pulmonary veins.
- Extralobar sequestration has its own pleura and has systemic venous return.
- Extralobar sequestration is commonly a congenital occurrence that may be associated with other congenital anomalies.
- Sequestrations may become infected.

Suggested Readings

Collin PP, Desjardins JG, Khan AH. Pulmonary sequestration. *J Pediatr Surg.* 1987;22(8):750-753.

DeParedes CG, Pierce WS, Johnson DG, Waldhausen JA. Pulmonary sequestration in infants and children: a 20-year experience and review of the literature. *J Pediatr Surg.* 1970;5(2):136-147.

Flye MW, Conley M, Silver D. Spectrum of pulmonary sequestration. *Ann Thorac Surg.* 1976;22(5):478-482.

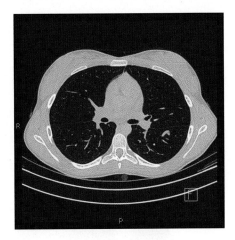
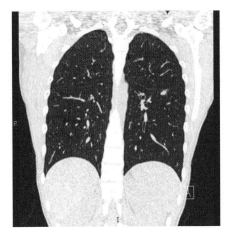
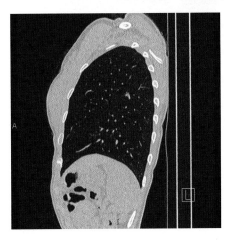
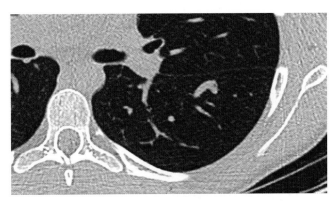

1. What is the percentage of this case in patients with hereditary hemorrhagic telangiectasia (HHT)?

2. What is the most common clinical manifestation of HHT?

3. What is the major risk of this case in patients with HHT?

4. What organs can be affected in patients with HHT?

5. What are the treatment options?

Case ranking/difficulty:

Category: Thorax

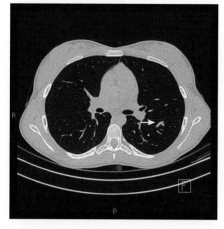

Non-contrast axial CT of the chest in lung window demonstrates opacity representing arteriovenous malformation in the superior segment of the left lower lobe (*arrow*).

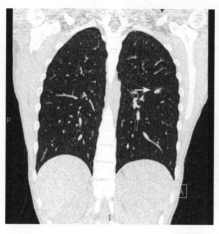

Non-contrast coronal CT of the chest in lung window demonstrates opacity representing arteriovenous malformation in the superior segment of the left lower lobe (*arrow*).

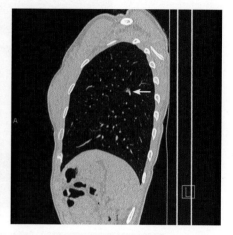

Non-contrast sagittal CT of the chest in lung window demonstrates opacity representing arteriovenous malformation in the superior segment of the left lower lobe (*arrow*).

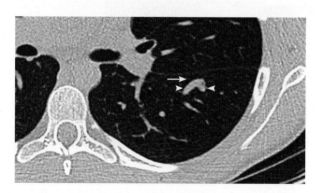

Non-contrast magnified axial CT of the chest in lung window demonstrates opacity representing arteriovenous malformation in the superior segment of the left lower lobe (*arrow*). The *simple arrowhead* points to the feeding artery and the *outlined arrowhead* points to the draining vein.

Pearls

- HHT, or Osler-Weber-Rendu disease consists of formation of abnormal blood vessels such as arteriovenous malformations and telangiectasias.
- The disease is genetic with autosomal dominant inheritance.
- Pulmonary arteriovenous malformation is present in 30% of patients with HHT. They are markers for HHT; 85 to 90% of people with pulmonary arteriovenous malformation have HHT.
- Pulmonary arteriovenous malformation is diagnosed by thin section non-contrast CT that demonstrates the feeding artery and the draining vein.
- Treatment of pulmonary arteriovenous malformation consists of transcatheter embolization.

Answers

1. Pulmonary arteriovenous malformation is present in 30% of patients with HHT.

2. Epistaxis is the most common manifestation of HHT.

3. Pulmonary arteriovenous malformation is a major risk factor for the development of brain abscess.

4. HHT is a genetic disorder that leads to abnormal blood vessel formation in many organs such as the lungs, liver, brain, skin, and the gastrointestinal system.

5. Treatment of pulmonary arteriovenous malformation consists of transcatheter embolization. Individuals with pulmonary arteriovenous malformation of 3 mm or larger, are at risk for stroke or TIA due to passage of small clots through the malformation.

Suggested Readings

Guttmacher AE, Marchuk DA, White, RI. Hereditary hemorrhagic telangiectasia. *N Engl J Med.* 1995;333(14):918-924.

Kjeldsen AD, Oxhøj H, Andersen PE, Elle B, Jacobsen JP, Vase P. Pulmonary arteriovenous malformations. Screening procedures and pulmonary angiography in patients with hereditary hemorrhagic telangiectasia. *Chest.* 1999;116(2):432-439.

Moussouttas M, Fayad P, Rosenblatt M, et al. Pulmonary arteriovenous malformations; cerebral ischemia and neurologic manifestations. *Neurology.* 2000;55:959-964.

3-year-old female with mass felt in the upper chest

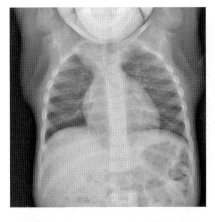
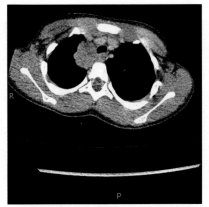
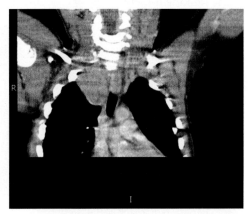
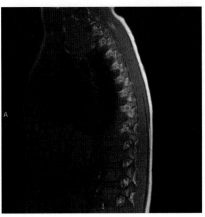
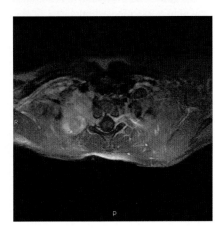
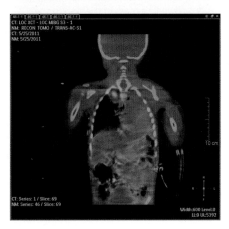

1. In which mediastinal compartment, is the mass seen in the images located?

2. What is the most common posterior mediastinal mass in children?

3. What is the most common location of this entity?

4. What is the radiopharmaceutical used in this SPECT/CT image?

5. What is the treatment of this case?

Case ranking/difficulty: **Category:** Thorax

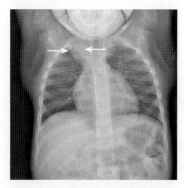

Frontal radiograph of the chest reveals a mass in the right upper mediastinum (*arrows*).

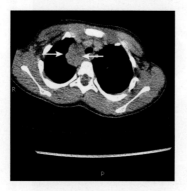

Axial CT of the chest reveals a mass in the right upper mediastinum (*arrows*).

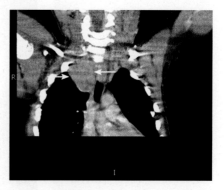

Coronal CT of the chest reveals a mass in the right upper mediastinum (*arrows*).

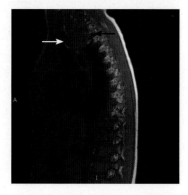

Sagittal MRI-T1 reveals a mass in the upper posterior mediastinum (*white arrow*). The mass extends to the right neural foramina between C7 and T1 (*black arrow*).

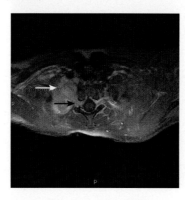

Contrast enhances axial MRI-T1, reveals a mass in the upper posterior mediastinum (*white arrow*). The mass extends to the right neural foramina between C7 and T1 (*black arrow*).

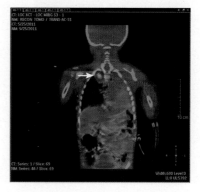

Coronal SPECT/CT reveals concentration of I-123-MIBG in the mass (*arrow*). The left lung is opacified due to malposition of the endotracheal tube in the right main stem bronchus (during the study, the patient was sedated).

Answers

1. The mass seen in the images is located in the upper and posterior mediastinum. Extension of the mass to the neural foramina between C7 and T1 is seen.

2. Neuroblastoma is the most common pediatric posterior mediastinal mass.

3. Pediatric neuroblastoma most commonly arises from the adrenal gland.

4. The radiopharmaceutical used is I-123-metaiodobenzylguanidine (mIBG) which is catecholamine analog.

5. Therapy includes radiation, chemotherapy, surgery, and stem cell transplantation.

- It most frequently originates in one of the adrenal glands, but can also develop in nerve tissues in any other location.
- mIBG, a catecholamine analog scintigraphy labeled with I-131 or I-123 scintigraphy, can add in the diagnosis of neuroblastoma.

Suggested Readings

Brisse HJ, McCarville MB, Granata C, et al. Guidelines for imaging and staging of neuroblastic tumors: consensus report from the International Neuroblastoma Risk Group Project. *Radiology*. 2011;261(1):243-257.

Melzer HI, Coppenrath E, Schmid I, et al. ^{123}I-MIBG scintigraphy/SPECT versus ^{18}F-FDG PET in paediatric neuroblastoma. *Eur J Nucl Med Mol Imaging*. 2011;38(9):1648-1658.

Pearls

- Neuroblastoma is the most common extracranial solid cancer in childhood.

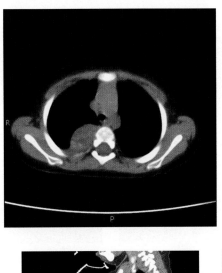
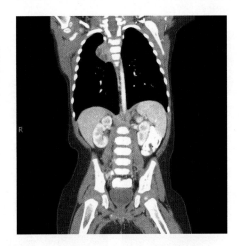
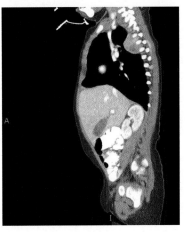
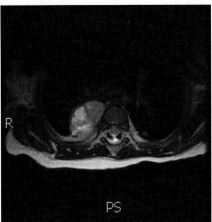

1. What are few of the diseases that this case can be associated with?

2. In which mediastinal compartment, is the mass seen in the images located?

3. What are the CT imaging features of this entity?

4. What are the most common metastatic sites of this entity?

5. What are the radiopharmaceuticals that are used for follow-up and staging of this entity?

Case ranking/difficulty:

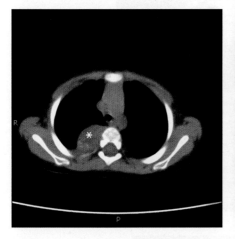

Axial non-contrast CT of the chest shows a posterior mediastinal mass in the upper right paraspinal region (*asterisk*). Calcification noted inside this tumor.

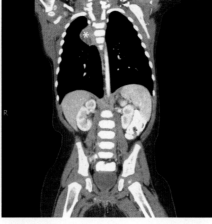

Coronal-contrast enhanced CT of the chest shows a posterior mediastinal mass in the right upper paraspinal region (*asterisk*) with heterogeneous enhancement. Areas of low attenuation noted inside the mass which may suggest necrosis.

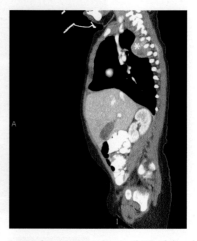

Sagittal-contrast enhanced CT of the chest shows a posterior mediastinal mass in the right upper paraspinal region (*asterisk*) with heterogeneous enhancement. Areas of low attenuation noted inside the mass which may suggest necrosis.

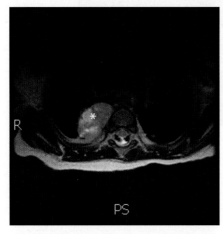

Axial MR-T2 of the spine shows a posterior mediastinal mass in the right upper paraspinal region (*asterisk*) with heterogeneous high signal. The mass did not extend to the neural formina.

Answers

1. Neuroblastoma may be associated with Von Recklinghausen disease, Beckwith-Wiedemann syndrome, DiGeorge syndrome, fetal alcohol syndrome, and Hirschsprung's disease.

2. This mass is a neuroblastoma that is located in the posterior mediastinal mass.

3. CT imaging features are heterogeneous enhancement. The tumor can cross the midline. It can encase vessels. Thirty percent of neuroblastomas demonstrate calcification on CT. It can metastasize to bone.

4. The most common metastatic sites of neuroblastoma are liver and bone.

5. I-123 MIBG and Tc-99m MDP are used for detecting metastatic lesions. MIBG is cathecolamine analog and MDP has affinity to bone.

Pearls

- Neuroblastoma is the most common extracranial pediatric neoplasm and the third most common pediatric malignancy after leukemia and central nervous system tumors.
- Neuroblastomas can arise from anywhere along the sympathetic chain.
- About two-thirds of all neuroblastomas start in the abdomen, developing in the nerve tissue of the adrenal glands (above the kidneys).
- Thoracic neuroblastoma accounts for 15% of all neuroblastimas. It is located in the posterior mediastinum and may invade the neural foramina.
- The tumor may demonstrate calcifications.
- Tumor can encase vessels.

Suggested Readings

Merten DF. Diagnostic imaging of mediastinal masses in children. *AJR Am J Roentgenol*. 1992;158:825-832.

Ribet ME, Cardot GR. Neurogenic tumors of the thorax. *Ann Thorac Surg*. 1994;58:1091-1095.

Slovis TL, Meza MP, Cushing B, et al. Thoracic neuroblastoma: what is the best imaging modality for evaluating extent of disease? *Pediatr Radiol*. 1997;27:273-275.

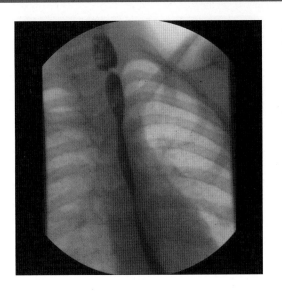 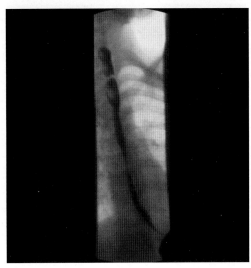

1. What is the diagnosis?

2. What are the clinical manifestations
   of the acute phase of this entity?

3. What are diseases that may be included
   in the differential?

4. Name a few agents that can cause this entity.

5. How is this entity treated?

Case ranking/difficulty: 🦠🦠

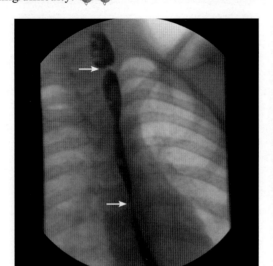 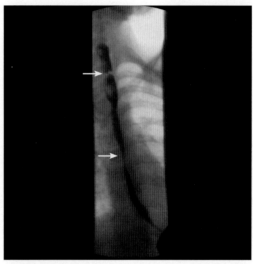

Esophagogram reveals two strictures (*arrows*). The lower stricture is longer than the upper one.

Answers

1. Two esophageal strictures are seen. With a history of ingestion of cleaning material, the diagnosis of lye ingestion should be made.

2. The acute phase of lye ingestion may present as abdominal pain, painful vomiting, oral mucosal erosive lesions, soft palate edema, and dysphagia.

3. The differential diagnosis may include esophagitis, achalasia, status post repair of esophageal atresia, esophageal motility disorders, and Schatzki ring.

4. Agents that can cause injury to the esophagus are substances containing bases such as lye, ammonia, electric dishwasher soap, detergent powders, and disc batteries.

5. The images show strictures which are sequela of caustic agent ingestion. This is treated by repeated esophageal dilatations.

Pearls

- Ingestion of corrosive agents may cause esophageal strictures.
- Burns in other body parts are also possible mainly in the skin and eyes.
- Severity of injury depends on the ingested material and the time of contact with the affected tissue.
- Treatment is by gastric lavage and bowel irrigation.
- Vomiting is inefficient and should not be induced.
- Adequate cardiopulmonary function should be ensured.
- Esophagogram is the imaging modality for the diagnosis. It reveals strictures at different levels.

Suggested Readings

Eyer F, Zilker T. Caustic injuries of the eye, skin and the gastrointestinal tract. *Ther Umsch*. 2009;66(5):379-386.

Janousek P, Jurovcík M, Grabec P, Kabelka Z. Corrosive oesophagitis in children following ingestion of sodium hydroxide granules–a case report. *Int J Pediatr Otorhinolaryngol*. 2005;69(10):1429-1432.

McKenzie LB, Ahir N, Stolz U, Nelson NG. Household cleaning product-related injuries treated in US emergency departments in 1990-2006. *Pediatrics*. 2010;126(3):509-516.

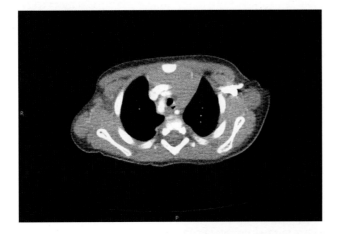
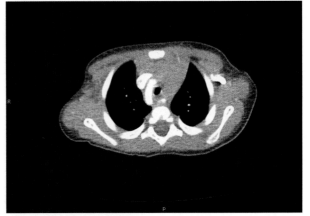
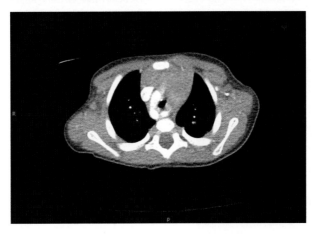

1. How many aortic arch pairs are normally formed during the embryogenesis?

2. What is the expected finding in a lateral chest radiograph of this entity?

3. What is the expected finding in a frontal chest radiograph of this entity?

4. In this entity, how many arteries are usually branching from the aortic arch?

5. What is the most distal artery branching from the aortic arch in this entity?

Case ranking/difficulty:

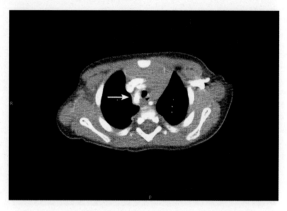 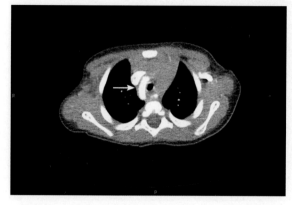

Axial CT angiography of the chest demonstrates a right aortic arch (*arrow*) with three vessels branching from the arch. A small common carotid trunk that immediately bifurcates into the left common carotid and right common carotid artery, right subclavian artery, and aberrant left subclavian artery that courses posterior to the esophagus.

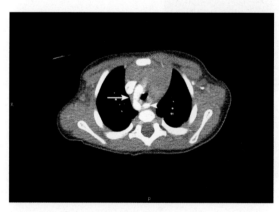

Axial CT angiography of the chest demonstrates a right aortic arch (*arrow*) with three vessels branching from the arch. A small common carotid trunk that immediately bifurcates into the left common carotid and right common carotid artery, right subclavian artery, and aberrant left subclavian artery that courses posterior to the esophagus (*arrowhead*).

Answers

1. Six aortic arch pairs are formed during the embryogenesis. Persistence or abnormal regression of the arch pairs can lead to the development of a variety of aortic arch malformations, some of which form complete vascular rings.

2. The aberrant left subclavian artery courses posterior to the esophagus causing the esophagus and the trachea to be displaced anteriorly.

3. Right aortic arch displaces the trachea to the left.

4. Four arteries are branching from a vascular ring with right aortic arch: Left common carotid, right common carotid, right subclavian, and aberrant left subclavian artery.

5. The most distal artery branching from a vascular ring with a right aortic arch is aberrant left subclavian artery.

Pearls

- Right aortic arch with aberrant left subclavian artery is one of the most common vascular rings.
- A ligamentum arteriosum (remnant of the ductus arteriosus) usually completes the ring that encircles the trachea and the esophagus.
- The commonly branching vessels from the right aortic arch by order are: left common carotid artery, right common carotid artery, right subclavian artery, and aberrant left subclavian artery that courses posterior to the esophagus.
- The ring may cause compression on the esophagus and trachea and leads to clinical symptoms such as stridor and/or dysphagia.

Suggested Readings

Carlton C, Lewis KN, Franco A. Right aortic arch with aberrant left subclavian vein. Unknown case #62. SPR web site December 12-26, 2011. <http://mirc.childrensmemorial.org/storage/ss12/docs/20111216171448953/MIRCdocument.xml/>.

Chan FP, Jaffe RB, Condon VR, Frush DP. Congenital great vessel abnormalities. In: Slovis T, ed. *Caffey's Pediatric Diagnostic Imaging*, 11th ed. Philadelphia, PA: Mosby/Elsevier; 2008:1591-1604.

Lowe GM, Donaldson JS, Backer CL. Vascular rings: 10-year review of imaging. *RadioGraphics*. 1991;11:637-646.

2-year-old male with stridor

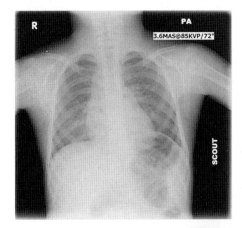
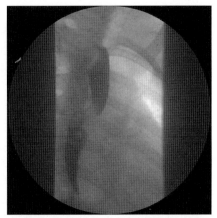
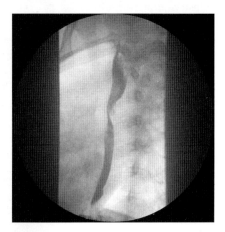
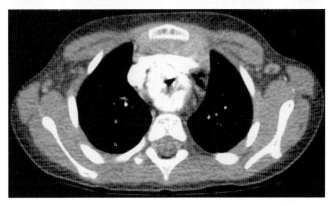

1. How is this entity formed during embryogenesis?

2. What vessel causes posterior esophageal impression as seen in the images?

3. What are the complications of this entity?

4. What are the associated anomalies of this entity?

5. How many pairs of pharyngeal arch arteries are formed during early embryogenesis?

Case ranking/difficulty:

Category: Thorax

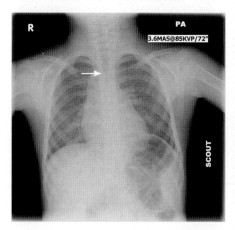

Frontal radiograph of the chest shows impression on the right lateral aspect of the trachea (*arrow*). The impression is due to a right aortic arch.

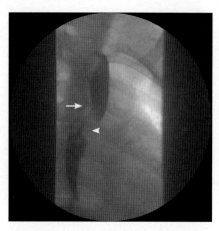

Frontal view of esophagogram shows impression on both sides of the esophagus. The impression on the right aspect of the esophagus (*arrow*) is due to right aortic arch and the impression on the left aspect of the esophagus (*arrowhead*) is due to the left aortic arch. The right sided impression is slightly higher that the left.

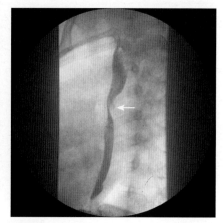

Lateral view esophagogram shows impression on the posterior aspect of the esophagus (*arrow*). The impression is caused by the dominant right aortic arch that passes behind the esophagus.

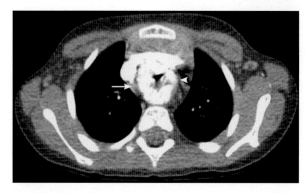

Axial view of CT of the chest shows right aortic arch (*arrow*) and left aortic arch (*arrowhead*).

Answers

1. During early embryogenesis, six pairs of pharyngeal arch arteries are formed. Most of them regress later on. Double aortic arch is formed when this process of regression and persistence does not occur normally, and the resulting vascular anatomy completely encircles the trachea and the esophagus.

2. The right aortic arch causes posterior esophageal impression, as seen on the lateral view of the esophagogram.

3. Complications of this entity may include tracheal compression, esophageal compression, stridor, and wheezing.

4. Associated anomalies of this entity may include coloboma, VACTERL, choanal atresia, and trisomy 21.

5. Six pairs of pharyngeal arch arteries are formed during early embryogenesis.

Pearls

- Double aortic arch is one of the two most common vascular rings.
- In 75% of cases, the right aortic arch is dominant and larger than the left.
- The right arch is located in a slightly higher level than the left arch.
- The smaller left arch passes anteriorly and to the left of the trachea in the usual position.
- Symptoms are caused by vascular compression of the airway, esophagus or both. Stridor, wheezing, persistent cough, and respiratory tract infection may be present.
- Treatment is surgical division of the vascular ring to alleviate the associated symptoms of tracheal and esophageal compression.

Suggested Readings

Backer CL, Ilbawi MN, Idriss FS, DeLeon SY. Vascular anomalies causing tracheoesophageal compression. Review of experience in children. *J Thorac Cardiovasc Surg.* 1989;97(5):725-731.

Picard E, Tal A. Tracheal compression caused by double aortic arch in two sisters. *Isr J Med Sci.* 1992;28(11):799-801.

Van Son JA, Julsrud PR, Hagler DJ, et al. Imaging strategies for vascular rings. *Ann Thorac Surg.* 1994;57(3):604-610.

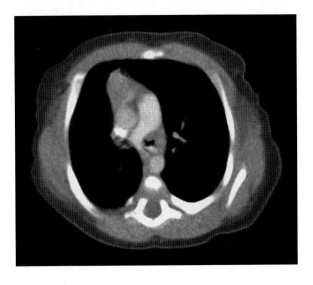 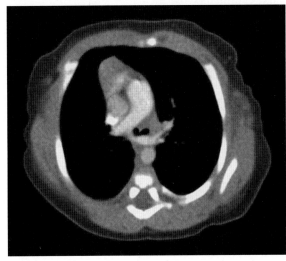

1. What are the findings?

2. Describe the abnormality of the pulmonary arteries in this case?

3. What is the course of the left pulmonary artery in this entity?

4. What are the complications of this entity?

5. What are the treatment options?

Case ranking/difficulty:

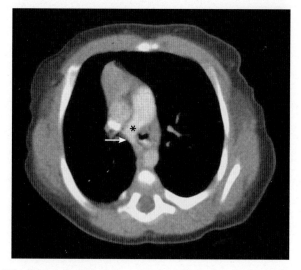 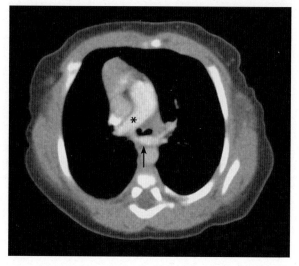

Axial CT at the level of the right pulmonary artery shows the left pulmonary artery branching from the right pulmonary artery (*asterisk*) and coursing between the trachea and the esophagus (*arrow*).

Answers

1. The case is a pulmonary sling that is created by anomalous origin of the left pulmonary artery from the posterior aspect of the right pulmonary artery.

2. The left pulmonary artery branches from the right pulmonary artery.

3. The course of the left pulmonary artery in this case is between the esophagus and the trachea.

4. Complication may include stenosis of the lower trachea, stenosis of the right mainstem bronchus, and obstructive emphysema of the right upper lobe.

5. Treatment includes treating pneumonia if present, intubation if patient is respiratory distressed, stabilization before surgery, and surgical correction.

Pearls

- Pulmonary sling is created when the left pulmonary artery originates from the posterior aspect of the right pulmonary artery.
- The anomalous left pulmonary artery courses over the right mainstem bronchus and then from right to left, posterior to the trachea or carina, and anterior to the esophagus, to reach the hilum of the left lung.

- This may be complicated by compression of the lower trachea producing airway symptomatology.
- Frontal chest radiographs demonstrate lower trachea compressed on its right side and deviated to the left.
- The lateral view of chest radiograph may reveal a density anterior to the esophagus and posterior to the trachea just above the carina. The trachea may be deviated anteriorly and the esophagus posteriorly.

Suggested Readings

Newman B, Cho YA. Left pulmonary artery sling-anatomy and imaging. *Semin Ultrasound CT MR*. 2010;31(2):158-170.

Sade RM, Rosenthal A, Fellows K, Castaneda AR. Pulmonary artery sling. *J Thorac Cardiovasc Surg*. 1975;69(3):333-346.

Tesler UF, Balsara RH, Niguidula FN. Aberrant left pulmonary artery (vascular sling): report of five cases. *Chest*. 1974;66(4):402-407.

12-year-old male with fever and peripherally inserted central catheter line placement

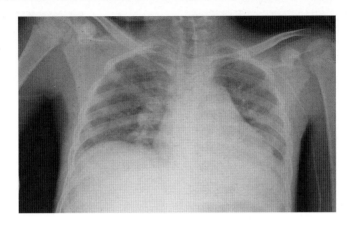

1. Where is the distal tip of the peripherally inserted central catheter (PICC) line as seen in the chest radiograph?

2. Name at least one venous structure in the chest that is considered to be the peripheral location for the distal tip of a PICC line.

3. Name a vascular structure where distal tip of a PICC line is considered to be malpositioned.

4. What is the anatomic landmark between peripheral and central venous locations?

5. Complications of malpositioned PICC line may include.

Case ranking/difficulty:

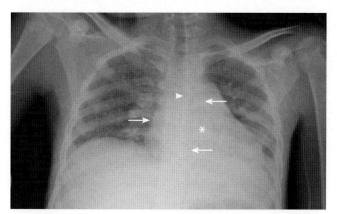

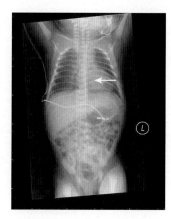

Frontal radiograph of the chest shows a PICC line coming from the left arm and its distal tip in the region of the main pulmonary artery. The *arrows* demonstrate the path of the PICC line through the right atrium and the right ventricle. The *arrowhead* points to an enteric tube. The *asterisk* demonstrates a retrocardiac opacity. There is obscuration of the left hemidiaphragm consistent with left lower lobe pneumonia.

Frontal radiograph of the chest and abdomen shows the PICC line coming from the left groin and its distal tip deviates to the left (*arrow*), in the right ventricle.

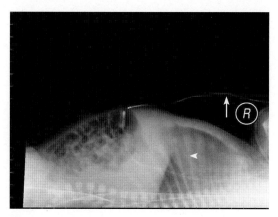

Cross table lateral view shows the PICC deviates anteriorly (*arrowhead*).

Pearls

- Position of the distal tip of a PICC line needs to be verified immediately after the insertion.
- Best position is the superior vena cava or the cavo-atrial junction.
- Any proximal central position distal to the first rib is also acceptable and considered central.
- PICC line tip distal to the right atrium is hazardous and may trigger complications.
- Among the known complications are: infections, arrhythmia, tamponade, and embolization.

Answers

1. The distal tip of the PICC line is in the main pulmonary artery.

2. Axillary vein is considered a peripheral location.

3. Right ventricle is not a good position for the PICC line. Complications such as arrhythmia may occur.

4. The axillary vein which is considered to be peripheral ends at the level of the first rib, where it continues as subclavian vein, considered to be central.

5. Complications of malpositioned PICC line may include clot formation and embolization, infection, cardiac tamponade, and arrhythmia.

Suggested Readings

Sneath N. Are supine chest and abdominal radiographs the best way to confirm PICC placement in neonates? *J Neonatal Nurs.* 2010;29(1):23-35.

Trerotola SO, Thompson S, Chittams J, Vierregger KS. Analysis of tip malposition and correction in peripherally inserted central catheters placed at bedside by a dedicated nursing team. *Vasc Interv Radiol.* 2007;18(4):513-518.

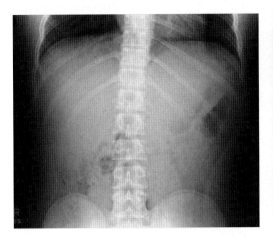 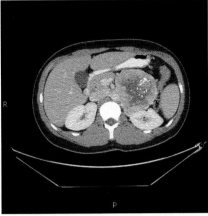 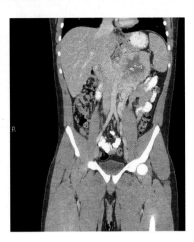

1. What are the findings?

2. Which diseases are associated with this entity?

3. What is the percentage of this entity that occurs in children?

4. What is the percentage of this entity that is bilateral?

5. What is secreted by this entity?

Case ranking/difficulty:

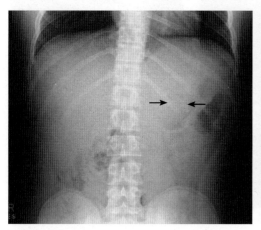

Frontal view of the abdomen reveals chunky calcifications in the left upper quadrant of the abdomen (*black arrows*).

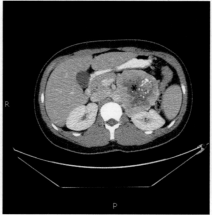

Axial CT of the abdomen obtained with intravenous contrast reveals a mass arising from the left adrenal gland (*asterisk*). The mass enhances in the periphery with central low attenuation. Chunky calcifications are seen in the mass.

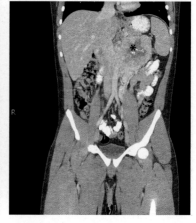

Coronal CT of the abdomen obtained with intravenous contrast reveals a mass arising from the left adrenal gland (*asterisk*). The mass enhances in the periphery with central low attenuation. Chunky calcifications are seen in the mass.

Answers

1. The CT scan demonstrates a mass in the left upper quadrant of the abdomen, enhancing peripherally with low attenuation center representing necrosis. Chunky calcifications are seen in the mass.

2. Pheochromocytomas may be isolated or associated with other disorders like multiple endocrine neoplasia (MEN) type 2A and 2B, Carney syndrome or phakomatosis like Von-Hippel-Lindau (VHL) disease and neurofibromatosis type I.

3. About 10% of pheochromocytoma cases occur in children.

4. About 10% of pheochromocytoma cases are bilateral.

5. Pheochromocytomas secrete excessive amounts of catecholamines like noradrenaline and adrenaline.

- Elevated catecholamines and metanephrines in plasma and elevated levels of urinary vanillylmandelic acid (VMA) in 24-hour urine collection help establish the diagnosis.
- Pheochromocytomas are very hyperintense on T2-weighted MRI.
- Pheochromocytomas may be heterogenous due to hemorrhage or necrosis.
- Pheochromocytomas can be located by nuclear study using iodine-123 labeled metaiodobenzylguanidine (MIBG).
- Many of the statistics related to pheochromocytomas follow 10% rule: 10% are bilateral, 10% are malignant, 10% are pediatric, 10% are extra-adrenal, 10% are extra-abdominal, 10% are familial, and 10% are silent.

Pearls

- Pheochromocytoma is a neuroendocrine tumor arising from chromaffin cells of the medulla of the adrenal glands or extra adrenal sympathetic chain.
- Clinically, patients may have episodic hypertensive crisis with visual changes.

Suggested Readings

Elsayes KM, Mukundan G, Narra VR, et al. Adrenal masses: MR imaging features with pathologic correlation. *Radiographics*. 2004;24(Suppl 1):S73-S86.

Johnson PT, Horton KM, Fishman EK. Adrenal mass imaging with multidetector CT: pathologic conditions, pearls, and pitfalls. *Radiographics*. 2009;29(5):1333-1351.

van Gils AP, Falke TH, van Erkel AR, et al. MR imaging and MIBG scintigraphy of pheochromocytomas and extra-adrenal functioning paragangliomas. *Radiographics*. 1991;11(1):37-57.

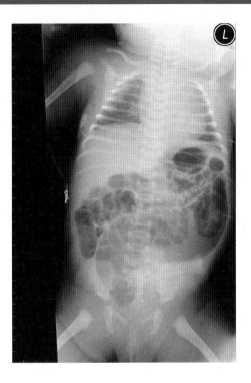

1. What are the findings?

2. What are the anomalies that may be associated with this entity?

3. What is the embryonic structure that the anus and the rectum develop from?

4. What anatomic structure is important in determining the severity of the lesion in this entity?

5. What are the treatment options?

Case ranking/difficulty:

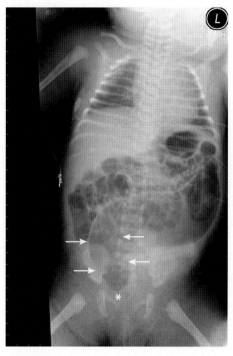

Frontal view of the abdomen demonstrates dilated descending colon and sigmoid (*arrows*). The region of the rectum is devoid of air (*asterisk*).

Pearls

- Imperforate anus or anal atresia is an anorectal malformation (ARM) where anal opening is absent. It is usually clinically obvious on physical examination. Newborn may not pass meconium and have abdominal distension or may pass meconium through fistula.
- Role of imaging is to determine the level of anal atresia, depict the fistulae if any, and preoperative planning.
- High lesion may be associated with rectourinary fistula in males and recto-cloacal or recto-vestibular fistulae in females.
- Cross table radiograph in prone position may show air in the rectal pouch at the level of obstruction. Less than 10 mm distance of the rectal pouch from perineum as measured on ultrasound is considered low lesion.
- However, radiograph and ultrasound are inaccurate as low lesion with meconium-filled pouch may appear high, and distended pouch or straining in a high lesion may appear as low lesion.
- Voiding cystourethrogram (VCUG) may help demonstrate fistulae. Cloaca is a condition where bladder, vagina, and colon form a common cavity with single perineal opening. In such a case, cloacogram helps demonstrate anatomy and fistulae.

Answers

1. Frontal view of the abdomen demonstrates dilated descending colon and sigmoid. The region of the rectum is devoid of air. Patient did not have an anal opening clinically consistent with anal atresia.

2. Imperforate anus is associated with an increased incidence of other anomalies, known as VACTERL association. (V-vertebral anomalies, A-anal anomalies, C-cardiac anomalies, T-tracheal anomalies, E-esophageal anomalies, R-renal anomalies, L-limb anomalies.)

3. The rectum and the anus develop from the dorsal potion of the hindgut or cloacal cavity.

4. Anal atresia can be low or high depending on relation of the rectal pouch to levator ani muscle. Pubococcygeal line on the lateral radiograph of pelvis represents the level of levator ani muscle.

5. Imperforate anus usually requires surgery for elimination of feces. Low lesions can be repaired immediately by anoplasty. High lesions require temporary colostomy prior to complete repair.

Suggested Readings

Fernbach SK, Poznanski AK. Pediatric case of the day. The three associated findings are (1) anorectal malformation; (2) sacral bony abnormality; (3) presacral mass. *Radiographics.* 1989;9(5):968-971.

Gupta AK, Bhargava S, Rohtagi M. Anal agenesis with recto-bulbar fistula. *Pediatr Radiol.* 1986;16(3):222-224.

Kohda E, Fujioka M, Ikawa H, Yokoyama J. Congenital anorectal anomaly: CT evaluation. *Radiology.* 1985;157(2):349-352.

3-year-old male with abdominal mass

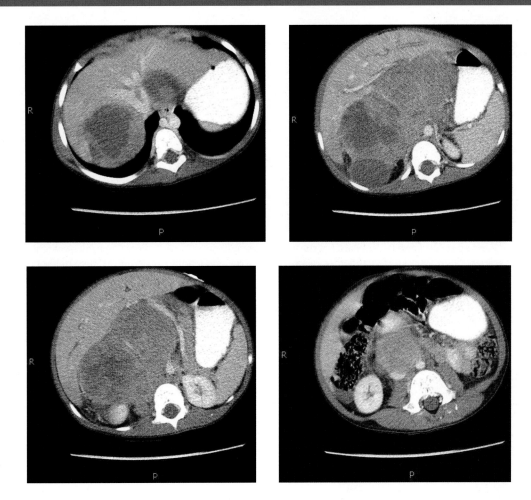

1. What is the differential diagnosis of the case?

2. What are the diseases that the case can be associated with?

3. What are the MRI findings of such a case?

4. What are the organs that such a tumor can originate from?

5. What is the percentage that this tumor demonstrates calcifications that can be seen in CT?

Case ranking/difficulty:

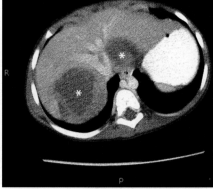

Axial CT at the level of the upper abdomen demonstrates a heterogeneous mass (*asterisks*) with areas of low attenuation that represent necrosis. The epicenter of the mass is in the right upper quadrant of the abdomen, in the right adrenal gland. The mass crosses the midline, encases, and displaces vessels.

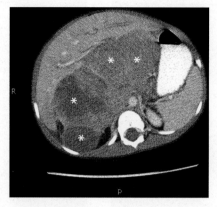

Axial CT at the level of the upper abdomen demonstrates a heterogeneous mass (*asterisks*) with areas of low attenuation that represent necrosis. The epicenter of the mass is in the right upper quadrant of the abdomen in the right adrenal gland. The mass crosses the midline, encases, and displaces vessels.

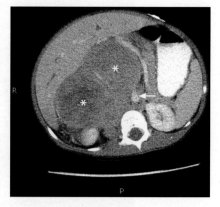

Axial CT at the level of the upper abdomen demonstrates a heterogeneous mass (*asterisks*) with areas of low attenuation that represent necrosis. The epicenter of the mass is in the right upper quadrant of the abdomen, in the right adrenal gland. The mass crosses the midline, encases, and displaces vessels. The aorta (*arrow*) is encased by the mass.

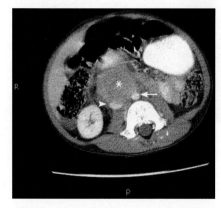

Axial CT at the level of the upper abdomen demonstrates a heterogeneous mass (*asterisk*) with areas of low attenuation that represent necrosis. The epicenter of the mass is in the right upper quadrant of the abdomen in the right adrenal gland. The mass crosses the midline, encases, and displaces vessels. The *arrow* points to the aorta and the *arrowhead* points to the inferior vena cava that is compressed by the mass.

Answers

1. Differential diagnosis includes neuroblastoma, Wilms' tumor, rhabdomyosarcoma, hepatoblastoma, and teratoma.

2. There has been association with a number of disorders, such as Hirschsprung disease, fetal alcohol syndrome, DiGeorge syndrome, Von Recklinghausen disease, and Beckwith-Wiedemann syndrome.

3. Neuroblastomas are typically hypointense on T1-weighted images and hyperintense on T2-weighted images. When contrast material is administered, the tumor exhibits inhomogeneous enhancement.

4. Neuroblastomas can arise from anywhere along the sympathetic chain, including the adrenal glands.

5. About 80 to 90% of neuroblastomas show stippled calcifications on CT.

Pearls

- Neuroblastoma is the most common extracranial pediatric neoplasm and the third most common pediatric malignancy after leukemia and central nervous system (CNS) tumors.
- Stippled calcifications are present in up to 30% of plain radiographs.
- CT can show the organ of origin, extent of the tumor, lymphadenopathy, metastases, and calcifications. About 80 to 90% of neuroblastomas show stippled calcifications on CT.

Suggested Readings

Chu CM, Rasalkar DD, Hu YJ, et al. Clinical presentations and imaging findings of neuroblastoma beyond abdominal mass and a review of imaging algorithm. *Br J Radiol.* 2011;84(997):81-91.

Sutton D. The radiological diagnosis of adrenal tumours. *Br J Radiol.* 1975;48(568):237-258.

Xu Y, Wang J, Peng Y, Zeng J. CT characteristics of primary retroperitoneal neoplasms in children. *Eur J Radiol.* 2010;75(3):321-328.

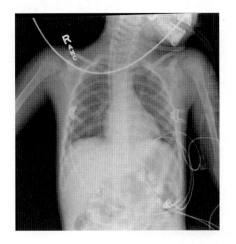
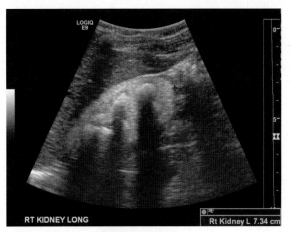
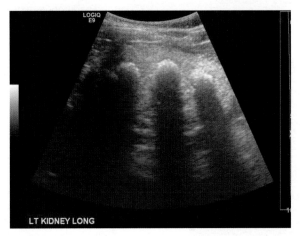

1. Describe the findings.

2. What is the differential diagnosis of the pattern seen in the sonogram?

3. What is the significance of echogenic cortex as seen in ultrasound?

4. What is the pathophysiology of the case?

5. What are the drugs that can lead to the shown entity?

Case ranking/difficulty:

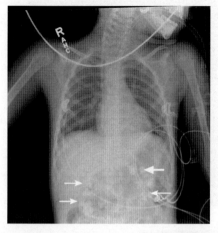

Frontal radiograph of the chest demonstrates bilateral calcifications in the visualized portions of the kidneys (*arrows*).

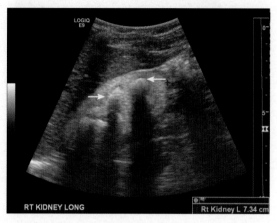

Longitudinal sonogram of the right kidney demonstrates echogenic cortex with multiple curved linear echogenicities that shadow (*arrows*) representing calcifications in the renal pyramids.

4. The distal nephron, primarily the collecting duct, is the site at which urine pH reaches its lowest values. Inadequate acid secretion and excretion produce a systemic acidosis.

5. Drugs that can lead to distal renal tubular acidosis include amphotericin B, lithium, and analgesics.

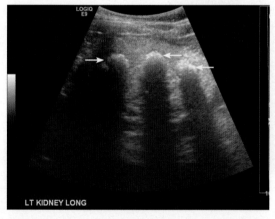

Longitudinal sonogram of the left kidney demonstrates echogenic cortex with multiple curved linear echogenicities that shadow (*arrows*) representing calcifications in the renal pyramids.

Answers

1. Bilateral calcifications are seen in the plain radiograph. The calcifications have the shape of the calyxes. The sonogram confirms the presence of calcifications by the shadows of curved linear echogenicities that are seen in the medullary region. This is consistent with medullary nephrocalcinosis. The cortex of the kidney is echogenic bilaterally.

2. Differential diagnosis includes renal tubular acidosis (type I-distal type), hyperparathyroidism, medullary sponge kidneys, milk-alkali syndrome, and hypercalciuria from any cause. The most common cause of hypercalciuria in the pediatric population is seen in preterm newborns in the neonatal intensive care unit due to excessive furosemide administration.

3. Echogenic cortex in renal ultrasound is a nonspecific finding and can be seen in any etiology of renal parenchymal disease.

Pearls

- Distal renal tubular acidosis is a disease that occurs when the kidneys cannot secrete acid, producing acidosis.
- Type I renal tubular acidosis is caused by a variety of conditions, including amyloidosis, sickle cell disease, systemic lupus erythematosus, Sjogren's syndrome, and use of certain drugs such as amphotericin B, lithium, and analgesics.
- During the disease, kidney stones and nephrocalcinosis are produced that can be seen in imaging.
- Differential diagnosis of medullary nephrocalcinosis includes medullary sponge kidney and hyperthyroidism.
- The echogenic cortex that is seen in the sonogram bilaterally is a non-specific finding and is consistent with renal parenchymal disease.

Suggested Readings

Courey WR, Pfister RC. The radiographic findings in renal tubular acidosis: analysis of 21 cases. *Radiology*. 1972;105(3):497-503.

Kessel D, Hall CM, Shaw DG. Two unusual cases of nephrocalcinosis in infancy. *Pediatr Radiol*. 1992;22(6):470-471.

Shultz PK, Strife JL, Strife CF, McDaniel JD. Hyperechoic renal medullary pyramids in infants and children. *Radiology*. 1991;181(1):163-167.

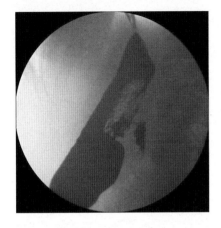 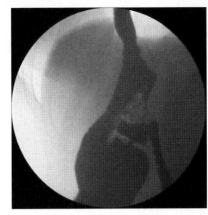 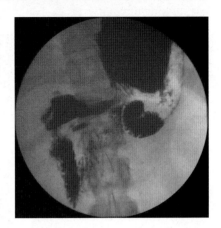

1. Describe the findings.

2. What is the etiology of the case?

3. What are the conditions that the case is associated with?

4. What are the typical CT findings?

5. What is the management of the case?

Case ranking/difficulty:

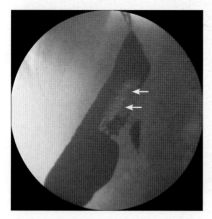 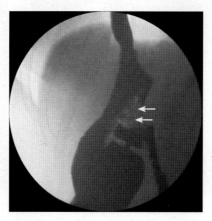

Upper gastrointestinal series in lateral view demonstrate amorphous filling defect (*arrows*) representing hair in the stomach.

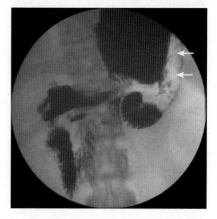

Upper gastrointestinal series in frontal view demonstrate amorphous filling defect (*arrows*) representing hair in the stomach.

Answers

1. Upper gastrointestinal series demonstrate amorphous filling defect representing hair in the stomach.

2. The etiology is the patient eating her own hair.

3. Trichobezoar is associated with mental retardation, PICA, and psychiatric disorders.

4. The typical CT finding of trichobezoar is a well-defined ovoid gastric mass with interspersed air.

5. The treatment of gastric trichobezoar is endoscopic removal of the hair from the stomach.

Pearls

- Trichobezoar is undigested material formed from hair trapped in the gastrointestinal system, most commonly the stomach.
- In children, trichobezoar is associated with pica, mental retardation or psychiatric disorders.
- Treatment consists of removal of the hair from the stomach through endoscopic intervention.

Suggested Readings

McCracken S, Jongeward R, Silver TM, et al. Gastric trichobezoar: sonographic findings. *Radiology*. 1986;161(1):123-124.

McGee AR, Lobb R. Trichobezoar; with a case report. *Radiology*. 1957;69(6):860-862.

Peake JD. Trichobezoar or hair ball; a case report. *Radiology*. 1948;51(6):816-819.

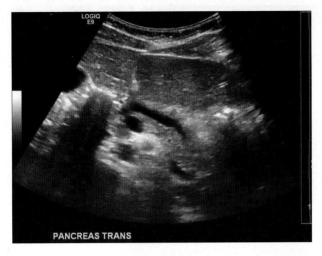
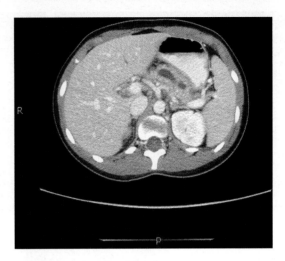
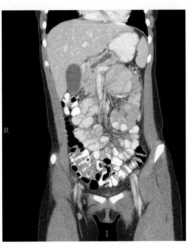
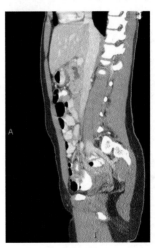

1. Describe the findings.

2. What is the etiology of this entity?

3. How patients may present clinically?

4. What are the CT features of this entity?

5. What are the goals of treatment?

Case ranking/difficulty:

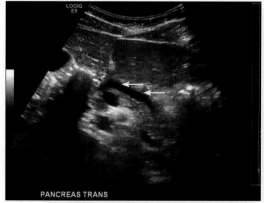

Sonogram of the upper abdomen demonstrates dilated pancreatic duct (*arrows*).

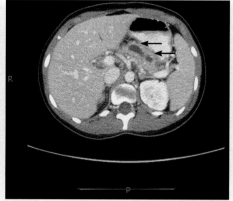

Axial CT of the abdomen following intravenous contrast administration reveals thickened pancreas with dilated pancreatic duct (*arrows*).

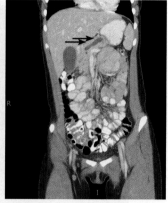

Coronal CT of the abdomen following intravenous contrast administration reveals thickened pancreas with dilated pancreatic duct (*arrows*).

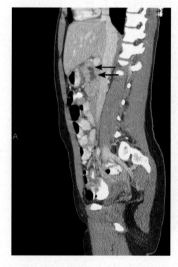

Sagittal CT of the abdomen following intravenous contrast administration reveals thickened pancreas with dilated pancreatic duct (*arrows*).

Answers

1. The pancreatic duct is dilated.

2. Etiologies of chronic pancreatitis include alcohol, gallstones, hypercalcemia in adults. In the pediatric population, the most common causes are trauma and idiopathic. Cystic fibrosis is also a cause of chronic pancreatitis.

3. Patients with chronic pancreatitis usually present with abdominal pain, steatorrhea resulting from malabsorption of the fats in food. Diabetes is a common complication.

4. CT features include dilatation of the main pancreatic duct; calcifications; changes in size, shape, and contour; pseudocysts; and bile duct changes.

5. The goals of treatment include alleviating pain, treating the underlying cause, restoring pancreatic function, managing complications such as pseudocysts, improving nutrition status, and enabling the patients to lead a reasonably good quality of life.

Pearls

- Diabetes is a common complication due to the chronic pancreatic damage and may require treatment with insulin.
- In the pediatric population, the most common cause of chronic pancreatitis are trauma and idiopathic.
- Cystic fibrosis may lead to chronic pancreatitis.
- CT findings include dilatation of the main pancreatic duct, calcifications, changes in size, shape, and contour, pseudocysts, and bile duct changes.

Suggested Readings

Matos C, Cappeliez O, Winant C, Coppens E, Devière J, Metens T. MR imaging of the pancreas: a pictorial tour. *Radiographics.* 2002;22(1):e2.

Vaughn DD, Jabra AA, Fishman EK. Pancreatic disease in children and young adults: evaluation with CT. *Radiographics.* 1999;18(5):1171-1187.

Visrutaratna P, Ukarapol N. Clinical image. Mediastinal pancreatic pseudocyst in chronic pancreatitis. *Pediatr Radiol.* 2010;40(7):1298.

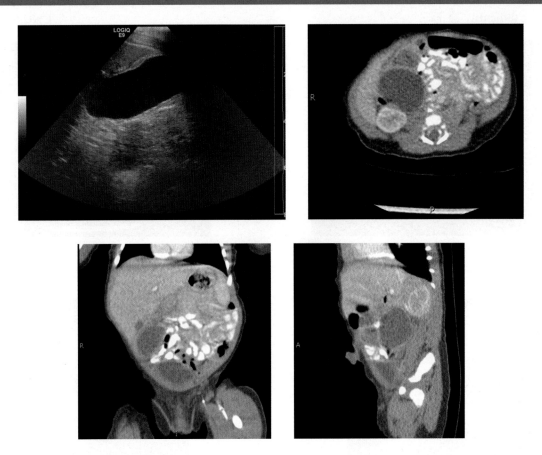

1. Describe the findings.

2. What is the most common site of this entity?

3. What is the most common portion of the small intestine that the shown entity is located?

4. What are the complications of the shown entity?

5. What may be included in the differential diagnosis?

Case ranking/difficulty: 🔴🔴

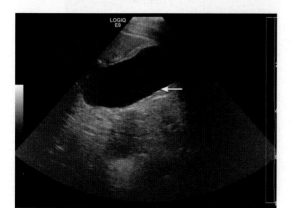

Sonogram of the abdomen demonstrates a cyst in the right upper quadrant of the abdomen (*arrow*).

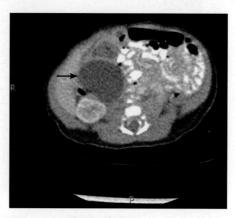

Axial CT of the abdomen with contrast demonstrates a cyst in the right upper quadrant of the abdomen (*arrow*).

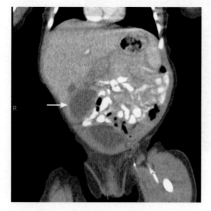

Coronal CT of the abdomen with contrast demonstrates a cyst in the right upper quadrant of the abdomen (*arrow*).

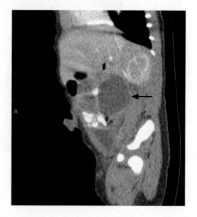

Sagittal CT of the abdomen with contrast demonstrates a cyst in the right upper quadrant of the abdomen (*arrow*).

Answers

1. There is a cyst in the right upper quadrant of the abdomen.

2. The small intestine is the most frequent site of gastrointestinal duplications, accounting for 44% of cases.

3. Most small-intestine duplications are located in the ileum.

4. Enteric duplications can serve as the focal point for volvulus or intussusceptions. Malignant development of this mucosal lining as well as cases of carcinoid tumors have been reported. Many lesions, however, are asymptomatic and the diagnosis is often made incidentally during a surgical procedure.

5. The differential diagnosis may include mesenteric cyst (lymphangioma), cystic teratoma, choledochal cyst, and an abscess.

Pearls

- Enteric duplications cysts are rare congenital malformations that may vary greatly in presentation, size, location, and symptoms.
- In CT, cysts appear as a structure of low attenuation with a wall that may enhance. In MRI, cyst has low signal in T1 and high signal in T2.

Suggested Readings

Berrocal T, Lamas M, Gutieérrez J, et al. Congenital anomalies of the small intestine, colon, and rectum. *Radiographics*. 1999;19(5):1219-1236.

Gul A, Tekoglu G, Aslan H, et al. Prenatal sonographic features of esophageal and ileal duplications at 18 weeks of gestation. *Prenat Diagn*. 2004;24:969-971.

Kleppel B. Congenital enteric duplication cyst; report of a case diagnosed roentgenologically. *Radiology*. 1958;70(4):570-573.

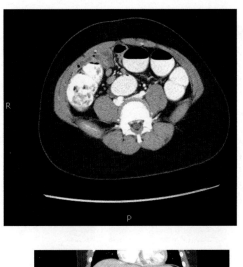 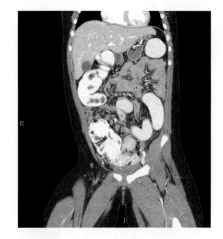

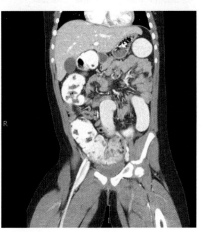 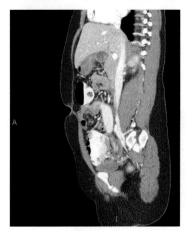

1. What are the imaging diagnostic features
   of the case?

2. What are the diseases that may be included
   in the differential diagnosis?

3. What is the most common cause of this case?

4. What is the main differential diagnosis?

5. What is the most common management of
   the case?

Case ranking/difficulty:

Category: Abdomen

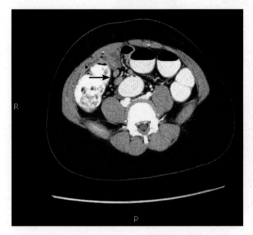

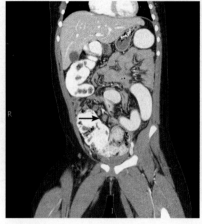

Axial CT of the abdomen with intravenous and rectal contrast demonstrates mesenteric lymph nodes slightly larger than a centimeter (*arrow*). The appendix was normal.

Coronal CT of the abdomen with intravenous and rectal contrast demonstrates mesenteric lymph nodes slightly larger than a centimeter (*arrow*). The appendix was normal.

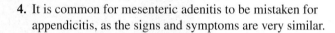

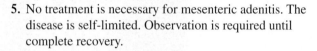

4. It is common for mesenteric adenitis to be mistaken for appendicitis, as the signs and symptoms are very similar.

5. No treatment is necessary for mesenteric adenitis. The disease is self-limited. Observation is required until complete recovery.

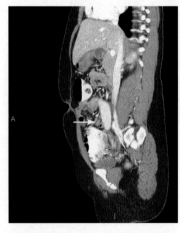

Sagittal CT of the abdomen with intravenous and rectal contrast demonstrates mesenteric lymph nodes slightly larger than a centimeter (*arrow*). The appendix was normal.

Answers

1. Diagnostic features include cluster of enlarged mesenteric lymph nodes in the right lower quadrant of the abdomen and normal appendix.

2. Among the diseases that may be included in the differential diagnosis are acute appendicitis, cholecystitis, inflammatory bowel disease, lymphoma, and urinary tract infections.

3. The most common cause of mesenteric adenitis is viral infection.

Pearls

- Inflammation of the mesenteric lymph nodes results in abdominal pain, tenderness, and fever.
- Mesenteric adenitis most commonly occurs in children and adolescents.
- The signs and symptoms of mesenteric adenitis can last from a few days up to a few weeks.
- It is common for mesenteric adenitis to be mistaken for appendicitis, as the signs and symptoms are very similar.
- Imaging modalities of choice are CT and ultrasound, with preference of ultrasound due to lack of ionizing radiation.
- In ultrasound, enlarged and hypoechoic cluster of lymph nodes are seen in the right lower quadrant of the abdomen.

Suggested Readings

Rao PM, Rhea JT, Novelline RA. CT diagnosis of mesenteric adenitis. *Radiology*. 1997;202(1):145-149.

Simanovsky N, Hiller N. Importance of sonographic detection of enlarged abdominal lymph nodes in children. *J Ultrasound Med*. 2007;26(5):581-584.

Simonovsky V. Ultrasound in the differential diagnosis of appendicitis. *Clin Radiol*. 1995;50(11):768-773.

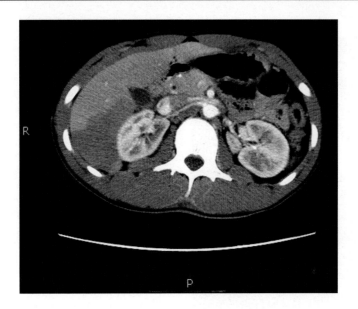

1. What are the findings?

2. Which organ is the most commonly injured in blunt abdominal trauma?

3. How will you grade the current injury?

4. What is grade 6 of hepatic injury as defined by the American Association for the Surgery of Trauma (AAST)?

5. What are the mechanisms of blunt abdominal injury?

Case ranking/difficulty:

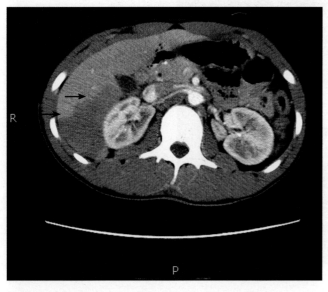

Axial CT of the abdomen with contrast in liver window demonstrates low attenuation in the right lobe of the liver (*arrows*) representing laceration.

Answers

1. There is low attenuation in the right lobe of the liver. In the context of trauma, this most likely represents laceration.

2. The spleen is the most commonly injured organ in blunt trauma of the abdomen.

3. This is grade 3 injury. There is parenchymal laceration more than 3 cm deep and less than 10 cm.

4. Grade 6 liver injury as defined by the AAST consists of hepatic avulsion.

5. Blunt force injuries to the abdomen can generally be explained by 3 mechanisms: rapid deceleration, crushed intra-abdominal contents, and sudden rise in intra-abdominal pressure.

Pearls

• Blunt abdominal trauma usually results from motor vehicle collisions, assaults, recreational accidents, or falls.
• Spleen is the most commonly injured organ in blunt abdominal trauma.
• CT scan criteria for staging liver trauma based on the AAST liver injury scale include the following:

  • Grade 1-Subcapsular hematoma less than 1 cm in maximal thickness, capsular avulsion, superficial parenchymal laceration less than 1 cm deep, and isolated periportal blood tracking.
  • Grade 2-Parenchymal laceration 1 cm to 3 cm deep and parenchymal/subcapsular hematomas 1 cm to 3 cm thick.
  • Grade 3-Parenchymal laceration more than 3 cm deep and parenchymal or subcapsular hematoma more than 3 cm in diameter.
  • Grade 4-Parenchymal/subcapsular hematoma more than 10 cm in diameter, lobar destruction, or devascularization.
  • Grade 5-Global destruction or devascularization of the liver.
  • Grade 6-Hepatic avulsion.

Suggested Readings

Körner M, Krötz MM, Degenhart C, et al. Current role of emergency US in patients with major trauma. *Radiographics*. 2008;28(1):225-242.

Sivit CJ. Abdominal trauma imaging: imaging choices and appropriateness. *Pediatr Radiol*. 2009;39(Suppl 2): S158-S160.

Yoon W, Jeong YY, Kim JK, et al. CT in blunt liver trauma. *Radiographics*. 2005;25(1):87-104.

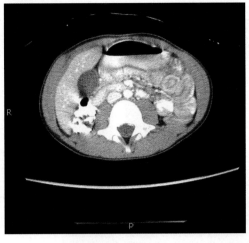
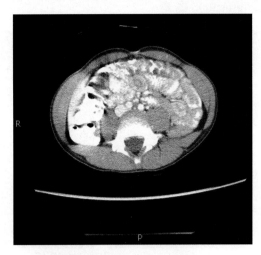
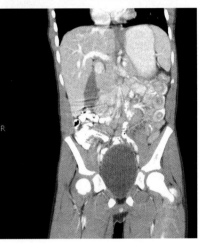
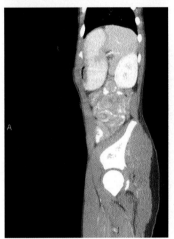

1. What are the findings that are seen in the images?

2. In which age group, are small bowel intussusceptions most likely to be present?

3. What are the causes for small bowel intussusceptions?

4. What are the CT and ultrasound features that differentiate the transient small bowel intussusceptions from the complicated ones that require surgery?

5. What is the management of transient small bowel intussusceptions?

Case ranking/difficulty:

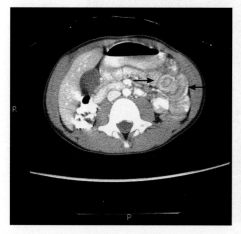 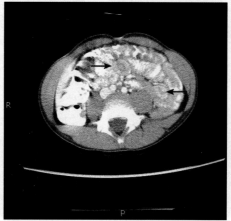 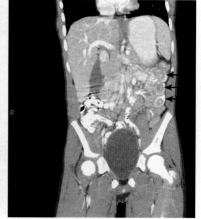

Axial CT of the abdomen reveals multiple small bowel intussusceptions (*arrows*).

Coronal CT of the abdomen reveals multiple small bowel intussusceptions (*arrows*).

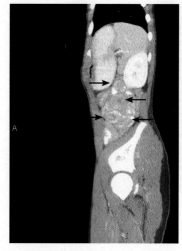

Sagittal CT of the abdomen reveals multiple small bowel intussusceptions (*arrows*).

Answers

1. Multiple small bowel intussusceptions are noted. There is no obstruction, no ascites, and no abscesses.

2. Small bowel intussusceptions are usually seen in older children, more than 4 years old.

3. Causes that may be a lead point to trigger intussusception are Henoch-Schonlein purpura, viral gastroenteritis, mesenteric lymphadenopathy, bowel lymphoma, and Meckel's diverticulum.

4. The CT and the ultrasound features that differentiate the transient small bowel intussusceptions from the complicated ones that require surgery are small size without wall swelling, short segment, preserved wall motion, and absence of the lead point.

5. Conservative management with ultrasound monitoring rather than an immediate operation is recommended for those patients with typical transient small bowel intussusceptions. Atypical US findings or clinical deterioration of the patient with persistent intussusception warrant surgical exploration.

Pearls

- Small bowel intussusceptions are usually seen in children older than 4 years old.
- Usually there is a cause that triggers the intussusception.
- Transient small bowel intussusceptions are typically asymptomatic or mildly symptomatic.
- Among the causes are acute viral gastroenteritis, mesenteric lymphadenopathy, Henoch-Schonlein purpura, bowel lymphoma, diverticulum, and others.
- Typical imaging findings of transient small bowel intussusception include small size without wall swelling, short segment, preserved wall motion, and absence of the lead point.
- Conservative management with ultrasound and clinical monitoring is the treatment of choice.

Suggested Readings

Catalano O. Transient small bowel intussusception: CT findings in adults. *Br J Radiol*. 1997;70(836):805-808.

Lvoff N, Breiman RS, Coakley FV, et al. Distinguishing features of self-limiting adult small-bowel intussusception identified at CT. *Radiology*. 2003;227(1):68-72.

Strouse PJ, DiPietro MA, Saez F. Transient small-bowel intussusception in children on CT. *Pediatr Radiol*. 2003;33:316-320.

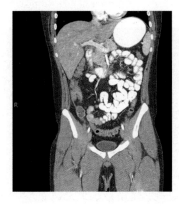 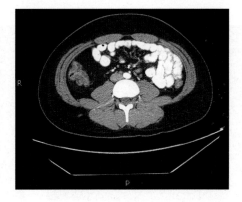 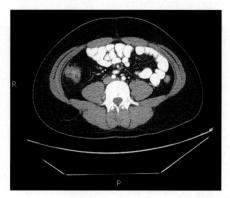

1. What are the findings?

2. What is the differential diagnosis of this case?

3. What are the complications?

4. What are the clinical manifestations of this case?

5. What are the treatment options?

Case ranking/difficulty:

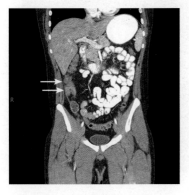

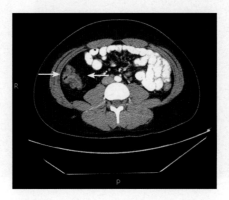

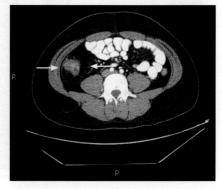

Coronal view of contrast CT of the abdomen reveals a thickened ascending colon wall with fatty stranding around the colon (*arrows*).

Axial view of contrast CT of the abdomen shows a thickened ascending colon wall with fatty stranding around the colon (*arrows*).

Answers

1. The right colon is thickened with fatty mesenteric stranding surrounding the thickened peri-colonic area. These signs indicate inflammation.

2. Differential diagnosis includes bacterial gastroenteritis, ulcerative colitis, amebiasis, giardiasis, and irritable bowel syndrome.

3. Complications of Crohn's disease include fistula and abscess formation, extra intestinal manifestations such as arthritis, perforation, and development of cancer.

4. Low-grade fever, prolonged diarrhea with abdominal pain, weight loss, and generalized fatigability are usually reported. Patients may have blood and pus in stools.

5. Treatment may include medications such as 5-aminosalicylic acid derivatives, mesalamine, steroids, 6-MP. Surgery is required if complications occur.

Pearls

- Crohn's disease is a transmural inflammatory process of the bowel.
- The disease can involve small bowel, colon, or both.
- Increasing frequency in children.
- Main complications are fistula and abscess formation.
- Extra intestinal manifestations are common.

Suggested Readings

Fidler JL, Guimaraes L, Einstein DM. MR imaging of the small bowel. *Radiographics*. 2009;29(6):1811-1825.

Hoeffel C, Crema MD, Belkacem A, et al. Multi-detector row CT: spectrum of diseases involving the ileocecal area. *Radiographics*. 2009;26(5):1373-1390.

Shanbhogue AK, Prasad SR, Jagirdar J, et al. Comprehensive update on select immune-mediated gastroenterocolitis syndromes: implications for diagnosis and management. *Radiographics*. 2010;30(6):1465-1487.

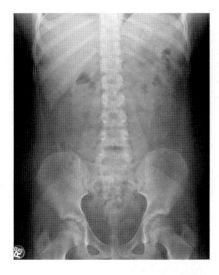

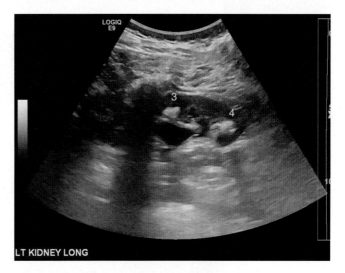

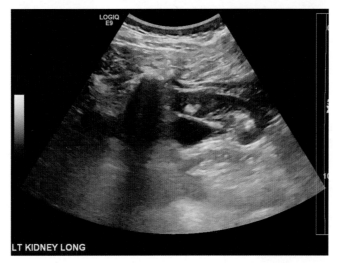

1. What are the findings?

2. What is the most common composition of this entity?

3. What is the etiology of the case?

4. Which bacteria may cause this entity?

5. What are the risk factors for the development of struvite stones?

Case ranking/difficulty:

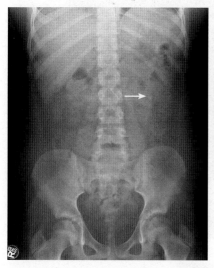

Frontal radiograph of the abdomen reveals a density in the lower pole of the left kidney (*arrow*) representing a calculus.

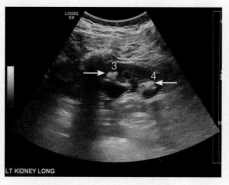 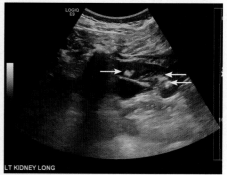

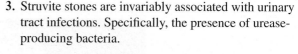

Longitudinal sonogram of the left kidney reveals two echogenic structures (*arrows*) in the calyces of the left kidney. Hydronephrosis is seen.

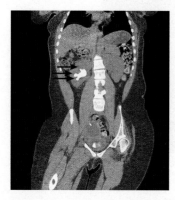

Coronal non-contrast CT of another patient demonstrates staghorn calculus of the right kidney. The calculus noted in the pelvis and in the calyces (*arrows*).

Answers

1. The ultrasound images reveal echogenic structures in the calyces, some shadow. Hydronephrosis of the left kidney is present. In the frontal abdominal radiograph, there is a density overlying the lower pole of the left kidney representing the stone. This represents a staghorn calculus. Branching of the stone into the cayces is seen.

2. Struvite-carbonate-apatite stones are 75% of all staghorn calculi.

3. Struvite stones are invariably associated with urinary tract infections. Specifically, the presence of urease-producing bacteria.

4. *Ureaplasma urealyticum, Proteus* species, *Providencia stuartii,* and *Aeromonas hydrophila* may produce struvite stone. *Escherichia coli* does not produce urease and is not associated with struvite stone formation.

5. Struvite stones may develop in patients with urinary tract infections due to prior urinary diversion or urologic surgery, presence of indwelling catheters, neurogenic bladder, vesicoureteral reflux, and other anatomic abnormalities.

Pearls

- Upper urinary tract stones that are branching to multiple calyces are classified as staghorn calculi.
- Approximately 75% are composed of a struvite-carbonate-apatite matrix.
- Struvite stones are invariably associated with urinary tract infections.

Suggested Readings

Griffith DP, Osborne CA. Infection (urease) stones. *Miner Electrolyte Metab.* 1987;13(4):278-285.

Kim JC. US and CT findings of xanthogranulomatous pyelonephritis. *Clin Imaging.* 2007;25(2):118-121.

Penter G, Arkell DG. The fragmented staghorn calculus: a radiological sign of pyonephrosis. *Clin Radiol.* 1989;40(1):61-63.

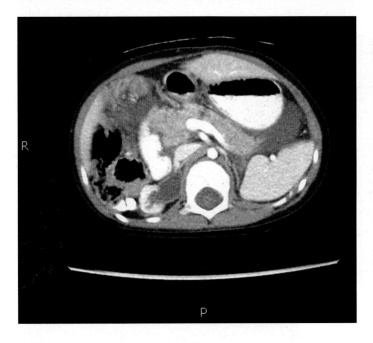 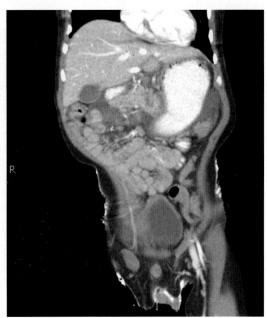

1. What are the findings?

2. What is the imaging modality of choice for the diagnosis of this case?

3. What is the percentage of this entity among cases of major abdominal trauma?

4. What are the laboratory findings that may assist in the diagnosis of this case?

5. What are the complications of this case?

Case ranking/difficulty:

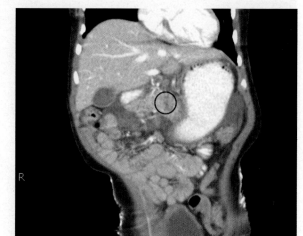

Axial contrast-enhanced CT of the abdomen reveals a low attenuating non-enhancing linear area in the pancreas that is perpendicular to the long axis of pancreatic body (*circle*). There is fluid in the lesser sac (*arrow*).

Coronal contrast-enhanced CT of the abdomen reveals a low attenuating non-enhancing linear area in the pancreas that is perpendicular to the long axis of pancreatic body (*circle*).

Answers

1. There is a low attenuating non-enhancing linear area in the pancreas that is perpendicular to the long axis of pancreatic body. There is fluid in the lesser sac.

2. CT is the imaging modality of choice for the diagnosis of pancreatic laceration.

3. Pancreatic injury occurs in less than 5% of cases of major abdominal trauma.

4. In pancreatic injury, there is increase in serum lipase and in serum amylase.

5. Complications of pancreatic injury are bleeding, pancreatic abscess, recurrent pancreatitis, fistula formation, pancreatic pseudo-cyst, thrombosis, and pseudoaneurysm.

Pearls

- Pancreatic injury occurs in less than 5% of cases of major abdominal trauma.
- CT is the modality of choice for the diagnosis.
- Pancreatic injury can range from minor contusions and hematoma to major lacerations or rupture.
- Imaging features of pancreatic injury include pancreatic edema or enlargement, peripancreatic or intrapancreatic fluid collection, and fluid collection in lesser peritoneal sac.
- Treatment varies according to severity from observation to surgical exploration.

Suggested Readings

Ahmed N, Vernick JJ. Pancreatic injury. *South Med J.* 2009;102(12):1253-1256.

Craig MH, Talton DS, Hauser CJ, Poole GV. Pancreatic injuries from blunt abdominal trauma. *Am Surg.* 1995;61:125-128.

Wright MJ, Stanski C. Blunt pancreatic trauma: a difficult injury. *South Med J.* 2000;93(4):383-385.

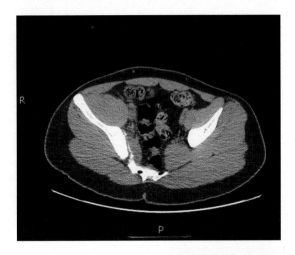
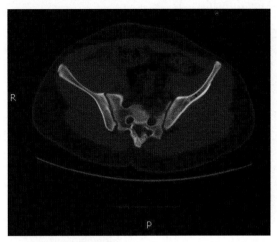
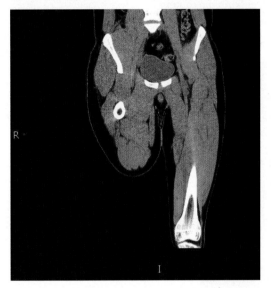

1. What are the findings?

2. What is the differential diagnosis?

3. What is the cause of hemophilia A?

4. What type of hereditary transmission has hemophilia?

5. What is the radiology psoas sign?

Case ranking/difficulty:

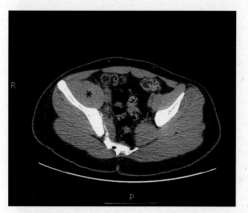

Axial non-contrast CT of the pelvis reveals thickening and enlargement of the right iliacus muscle (*asterisk*). In the context of hemophiliac patient and traumatic injury, this represents hematoma.

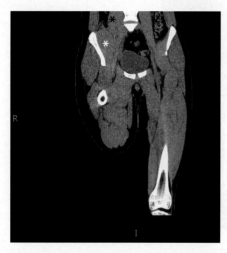

Coronal non-contrast CT of the pelvis reveals thickening and enlargement of the right psoas muscle (*black asterisk*) and the right iliacus muscle (*white asterisk*). In the context of hemophiliac patient and traumatic injury, this represents hematoma.

Answers

1. Non-contrast CT reveals thickening and heterogeneously enlarged right psoas and right iliacus muscles. In hemophiliac patient who had traumatic injury, this is hematoma until proven otherwise.

2. Differential diagnosis includes iliopsoas hematoma or abscess, infiltrating neoplasm, and leaking aneurysm.

3. Hemophilia A is caused by congenital absence of coagulation factor VIII.

4. Hemophilia has recessive X-linked hereditary pattern.

5. The psoas sign is loss of the sharp delineation of the psoas muscle border that is normally seen on a plain

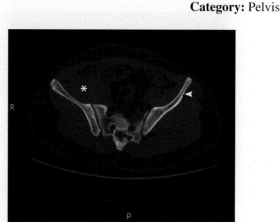

Axial non-contrast CT of the pelvis in bone window reveals thickening and enlargement of the right iliacus muscle (*asterisk*). In the context of hemophiliac patient and traumatic injury, this represents hematoma. There is small non-displaced fracture of the left iliac bone (*arrowhead*).

erect abdominal film. This sign is significant for intra-abdominal or retroperitoneal pathology, such as hemorrhage or inflammation.

Pearls

- Hemophilia A and B are inherited bleeding disorders caused by deficiencies of clotting factor VIII (FVIII) and factor IX (FIX), respectively.
- Both hemophilia A and B are X-linked recessive disorders.
- Iliopsoas bleeding is a common complication in a hemophiliac patient.
- The differential diagnosis of iliopsoas hematoma includes iliopsoas abscess and any infiltrating neoplasm in the muscle such as rhabdomyosarcoma in children.
- Treatment includes administration of the missing coagulation factors and in severe cases, establish homeostasis and surgical intervention if needed.

Suggested Readings

Domula M, Weissbach G, Lenk H, Meissner F. Iliopsoas hemorrhage in hemophilic children. *Folia Haematol Int Mag Klin Morphol Blutforsch*. 1985;112(6):834-844.

Graif M, Martinovitz U, Strauss S, Heim M, Itzchak Y. Sonographic localization of hematomas in hemophilic patients with positive iliopsoas sign. *AJR Am J Roentgenol*. 1987;148(1):121-123.

Lenchik L, Dovgan DJ, Kier R. CT of the iliopsoas compartment: value in differentiating tumor, abscess, and hematoma. *AJR Am J Roentgenol*. 1994;162(1):83-86.

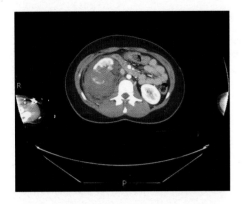 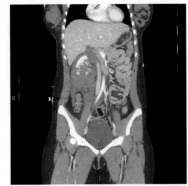 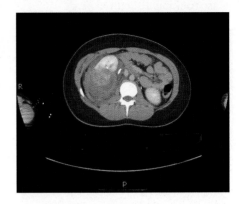

1. What are the findings?

2. What is the possible etiology of this entity?

3. What are the clinical symptoms?

4. According to the scale of the American Association of Surgeons in Trauma (AAST) organ injury severity, how will you grade this case?

5. How is grade I (according to the Renal Injury Scale of the American Association of Surgeons in Trauma) being treated?

Case ranking/difficulty:

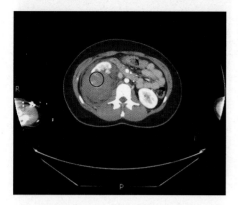

Axial contrast-enhanced CT of the abdomen demonstrates high-grade laceration/ fracture of the right kidney, involving the hilum, lower interpolar and posterior lower pole regions (*circle*). No definite vascular avulsions are visualized. Extensive retroperitoneal hematoma and urine, displacing the right kidney anterolaterally and appearing to stretch the normally opacified right renal artery are noted.

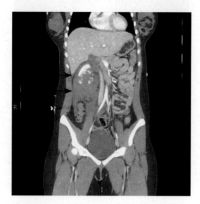

Coronal contrast-enhanced CT of the abdomen demonstrates high-grade laceration/fracture of the right kidney, involving the hilum, lower interpolar and posterior lower pole regions (*arrows*). No definite vascular avulsions are visualized. Extensive retroperitoneal hematoma and urine, displacing the right kidney anterolaterally and appearing to stretch the normally opacified right renal artery are noted.

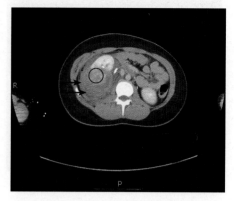

Axial contrast-enhanced CT of the abdomen demonstrates high-grade laceration/fracture of the right kidney, involving the hilum, lower interpolar and posterior lower pole regions (*arrows*). There is evidence of active bleeding (*circle*).

Answers

1. There is high-grade laceration/fracture of the right kidney, involving the hilum, lower interpolar and posterior lower pole regions. No definite vascular avulsions are visualized. Extensive retroperitoneal hematoma and urine, displacing the right kidney anterolaterally and appearing to stretch the normally opacified right renal artery. GU delayed phase demonstrates evidence for active bleeding.

2. Possible causes for renal injury are motor vehicle crash, fall, pedestrian struck, stab wounds, and sport injury.

3. Patient may present with flank or abdominal pain and hematuria. If there is severe blood loss, patient may have low blood pressure and even hypovolemic shock.

4. The injury extends through the renal cortex, medulla, and the hilum. There is active bleed, meaning injury to the renal artery or vein, but there is contained hematoma. The kidney is not completely shattered and there is no direct evidence of devascularization. According to the Renal Injury Scale of the American Association of Surgeons in Trauma, this is grade IV.

5. Approximately 82% of injuries may be classified as grade I and include parenchymal contusions and isolated subcapsular hematomas. No treatment is necessary. Observation and follow-up is necessary to assure spontaneous resolution.

Pearls

- Renal injury may result from any kind of trauma.
- In 80% of cases, the mechanism is direct blow.
- Severity of injury is graded into 5 levels from superficial cortical laceration to shattering of the kidney and devascularizing injuries to the renal pedicle (according to the American Association of Surgeons in Trauma organ injury severity scale).
- Therapeutic options depend on the severity of the injury. Most cases are very mild and require only observation.
- The only absolute indication for surgical exploration is life-threatening bleeding.
- CT is the modality of choice for diagnosis.

Suggested Readings

Ahmed S, Morris LL. Renal parenchymal injuries secondary to blunt abdominal trauma in childhood: a 10-year review. *Br J Urol*. 1982;54(5):470-477.

Cass AS. Blunt renal trauma in children. *J Trauma*. 1983;23(2):123-127.

Lee YJ, Oh SN, Rha SE, Byun JY. Renal trauma. *Radiol Clin North Am*. 2007;45(3):581-592.

5-month-old female with mass in the neck

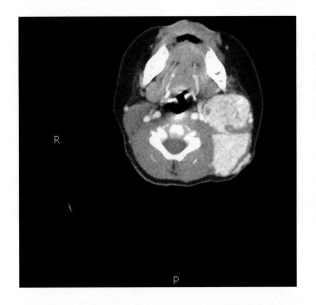 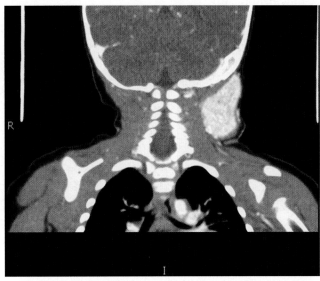

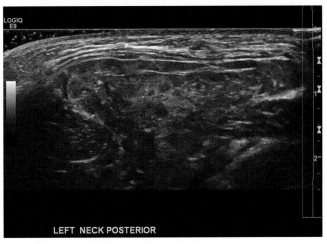 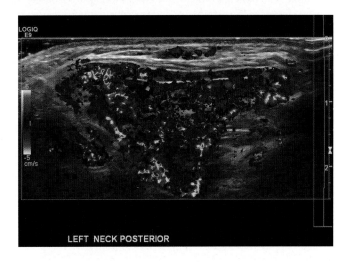

1. What are the findings?

2. What is the most common tumor in infants?

3. What is the best modality for the diagnosis of this entity?

4. What is the natural behavior of most infantile hemangiomas?

5. How are the majority of patients with this entity being treated?

Case ranking/difficulty:

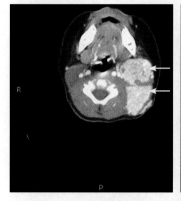

Axial contrast-enhanced CT of the neck revealing heterogeneous intensely enhancing mass is seen in the left suprahyoid neck underneath the left sternocleidomastoid muscle, which extends to the subcutaneous margin (*arrows*).

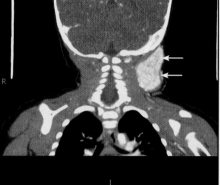

Coronal contrast-enhanced CT of the neck revealing heterogeneous intensely enhancing mass is seen in the left suprahyoid neck underneath the left sternocleidomastoid muscle, which extends to the subcutaneous margin (*arrows*).

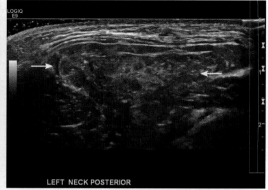

Sonogram of the neck shows heterogeneous hypoechoic structure in the left neck beneath the left ear in the same region of the mass seen in the CT (*arrows*).

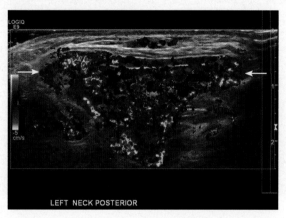

Doppler sonogram of the neck reveals heterogeneous hypoechoic structure in the left neck beneath the left ear in the same region of the mass seen in the CT (*arrows*). Intense flow noted in this structure.

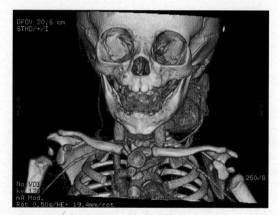

3D reconstruction demonstrates the hemangioma. The left internal jugular vein serves as a draining vessel.

Answers

1. There is heterogeneous enhancing subcutaneous mass in the left suprahyoid location of the neck. In ultrasound, the mass is hypoechoic and heterogeneous with intense vascular flow.

2. The most common tumor in infant is infantile hemangioma.

3. MRI is the imaging modality of choice to delineate the location and extent of both cutaneous and extracutaneous hemangiomas.

4. Most hemangiomas have proliferative phase and then they involute.

5. Most hemangiomas need only observation as they involute after the proliferative phase.

Pearls

- Hemangioma is the most common tumor in infants.
- In 20% of infants, lesions are multiple.
- CT and MRI show markedly enhancing lesion. It delineates the location and extent of both cutaneous and extracutaneous hemangiomas. In MRI, the lesion has high signal in T2 and is highly vascular.

Suggested Readings

Donnelly LF, Adams DM, Bisset GS 3rd. Vascular malformations and hemangiomas: a practical approach in a multidisciplinary clinic. *AJR Am J Roentgenol.* 2000;174(3):597-608.

Dubois J, Patriquin HB, Garel L, et al. Soft-tissue hemangiomas in infants and children: diagnosis using Doppler sonography. *AJR Am J Roentgenol.* 1998;171(1):247-252.

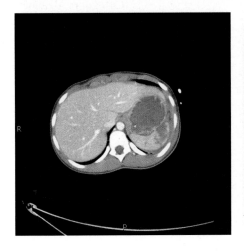 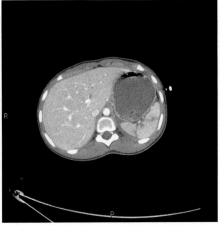 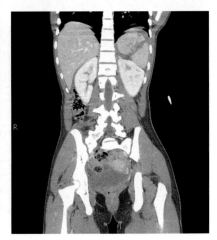

1. What are the findings?

2. What are the risk factors of this entity?

3. What is the most common affected organ in abdominal blunt trauma?

4. What grade will you give to this entity?

5. What are the treatment options?

Case ranking/difficulty:

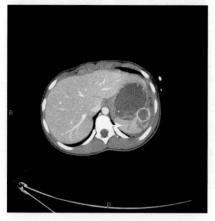

Axial contrast CT at the level of the upper abdomen. The lateral aspect of the spleen is devascularized (*circle*). Rupture noted in the medial aspect of the spleen (*arrow*).

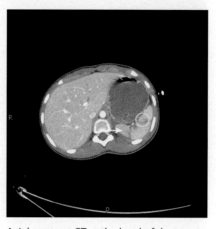

Axial contrast CT at the level of the upper abdomen. The lateral aspect of the spleen is devascularized. The lateral aspect of the spleen is lacerated (*circle*). Rupture noted in the medial aspect of the spleen (*arrow*).

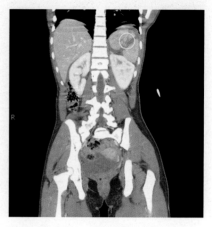

Coronal contrast CT of the abdomen. Rupture noted in the spleen (*circle*).

Answers

1. There are heterogeneous areas of low attenuation in the spleen. In the context of trauma, this represents splenic injury. There is perisplenic hematoma. There is devitalization of the lateral aspect of the spleen with rupture of the medial aspect. There is no active extravasation.

2. Risk factors include any type of abdominal trauma. Any disease with splenomegaly along with minor trauma can lead to splenic rupture. This includes infectious mononucleosis, malaria, or any other hematologic abnormality.

3. The spleen is the most commonly affected organ in blunt injury of the abdomen.

4. Our case represents grade IV splenic injury as there is laceration involving segmental vessels with major devascularization.

5. Initially patient hemodynamic stability needs to be confirmed. Treatment varies from just observation in mild cases to splenic angioembolization and/or splenectomy in severe cases.

Pearls

- Spleen is the most common affected organ in blunt injury of the abdomen.
- Penetrating abdominal trauma may also lead to splenic injury; however, less frequently seen than in blunt trauma.
- Other risk factors for splenic injury include diseases such as infectious mononucleosis, malaria, and any other disease with significant splenomegaly. The spleen becomes fragile and vulnerable for rupture.
- Severity of splenic injury is graded from I to V according to the classification system of the American Association for the Surgery of Trauma (AAST).

Suggested Readings

Keller MS, Vane DW. Management of pediatric blunt splenic injury: comparison of pediatric and adult trauma surgeons. *J Pediatr Surg*. 1995;30(2):221-224; discussion 224-225.

Madoff DC, Denys A, Wallace MJ, et al. Splenic arterial interventions: anatomy, indications, technical considerations, and potential complications. *Radiographics*. 2005;25(Suppl 1):S191-S211.

Moore EE, Cogbill TH, Jurkovich GJ, Shackford SR, Malangoni MA, Champion HR. Organ injury scaling: spleen and liver (1994 revision). *J Trauma*. 1995;38(3):323-324.

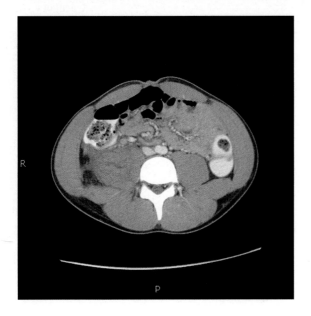
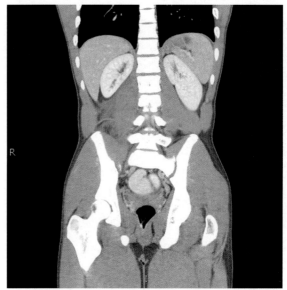

1. What are the findings?

2. What are the risk factors for the development of this entity?

3. What can be in the differential diagnosis?

4. What are the MRI findings of the shown entity?

5. What are the most likely treatment options for this case?

Case ranking/difficulty:

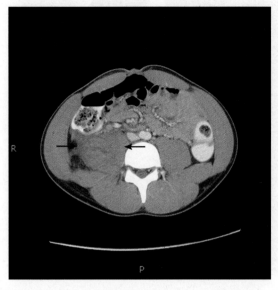

Axial contrast-enhanced CT of the abdomen reveals significant right psoas muscle enlargement (*arrows*). The psoas muscle appears heterogeneous with significant strandings of the retroperitoneal fat around the muscle.

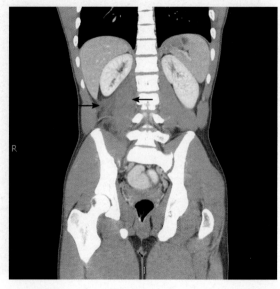

Coronal contrast-enhanced CT of the abdomen reveals significant right psoas muscle enlargement (*arrows*). The psoas muscle appears heterogeneous with significant strandings of the retroperitoneal fat around the muscle.

Answers

1. There is enlargement of the right psoas muscle which appears heterogeneous. Stranding of the fat around the right psoas is noted.

2. Risk factors include trauma, use of anticoagulants, coagulopathy, previous surgery, ruptured aneurysm, and spontaneous occurrence.

3. Differential diagnosis may include abscess, phlegmon, necrotic mass infiltrating the psoas or contusion, and hematoma.

4. MRI findings vary according to the age of the hemorrhage. There is increased T2 signal in acute bleed and markedly increased T1 signal in subacute bleed.

5. No drainable fluid collection noted. If the patient is hemodynamically stable, then just observation is required until the hematoma resorption.

Pearls

- Psoas hematoma is a relatively common occurrence.
- Trauma can cause diffuse hemorrhage and contusion.
- Psoas hematoma manifests as enlargement and heterogeneous appearance of the psoas muscle.
- Differential diagnosis includes acute bleed and infection (acute or chronic).
- The main risk factors in the pediatric population are trauma and coagulopathy.
- In adults, the risk factors are use of anticoagulants and post-surgical bleed.

Suggested Readings

Cuvelier C. Psoas hematoma. *N Engl J Med*. 2001;344:349.

Kwon OY, Lee KR, Kim SW. Spontaneous iliopsoas muscle haematoma. *Emerg Med J*. 2009;26(12):863.

Torres GM, Cernigliaro JG, Abbitt PL, et al. Iliopsoas compartment: normal anatomy and pathologic processes. *Radiographics*. 1995;15(6):1285-1297.

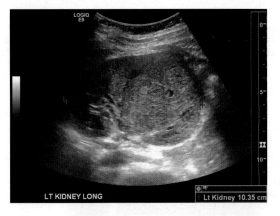
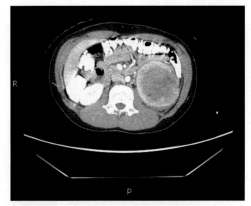
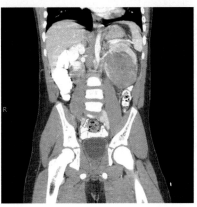
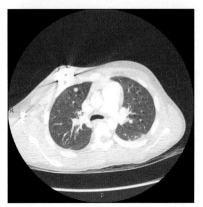

1. What are the findings?

2. What is the stage of the shown entity?

3. What is the differential diagnosis?

4. What are the sites of metastasis of this entity?

5. What are the sonographic findings of the shown entity?

Case ranking/difficulty:

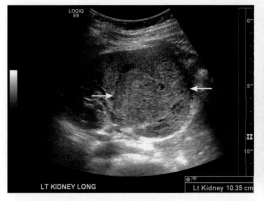
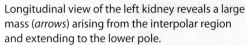

Longitudinal view of the left kidney reveals a large mass (*arrows*) arising from the interpolar region and extending to the lower pole.

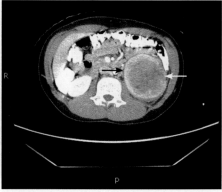

CT of the abdomen reveals a large mass occupying the left kidney (*arrows*). The mass is displacing the upper pole superiorly and medially. The visualized cortex engulfs the mass and forms the claw sign.

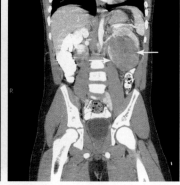

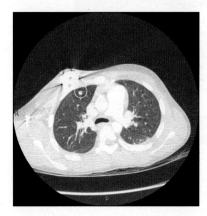

Lung window reveals a right upper lobe small nodule (*circle*) that turns out to be a metastatic lesion.

Answers

1. There is a mass arising from the left kidney. The mass displaces the left kidney superiorly and medially. The cortex of the left kidney engulfs the mass and forms the claw sign. A pulmonary nodule is noted in the right upper lobe.

2. This is stage IV. There is distant metastatic disease in the lung. The nodule in the right upper lobe was found to be a metastatic lesion.

3. The differential diagnosis of Wilms' tumor may include: Clear cell sarcoma of the kidney, Rhabdoid tumor of the kidney, mesoblastic nephroma, and renal medullary carcinoma.

4. Wilms' tumor may be complicated by a tumor thrombus to the renal vein, inferior vena cava, and right atrium. Metastasis to the liver, lungs, bone, and brain may occur. Lymph node metastases beyond abdomen or pelvis may also occur.

5. The sonographic finding of Wilms' tumor is an echogenic mass with the echogenicity slightly greater than the liver. The mass is inhomogeneous. The mass does not shadow.

Pearls

- Wilms' tumor affects children between 2 and 5 years of age. It is rare after the age of 6 years.
- Wilms' tumor accounts for 6 to 7% of all pediatric malignancies.
- The tumor is echogenic in ultrasound, slightly more than the liver.
- It has low attenuation compared to renal parenchyma in enhanced CT.
- Complications include tumor thrombus to the renal vein, inferior vena cava, and the right atrium.
- The tumor may metastasize to the lung, liver, bone, and brain.
- Treatment includes nephrectomy and chemotherapy. In advanced disease, radiation therapy is added.

Suggested Readings

Brasch RC, Randel SB, Gould RG. Follow-up of Wilms' tumor: comparison of CT with other imaging procedures. *AJR Am J Roentgenol.* 1981;137(5):1005-1009.

Hugosson C, Nyman R, Jacobsson B, Jorulf H, Sackey K, McDonald P. Imaging of solid kidney tumours in children. *Acta Radiol.* 1995;36(3):254-260.

Siddiqui AR, Cohen M, Moran DP. Abdominal masses in children: multiorgan imaging with 99mTc methylene diphosphonate. *AJR Am J Roentgenol.* 1982;139(1):35-38.

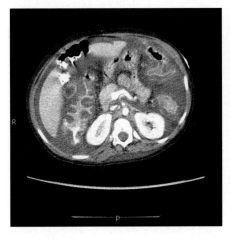 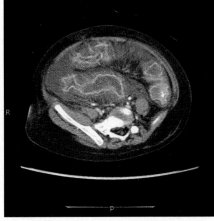 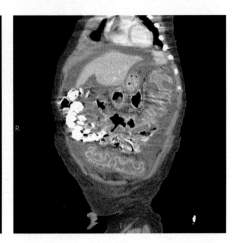

1. What is the diagnosis?

2. What are the risk factors for the development
   of this entity?

3. What is the micro-organism implicated
   with the disease?

4. What are the cross-sectional imaging findings
   of this entity?

5. What are the treatment options?

Case ranking/difficulty:

Category: Gastrointestinal

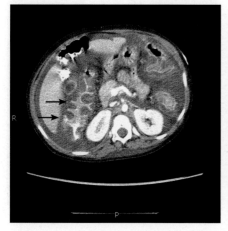

Axial CT reveals thickening and dilated colon in the region of the hepatic flexure (*arrows*). Ascites noted.

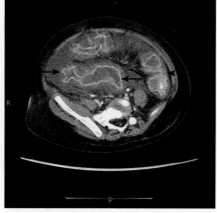

Axial CT reveals thickening and dilated colon in the region of the sigmoid colon (*arrows*) and the descending colon (*arrowhead*). Ascites noted.

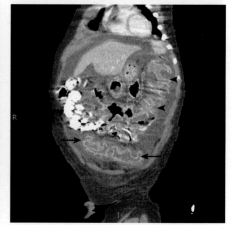

Coronal CT reveals thickening and dilated colon in the region of the sigmoid colon (*arrows*) and the descending colon (*arrowheads*). Ascites noted.

Answers

1. The diagnosis is pseudomembranous colitis.

2. Risk factors for the development of pseudomembranous colitis are use of broad spectrum antibiotics and clindamycin, old age, and immunosuppression such as HIV.

3. *Clostridium difficile* has been implicated with the disease.

4. The cross-sectional image findings of pseudomembranous colitis include dilated, thickened, and enhancing colonic wall. The colon is fluid-filled and ascites may be present. Findings are nonspecific and can be present with other etiologies of colitis.

5. Treatment includes metronidazole if *Clostridium difficile* has been implicated. Hydration and supportive therapy are essential. If there is toxic megacolon and perforation, then surgical intervention with colectomy is performed.

Pearls

- *Clostridium difficile* is the most common cause of the disease.
- Mostly the disease is due to the recent use of clindamycin and a broad spectrum of antibiotics.
- Clinical findings are non-bloody diarrhea, abdominal pain, and fever.
- Risk factors include broad spectrum antibiotics, old age, and immunosuppression such as HIV disease.
- CT shows dilated and fluid-filled colon with thickened enhancing wall. Ascites is usually present.
- Enema should not be performed due to the risk of toxic megacolon and perforation.
- Treatment with metronidazole, hydration, and surgery in cases of toxic megacolon and perforation.

Suggested Readings

Bartlett JG, Gerding DN. Clinical recognition and diagnosis of *Clostridium difficile* infection. *Clin Infect Dis.* 2008;46(Suppl 1):S12-S18.

Chen N, Shih SL. Images in clinical medicine. *Pseudomembranous colitis. N Engl J Med.* 2011;364(5):e8.

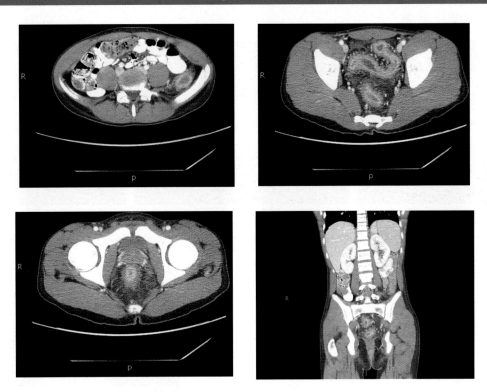

1. What is the diagnosis?

2. Based on the CT, how will you differentiate between this entity and Crohn's disease?

3. Enumerate few of the extracolonic manifestations of this entity?

4. What are the complications of this entity?

5. What is considered to be the etiology of this entity?

Case ranking/difficulty:

Category: Gastrointestinal

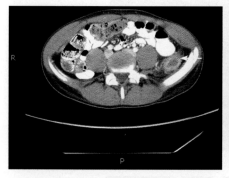

Axial-enhanced CT of the abdomen reveals inflammation of the descending colon (*arrow*).

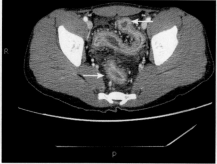

Axial-enhanced CT of the abdomen reveals inflammation of the descending colon and the rectosigmoid area (*arrows*).

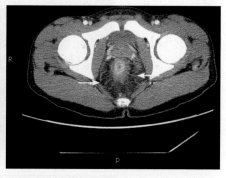

Axial-enhanced CT of the abdomen reveals inflammation of the rectum (*arrows*).

Answers

1. The diagnosis is ulcerative colitis.

2. In ulcerative colitis, the inflammation starts in the rectum and extends proximally in a continuous manner while in Crohn's disease, skip lesions are seen.

3. Extra-colonic manifestation of ulcerative colitis may include sacroiliitis, joint synovitis, iridocyclitis, pyoderma gangrenosum, and aphthous stomatitis.

4. The complications of ulcerative colitis are: colonic adenocarcinoma, sclerosing cholangitis, cholangiocarcinoma, pseudomembranous colitis, and toxic megacolon.

5. The exact etiology is unknown. Few causes may apply such as autoimmune disease or immune-mediated disease, environmental and dietary factors may be involved. It is also considered that patients have genetic susceptibility.

Coronal-enhanced CT of the abdomen reveals inflammation of the descending colon (*arrows*).

Pearls

- Ulcerative colitis is chronic inflammatory disease of the colon.
- The inflammation starts in the rectum and extends proximaly in a continuous manner.
- CT reveals thickening of the wall of the affected colon with pericolonic stranding of the fat.
- Long standing diseased colon may show narrowed colon with loss of the haustral folds in barium enema.
- Long standing disease is a risk for development of colonic adenocarcinoma.
- Extra colonic manifestation such as arthritis may be seen.

Suggested Readings

da Luz Moreira A, Vogel JD, Baker M, Mor I, Zhang R, Fazio V. Does CT influence the decision to perform colectomy in patients with severe ulcerative colitis? *J Gastrointest Surg*. 2009;13(3):504-507.

Johnson KT, Hara AK, Johnson CD. Evaluation of colitis: usefulness of CT enterography technique. *Emerg Radiol*. 2009;16(4):277-282.

Sallam BM, Pilch-Kowalczyk A, Gruszczynska K, Baron J, Pugliese F. Diagnostic performance of CT colonography in a population with high prevalence of large bowel disease. *Med Sci Monit*. 2007;13(Suppl 1):105-110.

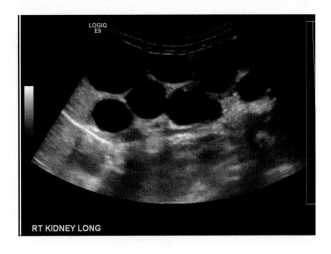

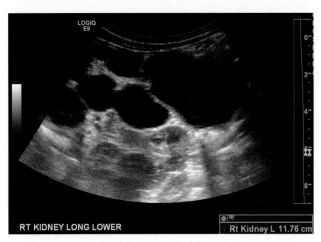

1. What are the findings?

2. The findings are unilateral. What is the most likely diagnosis?

3. What are the entities that may be included in the differential diagnosis?

4. What is the frequency of this entity in the United States?

5. What are the treatment options?

Case ranking/difficulty:

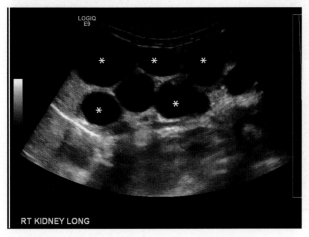

Longitudinal sonogram of the right kidney reveals non-communicating cysts in the right kidney (*asterisks*). There is no renal parenchyma (this kidney is not functioning).

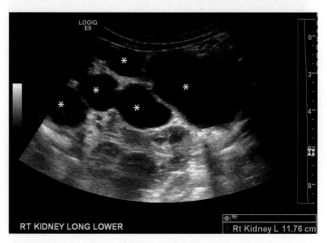

Longitudinal sonogram of the right kidney reveals non-communicating cysts in the right kidney (*asterisks*). There is no renal parenchyma (this kidney is not functioning). The kidney is large for a 3-month old infant.

Answers

1. The right kidney is large (11.76 cm). It is enlarged for 3-month-old infant. Multiple non-communicating anechoic structures noted. If these structures were to communicate it would have represented hydronephrosis. Non-communicating anechoic structures represent cysts. Cortex in the right kidney not seen, meaning that the right kidney is not functional.

2. The diagnosis is multicystic dysplastic kidney. Polycystic kidney disease is bilateral.

3. The differential diagnosis may include hydronephrosis, ureteropelvic junction obstruction, and polycystic kidney disease.

4. Frequency of multicystic dysplastic kidney disease is 1 in every 2400 live births.

5. The condition is not treatable. Periodic follow-up is recommended to assure normal function of the contralateral kidney.

Pearls

- Multicystic dysplastic kidney (MCDK) is a congenital maldevelopment in which the renal cortex is replaced by numerous cysts of multiple sizes.
- The calyceal drainage system is absent.
- Sonography demonstrates absence of renal cortex with multiple non-communicating cysts.

Suggested Readings

Kiyak A, Yilmaz A, Turhan P, Sander S, Aydin G, Aydogan G. Unilateral multicystic dysplastic kidney: single-center experience. *Pediatr Nephrol*. 2009;24(1):99-104.

Merrot T, Lumenta DB, Tercier S, Morisson-Lacombes G, Guys JM, Alessandrini P. Multicystic dysplastic kidney with ipsilateral abnormalities of genitourinary tract: experience in children. *Urology*. 2006;67(3):603-607.

Spence HM. Congenital unilateral multicystic kidney: an entity to be distinguished from polycystic kidney disease and other cystic disorders. *J Urol*. 1955;74(6):693-706.

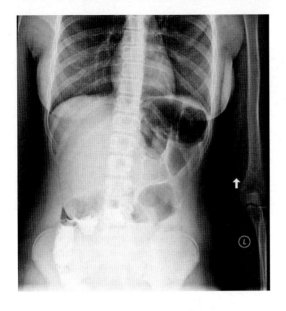
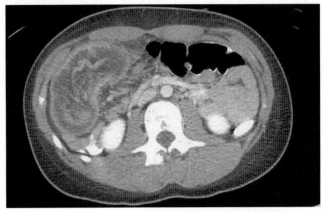
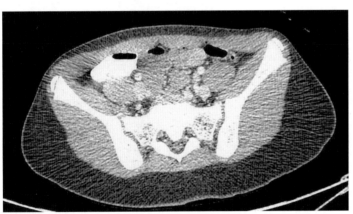
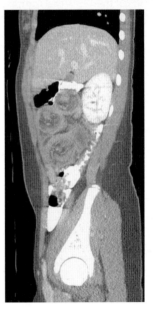

1. What complication of Peutz-Jeghers syndrome is shown in the CT?

2. What type of polyps is seen in Peutz-Jeghers syndrome?

3. Why treatment of intussusception is urgent?

4. What is the inheritance mode of Peutz-Jeghers syndrome?

5. What percentage of patients with Peutz-Jeghers syndrome develop intussusception or obstruction during their life time?

Case ranking/difficulty:

Category: Gastrointestinal

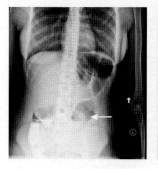
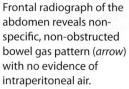

Frontal radiograph of the abdomen reveals non-specific, non-obstructed bowel gas pattern (*arrow*) with no evidence of intraperitoneal air.

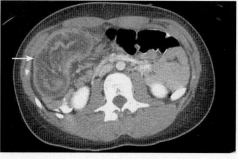

Axial contrast CT of the abdomen at the level of the right lower quadrant reveals small bowel-intussusception visualized with mesenteric fat, vessels, lymph nodes (*arrow*).

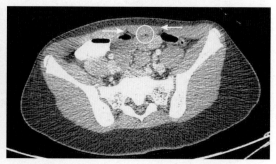

Axial contrast CT of the abdomen at the level of the left lower quadrant reveals traces of free intraperitoneal air (*arrows*) which is secondary to either previous surgery or necrotic bowel.

Answers

1. Small bowel intussusception is shown.

2. The polyps seen in Peutz-Jeghers syndrome are hamartomas.

3. The treatment of intussusception is urgent due to the risk of vascular compromise and necrosis.

4. The inheritance mode of Peutz-Jeghers syndrome is autosomal-dominant.

5. Approximately 50% of patients with Peutz-Jeghers syndrome experience intussusception and/or obstruction during their life time.

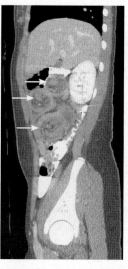

Sagittal contrast CT of the abdomen demonstrates enhancing vessels that are visualized within mesenteric fat pulled into the intussusception (*arrows*).

Pearls

- Peutz-Jeghers syndrome is an autosomal-dominant syndrome with variable inheritance consisting of hamartomatous polyps within the GI tract, especially the small bowel, as well as pigmented mucocutaneous lesions.
- The polyps in Peutz-Jeghers syndrome may lead to intussusception, mostly ileo-ileal.
- Intussusception is an emergent condition requiring rapid evaluation to prevent worsening obstruction, necrosis, and/or perforation.
- Radiography reveals non-specific bowel gas pattern. At times, the crescent sign is seen.
- CT and ultrasound reveal intussusception with a loop of bowel within a loop, referred to as the target sign. Fat density may be seen inside the bowel representing mesenteric fat.

Suggested Readings

Hinds R, Philp C, Hyer W, Fell JM. Complications of childhood Peutz-Jeghers syndrome: implications for pediatric screening. *J Pediatr Gastroenterol Nutr.* 2004;39:219-220.

Kopacova M, Tacheci I, Rejchrt S, Bures J. Peutz-Jeghers syndrome: diagnostic and therapeutic approach. *World J Gastroenterol.* 2009;15(43):5397-5408.

Rufener S, Koujok K, McKenna B, Walsh M. Small bowel intussusception secondary to Puetz-Jeghers polyp. *Radiographics.* 2008;28:284-288.

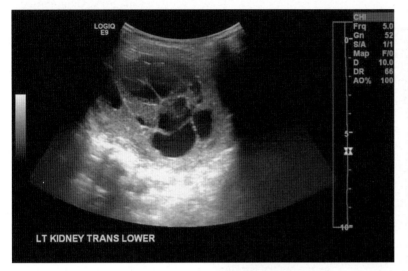

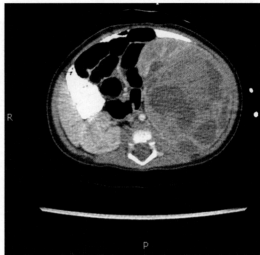

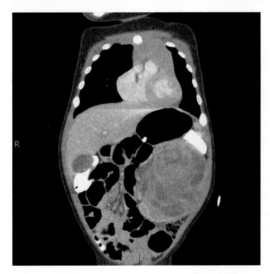

1. What is the most frequent benign renal tumor of childhood?

2. What is the typical age range that this entity occurs?

3. Describe the imaging characteristics of this entity.

4. Which gender is more affected by this entity?

5. What is the differential diagnosis?

Case ranking/difficulty: **Category:** Genitourinary

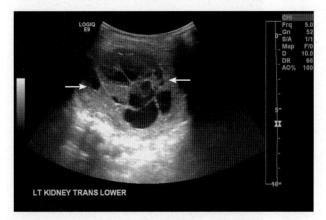

Transverse sonogram view of the left kidney reveals a mass in the left kidney (*arrows*). Medullary pyramids are displaced. The anechoic structures in the mass represent areas of necrosis.

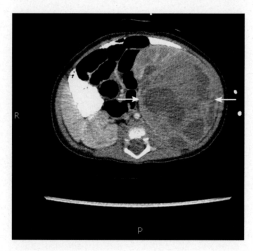

Axial CT of the left kidney reveals heterogeneous enhancing mass arising from the left kidney (*arrows*). Areas of low attenuation are seen representing necrosis.

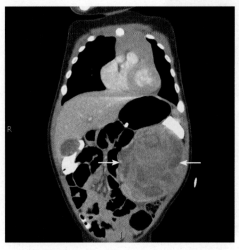

Coronal CT of the left kidney reveals heterogeneous enhancing mass arising from the left kidney (*arrows*). Areas of low attenuation are seen representing necrosis.

Pearls

- Mesoblastic nephroma is the most common renal tumor identified in the neonatal period and the most frequent benign renal tumor in childhood.
- Mesoblastic nephroma represents 3% of pediatric renal neoplasms.
- The tumor may spread to the other kidney or to nearby tissues.
- Large abdominal mass may be seen with mass effect on the neighboring organs.
- Cystic components and hemorrhage are usually identified in ultrasound and CT.

Answers

1. Mesoblastic nephroma is the most frequent benign renal tumor of childhood.

2. Typical age range of occurrence is between birth and 3 months.

3. The mass is usually large and solid with cystic components and hemorrhage that can be present.

4. Congenital mesoblastic nephroma is more common in males.

5. Differential diagnosis may include multicystic dysplastic kidney, Wilms' tumor, and neuroblastoma.

Suggested Readings

Chaudry G, Perez-Atayde AR, Ngan BY, Gundogan M, Daneman A. Imaging of congenital mesoblastic nephroma with pathological correlation. *Pediatr Radiol.* 2009;39(10): 1080-1086.

Sheth MM, Cai G, Goodman TR. AIRP best cases in radiologic pathologic correlation: congenital mesoblastic nephroma. *Radiographics.* 2012;32(1):99-103.

Silver IM, Boag AH, Soboleski DA. Best cases from the AFIP: Multilocular cystic renal tumor: cystic nephroma. *Radiographics.* 2008;28(4):1221-1225; discussion 1225-1226.

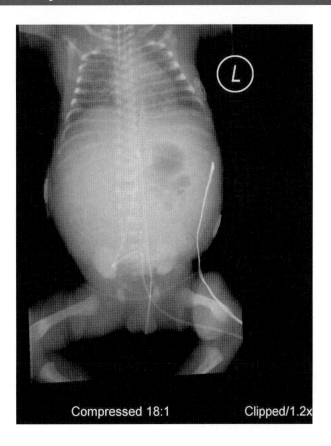

Compressed 18:1   Clipped/1.2x

1. What are the findings?

2. What is the differential diagnosis?

3. What is the diagnosis?

4. What are the risk factors for this condition?

5. What are the other entities that the case may be
   associated with?

Case ranking/difficulty:

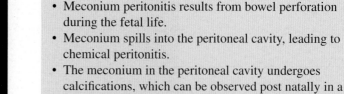

Frontal view of abdominal radiograph shows abdominal calcifications (*arrows*). The *circle* points to the distal tip of the umbilical arterial catheter.

Pearls

- Meconium peritonitis results from bowel perforation during the fetal life.
- Meconium spills into the peritoneal cavity, leading to chemical peritonitis.
- The meconium in the peritoneal cavity undergoes calcifications, which can be observed post natally in a plain abdominal radiograph.
- The calcifications can be seen on antenatal sonography.
- Meconium peritonitis is a benign condition.
- Infants with cystic fibrosis are at increased risk for meconium peritonitis.
- Atresia of the distal small bowel can also lead to bowel perforation and meconium peritonitis.

Suggested Readings

Lang I, Daneman A, Cutz E, Hagen P, Shandling B. Abdominal calcification in cystic fibrosis with meconium ileus: radiologic-pathologic correlation. *Pediatr Radiol.* 1997;27(6):523-527.

Swischuk LE. *Imaging of the Newborn, Infant, and Young Child.* 4th ed. Philadelphia: Lippincott, Williams & Wilkins; 1997.

Tseng JJ, Chou MM, Ho ES. Meconium peritonitis in utero: prenatal sonographic findings and clinical implications. *J Chin Med Assoc.* 2003;66(6):355-359.

Answers

1. Calcifications are seen.

2. Differential diagnosis may include in utero neuroblastoma, in utero teratoma, and meconium peritonitis.

3. The diagnosis is meconium peritonitis.

4. Cystic fibrosis is a risk factor. Newborns with meconium peritonitis will develop cystic fibrosis.

5. Meconium peritonitis may be associated with meconium ileus, microcolon, ileal atresia, and jejunal atresia.

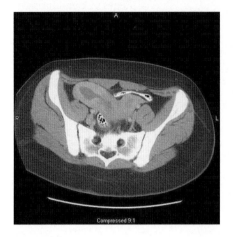 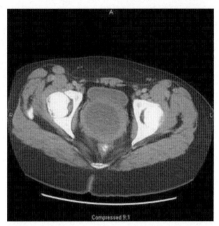 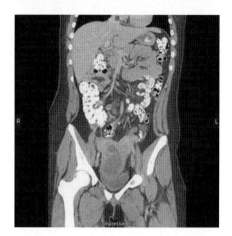

1. What is the morphology of the uterus as seen in the images?

2. Name the entities that may be included in the differential diagnosis.

3. What is the most common etiology of the case?

4. What are the associated abnormalities?

5. What are the treatment options?

Case ranking/difficulty: **Category:** Genitourinary

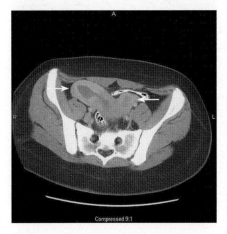

Axial CT of the pelvis demonstrates the uterus with the two cornuates (*arrows*).

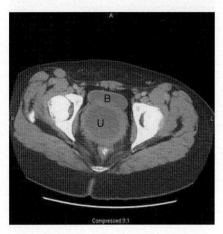

Axial CT of the pelvis demonstrates large fluid filled uterus (*U*). Bladder (*B*) is seen anterior to the uterus.

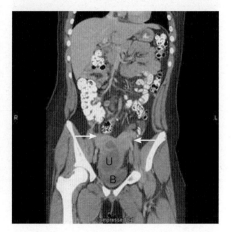

Coronal CT of the uterus shows the two cornuates (*arrows*) and the uterus (*U*) filled with fluid, hydrometrocolpos. The bladder (*B*) is seen beneath the uterus.

Answers

1. There is hydrometrocolpos that developed in bicornuate uterus.

2. Differential diagnosis may include pelvic rhabdomyosarcoma, pelvic abscess, and fallopian tube torsion.

3. Imperforate hymen is the most common etiology of hydrometrocolpos.

4. Associated abnormalities may include urogenital sinus, cloacal anomalies, imperforate anus, intestinal aganglionosis, and cardiac anomalies.

5. Treatment options include drainage, septum excision, dilatation of stenotic segment, and stenting.

Pearls

- Hydrometrocolpos is a rare congenital condition, which may occur in association with other malformations.
- Excessive mucus secretions accumulate from a genital tract obstruction, resulting in cystic dilatation of the vagina and uterus.
- The obstruction is frequently caused by imperforate hymen, and less commonly by other causes of vaginal stenosis, such as transverse septum.
- In our case, bicornuate uterus is most likely the cause of obstruction in the genital tract leading to the hydrometrocolpos.

Suggested Readings

Donnelly LF. Diagnostic imaging. *Pediatrics*. Philadelphia, PA: Amirsys; 2005.

Spencer R, Levy DM. Hydrometrocolpos report of three cases and review of the literature. *Ann Surg*. 1962;155(4):558-571.

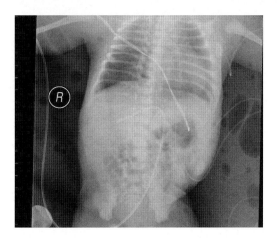
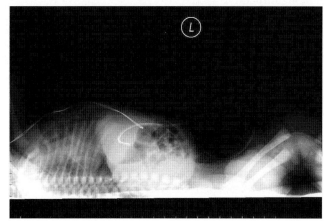

1. In the provided images, where is the distal tip of the umbilical venous catheter located?

2. What are the contraindications for insertion of umbilical venous line?

3. Where should be the normal position of the distal tip of umbilical arterial line?

4. Where should be the normal position of the distal tip of umbilical venous line?

5. What are the complications of umbilical catheters placement?

Case ranking/difficulty: 🐾 🐾   **Category:** Abdomen

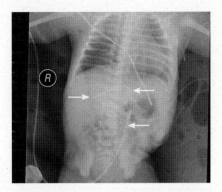

Frontal radiograph of the chest and abdomen shows an umbilical venous line (*arrows*). The distal tip deviates to the right and is located in the right portal vein. Note is made that the film is technically rotated to the left so that the umbilicus (entry port of the venous line) does not appear central.

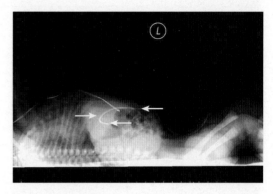

Cross-table lateral radiograph of the chest and abdomen shows an umbilical venous line (*arrows*) with the distal tip located in the right portal vein.

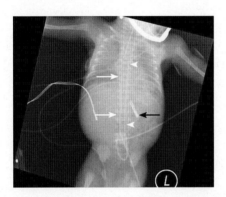

Frontal radiograph of the chest and abdomen demonstrates normal position of the umbilical arterial line (*arrowheads*) and the umbilical venous lines (*white arrows*). The distal tip of the umbilical arterial line should be between the levels T4 and T10. The distal tip of the umbilical venous line should normally be in the right atrium. The *black arrow* points to the distal tip of the enteric tube.

Pearls

- Distal tip of umbilical venous line should be kept in the right atrium.
- Distal tip of umbilical arterial line should be kept in the aorta between the levels of T4 and T10.
- In frontal chest radiograph, assuming that the film was symmetrically taken, the umbilical venous line is in the right side of the spine and umbilical arterial line is in the left side of the spine.
- Umbilical arterial catheters initially course caudally and then cranially. It forms a loop in the lower abdomen as the umbilical artery branches from the external iliac artery.
- Umbilical venous catheter travels straight in right, posterior, and cranial direction.

Answers

1. The distal tip of the umbilical venous catheter is in the right portal vein.

2. Contraindications include necrotizing enterocolitis, omphalitis, and peritonitis.

3. Normal position of the distal tip of the umbilical arterial line should be in the aorta between the levels of T4 and T10.

4. Normal position of the distal tip of umbilical venous line should be right atrium.

5. Complications may include omphalitis, cardiac tamponade and arrhythmia, vessel perforation, and embolism.

Suggested Readings

Hermansen MC, Hermansen MG. Intravascular catheter complications in the neonatal intensive care unit. *Clin Perinatol.* 2005;32(1):141-156, vii.

O'Gorman CS. Insertion of umbilical arterial and venous catheters. *Ir Med J.* 2005;98(5):151-153.

Schlesinger AE, Braverman RM, DiPietro MA. Pictorial essay. Neonates and umbilical venous catheters: normal appearance, anomalous positions, complications, and potential aid to diagnosis. *AJR Am J Roentgenol.* 2003;180(4):1147-1153.

4-week-old male with distended abdomen and centralized bowel loops in abdominal radiograph

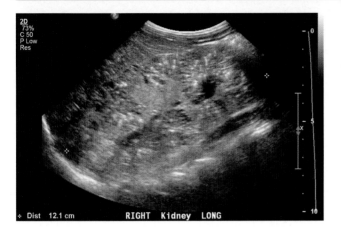 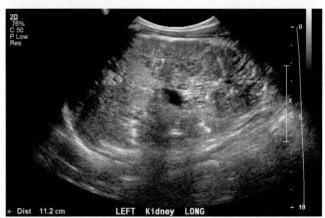

1. What is the hereditary pattern of this entity?

2. Which organ is mostly affected in this entity other than the kidney?

3. What are the complications of the entity?

4. What are the sonographic findings of this entity?

5. What is the etiology of this entity?

Case ranking/difficulty:

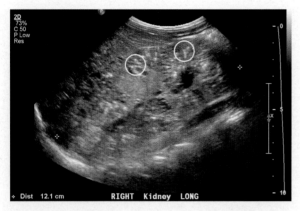

Longitudinal sonogram of the right kidney shows large kidney for age. Tiny echogenic foci seen throughout the entire kidney (*circles*) representing tiny cysts. The kidney is very echogenic.

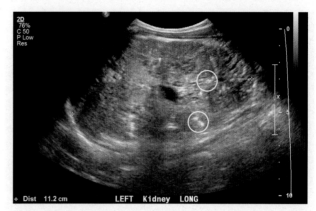

Longitudinal sonogram of the left kidney shows large kidney for age. Tiny echogenic foci seen throughout the entire kidney (*circles*) representing tiny cysts. The kidney is very echogenic.

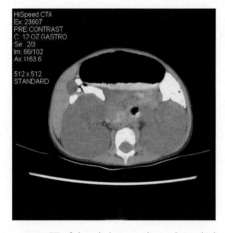

Axial non-contrast CT of the abdomen shows large kidneys.

Answers

1. The hereditary pattern of autosomal recessive polycystic kidney disease is autosomal recessive.

2. Autosomal recessive polycystic kidney disease affects mainly the kidneys and the liver.

3. Complications may include renal failure, periportal fibrosis, cirrhosis, and dilatation of the intra hepatic biliary ducts.

4. Sonographic findings include large and echogenic kidneys with bilateral echogenic foci. There is loss of the normal corticomedullary differentiation and pelvicalyceal distortion.

5. The disease is congenital.

Pearls

- Autosomal recessive polycystic kidney disease (ARPKD) is the most common heritable cystic renal disease manifesting in infancy and childhood.
- ARPKD is a disease of tubular malformation and ectasia. In the kidney, the disorder manifests as nonobstructive collecting duct ectasia.
- This results in multiple renal cysts and manifests as progressive renal failure.
- The two organs involved in autosomal recessive polycystic kidney disease are kidneys and liver with variable severity.
- CT and MRI are better to assess the degree of liver disease. Sonography is better for assessment of kidney disease.
- Kidneys are large with multiple tiny cysts that are not visualized. They manifest as multiple echogenic foci in ultrasound.
- Plain abdominal radiograph shows centralization of bowel loops due to large kidneys.

Suggested Readings

Blickman JG, Bramson RT, Herrin JT. Autosomal recessive polycystic kidney disease: long-term sonographic findings in patients surviving the neonatal period. *Am J Roentgenol.* 1995;164(5):1247-1250.

Longeran GJ, Rice RR, Suarez ES. Autosomal recessive polycystic kidney disease: radiologic-pathologic correlation. *Radiographics.* 2000;20:837-855.

Slovis TL, Bernstein J, Gruskin A. Hyperechoic kidneys in the newborn and young infant. *Pediatr Nephrol.* 1993;7(3):294-302.

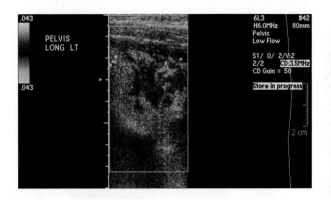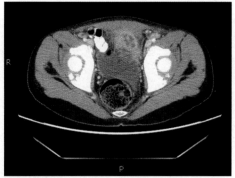
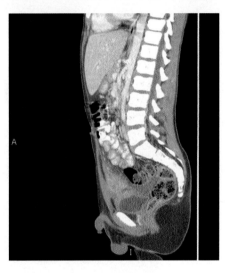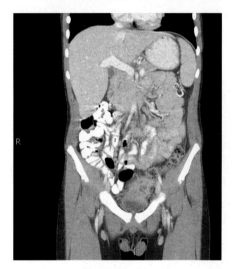

1. What are the findings?

2. What are the anatomical structures that the abnormal structures in the images connect during the fetal life?

3. Why is it important to remove this abnormal structure surgically?

4. What are the treatment options?

5. What are few of the diseases that may be associated with this entity?

Case ranking/difficulty:

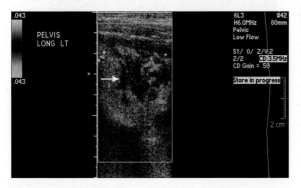

Longitudinal sonogram of the pelvis above the bladder shows heterogeneous mass. The mass is hypoechoic in its center (*arrow*) and echogenic peripherally, representing liquefying phlegmon.

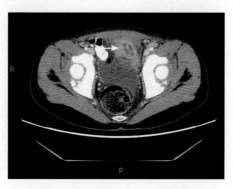

Axial CT at the level slightly above the bladder reveals heterogeneous density representing a phlegmon. In its center, there is fluid collection with enhancing wall representing an abscess (*arrow*).

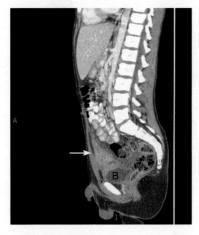

Sagittal midline CT of the pelvis shows heterogeneous density above the anterior superior wall of the bladder (*arrow*) representing a phlegmon turning into an abscess. B-bladder.

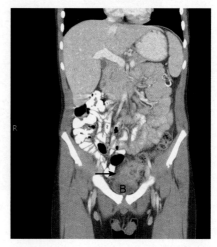

Coronal midline CT of the pelvis shows heterogeneous density above the anterior superior wall of the bladder (*arrow*) representing a phlegmon turning into an abscess. B-bladder.

Answers

1. There is inflammation in the space of Retzius.

2. The infected structure is the urachus. It connects the umbilicus with the anterosuperior wall of the bladder.

3. If the urachus is not surgically removed, there is a risk for development of adenocarcinoma.

4. Treatment of the entity shown in the images includes intravenous antibiotics, drainage, and surgical intervention.

5. Urachal remnant may be associated with some congenital anomalies. They may include Prune belly syndrome, bladder duplication, and bladder outlet obstruction.

Pearls

- The urachus connects the dome of the bladder to the umbilicus during fetal life.
- Failure of the urachus to obliterate leads to formation of diverticulum, cysts, sinus, or fibrous remnants.
- May lead to infections and abscess formation.
- Readily seen in sagittal cross-sectional imaging.
- Uncomplicated urachal remnants need to be surgically removed as there is risk of malignant transformation during adulthood.

Suggested Reading

Berrocal T, López-Pereira P, Arjonilla A, Gutiérrez J. Anomalies of the distal ureter, bladder, and urethra in children: embryologic, radiologic, and pathologic features. *Radiographics*. 2002;22:1139-1164.

4-month-old male with umbilical discharge

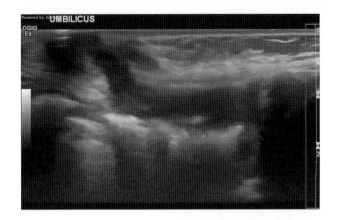
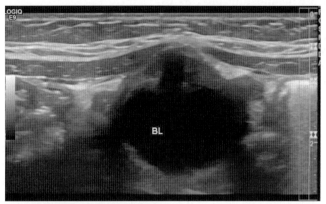
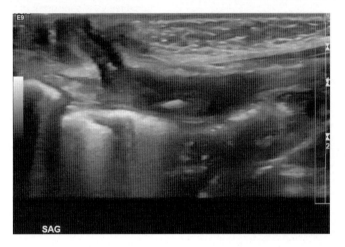

1. What is the name of the anatomic space that the pathologic structure seen in the images is located?

2. What are the findings?

3. What is the treatment?

4. Why is excision of this entity necessary?

5. Which entities may be included in the associated congenital anomalies?

Case ranking/difficulty: 🐾 🐾   Category: Genitourinary

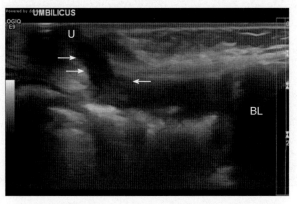

Longitudinal view sonogram of the anterior lower abdomen shows anechoic tubular structure connecting the bladder with the umbilicus (*arrows*). BL, bladder; U, umbilicus.

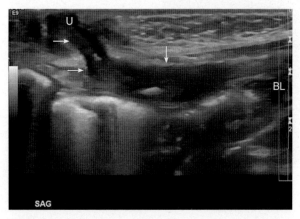

Longitudinal view sonogram of the anterior lower abdomen shows anechoic tubular structure connecting the bladder with the umbilicus (*arrows*). BL, bladder; U, umbilicus.

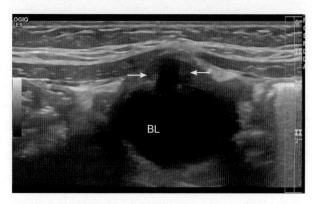

Transverse view sonogram of the bladder shows bulging of the anterior bladder wall (*arrows*; BL, bladder).

Pearls

- The urachus connects the dome of the bladder to the umbilicus during fetal life.
- Absence of complete obliteration of the urachus is a congenital abnormality.
- Sonogram shows anechoic tubular structure connecting the bladder to the umbilicus.
- Vesicoureterography may show contrast between the bladder and the umbilicus.
- Urachal lesions noted early in childhood should be excised to prevent problems in adulthood.
- Adults with urachal remnants are at risk for development of adenocarcinoma of the dome of the bladder.

Suggested Reading

Berrocal T, López-Pereira P, Arjonilla A, Gutiérrez J. Anomalies of the distal ureter, bladder, and urethra in children: embryologic, radiologic, and pathologic features. *Radiographics*. 2002;22:1139-1164.

Answers

1. The urachus is located in the space of Retzius.

2. The finding is an anechoic structure connecting the bladder to the umbilicus.

3. Treatment includes antibiotics to treat/or prevent infections and surgical excision.

4. Excision of patent urachus is necessary to prevent development of adenocarcinoma in adulthood.

5. Associated congenital anomalies may include bladder duplication, bladder outlet obstruction, and Prune belly syndrome.

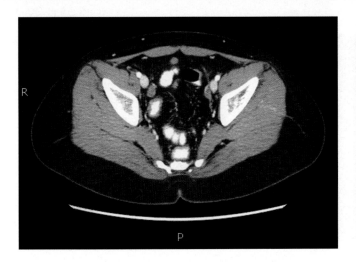 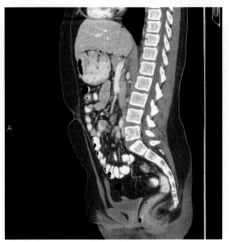

1. What is the name of the anatomical space where the abnormal structure is seen?

2. The abnormal structure seen in the images connects with . . .

3. Why the abnormal structure seen in the images need to be surgically removed?

4. What are the complications of the abnormal structure seen in the images?

5. What are the associated anomalies with the shown entity?

Case ranking/difficulty: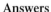

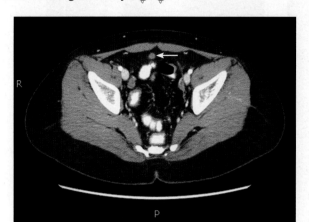

Axial CT of the abdomen shows urachal diverticulum (*arrow*).

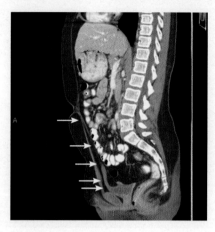

Sagittal CT of the abdomen, midline cut, demonstrates a diverticulum arising from the anterior superior aspect of the bladder and extends cranially as a fibrous band towards the umbilicus (*arrows*).

Answers

1. The urachal diverticulum is located in the space of Retzius.

2. During the fetal life, the urachus connects the dome of the bladder to the umbilicus.

3. Urachal remnants need to be surgically removed because of the increased risk of development of adenocarcinoma during adulthood.

4. Complications of the abnormal structure seen in the images may include urinary tract infection, umbilical discharge, malignant transformation, and hematuria.

5. Associated anomalies with the shown entity may include bladder duplication, bladder outlet obstruction, and Prune belly syndrome.

Pearls

- The urachus connects the dome of the bladder to the umbilicus during fetal life.
- Urachal diverticulum often exists with other congenital anomalies such as Prune belly syndrome and bladder outlet obstruction.
- Urachal diverticulum may lead to an incomplete filling and emptying of the bladder.
- Radiographically, the bladder is seen elongated with a pointed vertex.
- Urachal lesions noted early in childhood should be excised to prevent problems in adulthood.
- Adults with urachal remnants are at risk of development of adenocarcinoma of the dome of the bladder.

Suggested Reading

Berrocal T, López-Pereira P, Arjonilla A, Gutiérrez J. Anomalies of the distal ureter, bladder, and urethra in children: embryologic, radiologic, and pathologic features. *Radiographics*. 2002;22:1139-1164.

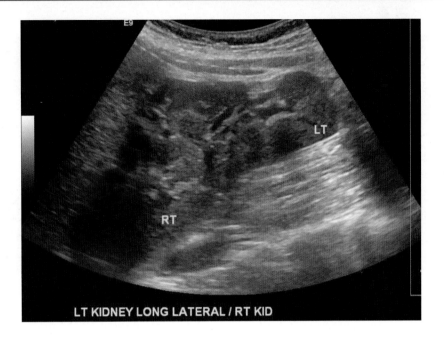

LT KIDNEY LONG LATERAL / RT KID

1. What is the etiology of this entity?

2. Describe the more common side and direction that this entity appears.

3. Describe the way fusion occurs in this entity.

4. Enumerate few complications of this entity.

5. What is the frequency of occurrence of this entity?

Case ranking/difficulty:

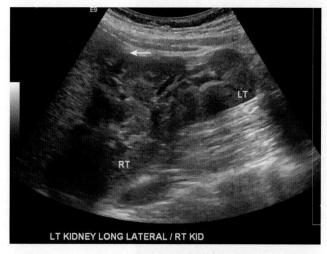

LT KIDNEY LONG LATERAL / RT KID

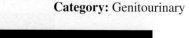

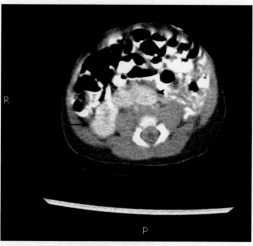

Longitudinal sonogram shows the left kidney fused to the lower pole of the right kidney in the right hemi abdomen. There is posterior "notch" between the two fused kidneys (*arrow*).

Axial CT reveals crossed fused ectopia. The left kidney (*black arrowhead*) is on the right side and fused to the lower pole of the right kidney (*black arrow*).

Answers

1. The etiology of crossed fused ectopia is congenital.

2. The more common appearance of crossed fused ectopia is left to right.

3. More commonly, the upper pole of the ectopic kidney is fused to the lower pole of the normally located kidney.

4. Complications may include ureteropelvic obstruction, trauma, calculi, hypertension, and urinary tract infection.

5. The frequency of occurrence of the entity shown is 1 out of 1,000 births.

Pearls

- Cross fused ectopia is a congenital anomaly, defined by a kidney that is located on the opposite side of midline from its ureter.
- The crossed kidney usually lies inferiorly to the normal kidney.
- The left to right ectopia is three times more common than the right to left.
- Patients generally present in adulthood with symptoms of urinary tract infection or calculi thought to be secondary to stasis.
- Complications include a high insertion of the ureter into the renal pelvis leading to ureteropelvic junction obstruction, as well as trauma to the inferiorly located kidney.
- The blood supply to the crossed kidney is usually anomalous. The ureters usually open normally in the bladder and are not ectopic.

Suggested Readings

Dyer RB, Chen MY, Zagoria RJ. Classic signs in uroradiology. *Radiographics*. 2004;24:S247-S280.

Gay SB, Armistead JP, Weber ME, Williamson BR. Left infrarenal region: anatomic variants, pathologic conditions, and diagnostic pitfalls. *Radiographics*. 1991;11:549-570.

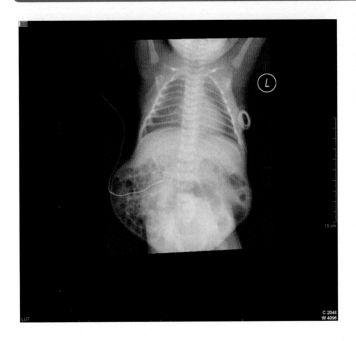 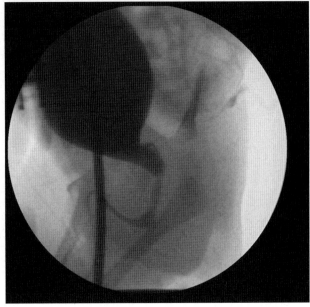

1. What are the findings?

2. What are the clinical features of this entity?

3. What is the frequency of this entity?

4. Which gender of this entity predominates?

5. What are the treatment options?

Case ranking/difficulty: 🐾 🐾

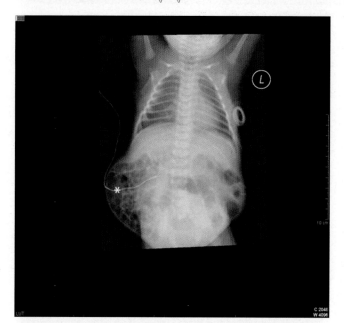

Frontal radiograph of the chest and abdomen demonstrates bowel loops protruding beyond the normal margins of the abdomen (*asterisk*).

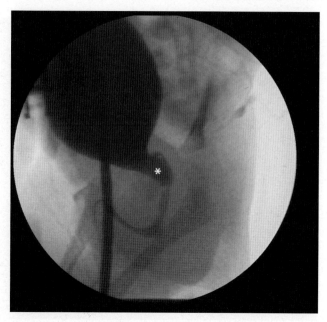

Voiding cystoureterography, during the voiding phase, demonstrates dilation of the posterior urethra (*asterisk*).

Answers

1. The bowel loops are protruding beyond the contours of the abdomen and there is dilated posterior urethra.

2. Features of Prune belly syndrome include partial or complete absence of abdominal muscles, cryptorchidism, and genitourinary abnormalities such as hydronephrosis and vesicoureteral reflux.

3. Frequency of the disease is approximately 1:40,000 live births.

4. The disease affects mostly males.

5. Treatment of the disease includes vesicostomy, remodeling of the abdominal wall and urinary tract, and orchiopexy in boys.

Pearls

- Prune belly syndrome is a rare congenital anomaly affecting 1 in 40,000 births, mainly males.
- Prune belly syndrome has the triad of:
  1. Partial or complete lack of abdominal muscles
  2. Undescendent testicles in males
  3. Genitourinary abnormalities (large ureters, hydronephrosis, vesicoureteral reflux)
- To confirm Prune belly syndrome, radiography is used to evaluate the abdomen and chest initially. For urinary tract evaluation, renal US and voiding cystourethrography are performed.
- The prostatic urethra is long and dilated as a result of prostatic hypoplasia. In voiding cystourethrography, it can mimic posterior urethral valve.

Suggested Readings

Aaronson A. Posterior urethral valve masquerading as the prune belly syndrome. *Br J Urol.* 1983;55:508-512.

Eagle JF, Barrett GS. Congenital deficiency of abdominal musculature with associated genitourinary abnormalities: a syndrome. Report of 9 cases. *Pediatrics.* 1950;6(5):721-736.

Henderson PR, Franco A. Prune Belly Syndrome. SPR web site Unknown case #24, 2010. <http://mirc.childrensmemorial.org/storage/ss12/docs/20100210155654640/MIRCdocument.xml>.

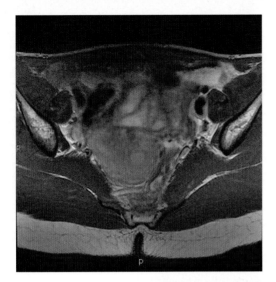

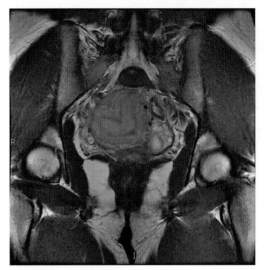

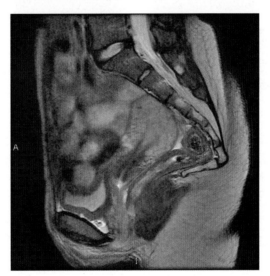

1. What are the findings?

2. What is the morphology of the uterus as seen in the sagittal view?

3. What is the embryonic structure leading to the shown anomaly?

4. Name at least three entities in the differential diagnosis.

5. What is the treatment of this entity?

Case ranking/difficulty:

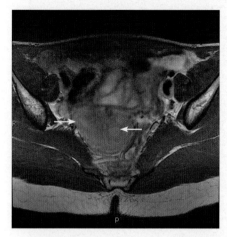

MRI-T2 axial image shows two endometrial cavities in the upper uterine segment (*arrows*).

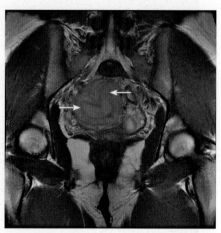

MRI-T2 coronal image shows the upper portion of the uterus divided into two endometrial cavities (*arrows*) that join in the lower uterine segment. The fundal contour remains flat.

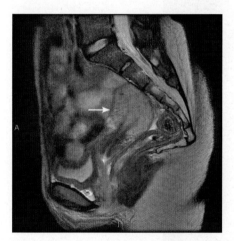

MRI-T2 sagittal shows retroverted uterus (*arrow*).

Answers

1. The uterine fundus is normal. Uterus is retroverted. Septated endometrial cavity is noted.

2. The sagittal plan demonstrates retroverted uterus.

3. The anomaly described in the images is a result of developmental anomaly of the Mullerian duct during embryogenesis.

4. Didelphys uterus, arcuate uterus, and bicornuate uterus.

5. Treatment consists of transvaginal hysteroscopic resection of the septum.

Pearls

- A septate uterus is a congenital malformation of the uterine cavity.
- The uterus is formed during embryogenesis by fusion of the two Mullerian ducts. Normally there is resorption of the partition between the two ducts and a single cavity is created. If the resorption is incomplete, a septate uterus is formed.
- In a septate uterus, the outer uterine fundus is normal.
- There is a wedge-shaped septal partition of the inner uterine cavity. The septum divides the inner uterine cavity into two endometrial cavities. The division may be partial or complete.
- Magnetic resonance imaging is the modality of choice for the diagnosis, although sonography and hysterography can be used too.
- It is important to differentiate between the different forms of Mullerian duct anomalies, such as bicornuate uterus or arcuate uterus, based on imaging, as the treatment is different.

Suggested Readings

Buttram VC, Gibbons WE. Müllerian anomalies: a proposed classification (an analysis of 144 cases). *Fertil Steril.* 1979;32(1):40-46.

Heinonen PK. Complete septate uterus with longitudinal vaginal septum. *Fertil Steril.* 2006;85(3):700-705.

Troiano RN, McCarthy SM. Mullerian duct anomalies: imaging and clinical issues. *Radiology.* 2004;233(1):19-34.

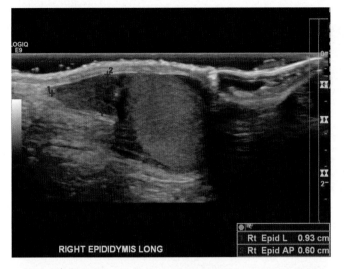

RIGHT EPIDIDYMIS LONG

| Rt Epid L | 0.93 cm |
| Rt Epid AP | 0.60 cm |

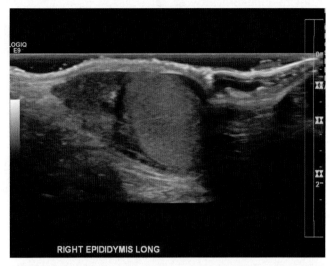

RIGHT EPIDIDYMIS LONG

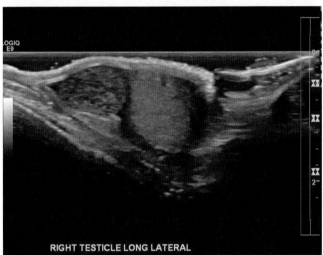

RIGHT TESTICLE LONG LATERAL

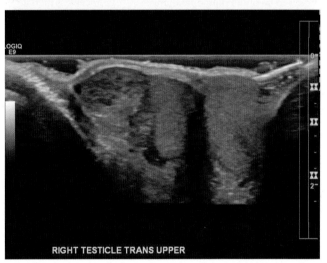

RIGHT TESTICLE TRANS UPPER

1. What are the findings?

2. What are the presenting clinical signs of this case?

3. The appendix testis is a remnant of which embryonic structure?

4. The appendix epididymis is a remnant of which embryonic structure?

5. What are the treatment options?

Case ranking/difficulty:

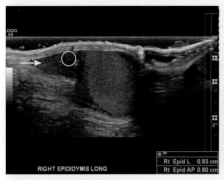

Longitudinal sonogram of the right scrotum shows enlarged right testicular appendage (*circle*) between the right testicle and the right epididymis (*arrow*). The measurement meant to be of the right epididymis; however, the technologist included the testicle appendage in the measurement.

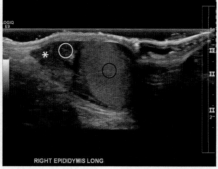

Longitudinal sonogram of the right scrotum shows enlarged right testicular appendage (*white circle*) between the right testicle and the right epididymis (*asterisk*). The right testicle is marked by *black circle*.

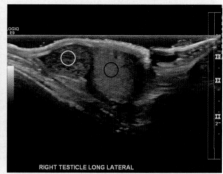

Longitudinal sonogram of the right scrotum shows enlarged right testicular appendage (*white circle*) that has heterogeneous appearance. The right testicle is marked by *black circle*.

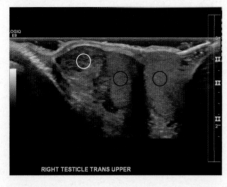

Transverse sonogram of the scrotum shows enlarged right testicular appendage (*white circle*) that has heterogeneous appearance. Both testicles are marked by *black circles*.

Answers

1. There is enlargement and heterogeneous appearance of the right testicular appendage.

2. Pain and swelling of the scrotum may be present. Erythema may be present. Nausea and vomiting may be seen in testicular torsion, but not in torsion of the testicular appendage. In light-skinned individuals, the palpable, infracted, tender appendage may be visible at the upper pole of the testis. This "blue-dot" sign is reported to occur in up to 21% of patients presenting with appendiceal torsion.

3. The appendix testis is a remnant of the paramesonephric (Müllerian) duct.

4. The appendix epididymis is a remnant of the mesonephric (Wolffian) duct.

5. Treatment of torsion of the testicular appendage is conservative such as pain relief, scrotal support, and reduced activity for few days. Surgery is not required.

Pearls

- Testicular appendage is a remnant of the Mullerian duct.
- Epididymal appendage is a remnant of the Wolffian duct.
- Torsion of the testicular appendage is more common than testicular torsion.
- Ultrasound is the imaging modality of choice.
- In ultrasound, the testicular appendage appears enlarged and heterogeneous with no flow.
- Treatment is conservative.

Suggested Readings

Johnson KA, Dewbury KC. Ultrasound imaging of the appendix testis and appendix epididymis. *Clin Radiol.* 1996;51:335-337.

Sellars MEK, Sidhu PS. Ultrasound appearances of the testicular appendages: pictorial review. *Eur Radiol.* 2003;13:127-135.

Wallace AD, Hollman AS. Colour Doppler ultrasound of the paediatric scrotum. *Imaging.* 1996;8:324-334.

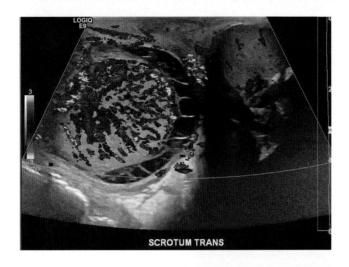

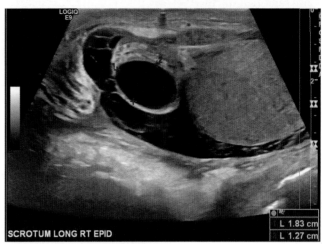

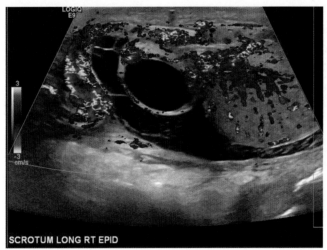

1. How do patients with this entity present clinically?

2. What are the risk factors of this entity?

3. What are the sonographic findings for this entity?

4. What are the micro-organisms that can cause this entity?

5. What are the treatment options?

Case ranking/difficulty:

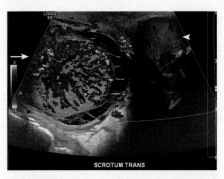

Transverse view sonogram of the scrotum demonstrates increased flow to the right testicle (*arrow*). The left testicle (*arrowhead*) appears normal. Septated complex right hydrocele is noted.

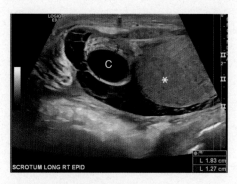

Longitudinal view sonogram of the right scrotum shows large epididymal cyst (*C*). There is low echogenicity in the upper pole of the right testicle representing edema (*asterisk*). Large septated complex hydrocele is noted.

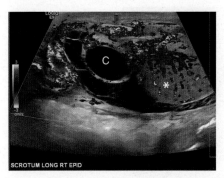

Longitudinal view sonogram of the right scrotum shows large epididymal cyst (*C*). There is low echogenicity in the upper pole of the right testicle representing edema (*asterisk*). Increased flow seen in the right scrotum. Large septated complex hydrocele is noted.

Pearls

- Swelling and pain are the most common signs and symptoms of epididymo-orchitis.
- Sonogram is the imaging modality of choice for the diagnosis.
- Hydrocele may be present.
- Most commonly epididymo-orchitis is caused by bacteria.
- The mumps virus may cause orchitis.
- The main sonographic differential diagnosis is torsion/ detorsion, as after spontaneous detorsion, blood flow is accentuated within the testicle.
- Treatment with antibiotics.

Answers

1. The diagnosis is acute epididymo-orchitis. Patients present with fever, swelling, erythema, and tenderness in the affected side of the scrotum.

2. Risk factors may include catheter insertion into the bladder, urinary tract infection, sexual activity, and mumps.

3. Sonographic findings include enlarged affected epididymis, heterogeneous echotexture of the affected testicle, hydrocele, and increased vascular flow to the affected side.

4. Micro-organisms are *Escherichia coli*, *Staphylococcus*, *Neisseria gonorrhoeae*, and mumps virus.

5. Treatment includes antibiotics, antipyretics, and analgesics.

Suggested Readings

Aso C, Enríquez G, Fité M, et al. Gray-scale and color Doppler sonography of scrotal disorders in children: an update. *Radiographics*. 2005;25:1197-1214.

Woodward PJ, Schwab CM, Sesterhenn IA. From the archives of the AFIP: extratesticular scrotal masses: radiologic-pathologic correlation. *Radiographics*. 2003;23:215-240.

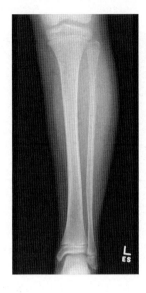
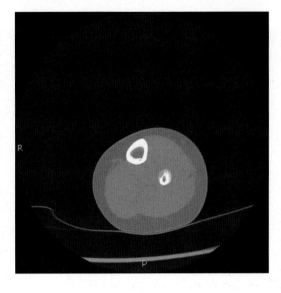
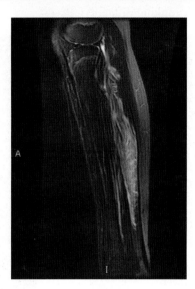

1. What is the differential diagnosis?

2. What type of periosteal reaction is associated with this case?

3. What is the most common location of the shown entity?

4. What is the most common presentation of the shown entity on conventional radiographs?

5. What is the age range of peak presentation of the case?

Case ranking/difficulty: **Category:** Lower extremities

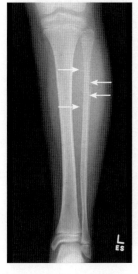

Frontal view of the left leg demonstrates periosteal reaction of the proximal fibula (*arrows*).

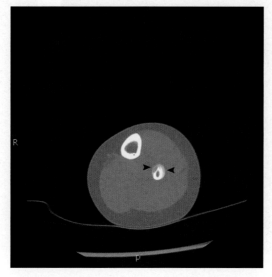

Axial CT of the left leg demonstrates periosteal reaction of the proximal left fibula (*arrowheads*).

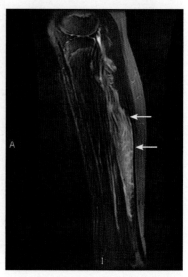

Sagittal T2-MRI of the proximal left fibula demonstrates high signal in the proximal fibula with periosteal reaction (*arrows*).

Answers

1. Differential diagnosis includes Ewing sarcoma, osteosarcoma, rhabdomyosarcoma, neuroblastoma, lymphoma, and other neoplasms of the bone.

2. The classic description of lamellated or "onion skin" type periosteal reaction is often associated with this lesion.

3. The diaphyses of the femur are the most common sites, followed by the tibia and the humerus.

4. On conventional radiographs, the most common osseous presentation is a permeative lytic lesion with periosteal reaction. The classic description of lamellated or "onion skin" type periosteal reaction is often associated with this lesion.

5. Ewing sarcoma is more common in males and usually presents in childhood or early adulthood, with a peak between 10 and 20 years of age.

Pearls

- Ewing sarcoma is a highly malignant primary bone tumor that is derived from red bone marrow.
- It can occur anywhere in the body, but most commonly in the pelvis and proximal long tubular bones, especially around the growth plates.
- Metastatic disease is present in 30% of patients at presentation.
- CT and MRI are useful for evaluation of soft tissue extension and of the disease and metastatic spread.

Suggested Readings

Ewing J. Classics in oncology. Diffuse endothelioma of bone. James Ewing. Proceedings of the New York Pathological Society, 1921. [reprint]. *CA Cancer J Clin.* 1972;22(2):95-98.

Kaste SC. Imaging pediatric bone sarcomas. *Radiol Clin North Am.* 2011;49(4):749-765, vi-vii.

Small RM, Friedlaender EY. Picture of the month. Ewing sarcoma. *Arch Pediatr Adolesc Med.* 2011;165(5): 465-466.

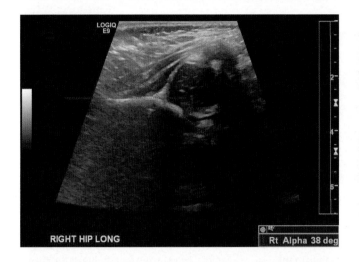

RIGHT HIP LONG — Rt Alpha 38 deg

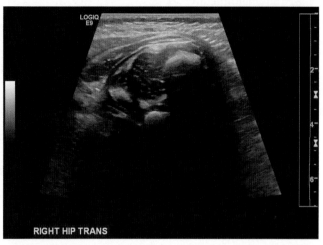

RIGHT HIP TRANS

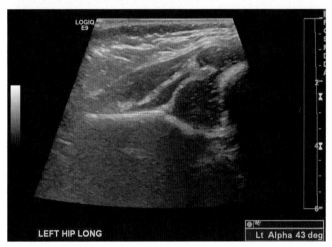

LEFT HIP LONG — Lt Alpha 43 deg

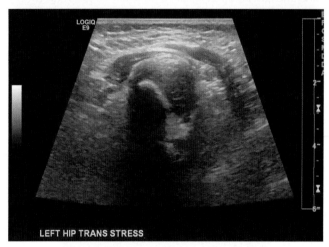

LEFT HIP TRANS STRESS

1. What are the findings?

2. What is the alpha angle in sonogram of the hips?

3. What is the normal value of the alpha angle?

4. Which of the delivery presentations is more prone for the development of this entity?

5. What are the risk factors for the development of this entity?

Case ranking/difficulty: **Category:** Pelvis

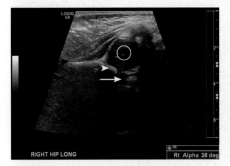

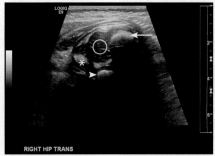

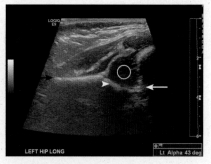

Coronal sonogram of the right hip demonstrates alpha angle of 38 degrees (normal more than 60 degrees). This represents dysplastic hip. The coverage of the femoral head by the acetabulum is less than 50%. The *white arrow* points to the triradiate cartilage. The *white arrowhead* points to the acetabular roof. The *black arrow* points to the vertical cortex of the ilium. The *circle* points to the cartilaginous femoral head.

Transverse view of the right hip demonstrates that the cartilaginous femoral head (*circle*) is not well centered throughout the triradiate cartilage (*white arrowhead*). The *asterisk* points to the acetabular roof. The *arrow* points to the greater trochanter of the right femur.

Coronal sonogram of the left hip demonstrates alpha angle of 43 degrees (normal more than 60 degrees). This represents dysplastic hip. The coverage of the femoral head by the acetabulum is less than 50%. The *white arrow* points to the triradiate cartilage. The *white arrowhead* points to the acetabular roof. The *black arrow* points to the vertical cortex of the ilium. The *circle* points to the cartilaginous femoral head.

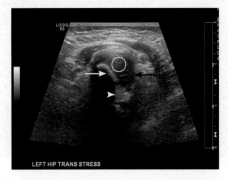

Transverse view of the left hip demonstrates that the cartilaginous femoral head (*circle*) is not well centered throughout the triradiate cartilage (*white arrowhead*). *White arrow* points to the acetabular roof. *Black arrow* points to the cartilaginous femoral head.

presentation, multiple gestation, first pregnancy, high birth weight, oligohydramnios, and postural and non-postural abnormalities including club-foot deformity and congenital torticollis.

Answers

1. Alpha angle less than 60 degrees; coverage of the femoral heads by the acetabulum is less than 50 percent; the acetabular edge is rounded; and in transverse view, the femoral heads are not well centered throughout the triradiate cartilage.

2. Alpha angle is the angle formed by the acetabular roof and the vertical cortex of the ilium.

3. The normal value of the alpha angle is greater than or equal to 60 degrees.

4. Infants born in breech presentations are more prone to develop hip dysplasia.

5. Risk factors for developmental dysplasia of the hips include female sex, a familial history, breech

Pearls

- The femoral head of the newborn normally ossifies at approximately 6 months of age. Until this time, sonography is the best imaging tool, as the femoral head is cartilaginous and its relation to the acetabulum cannot be assessed by plain radiographs.
- When femoral head ossifies, the best tool for diagnosis is plain radiographs of the hip and pelvis. Sonography becomes inadequate for evaluation of developmental hip dysplasia.
- Lines and angles are drawn to assess the relationship between the femoral head and the acetabulum in ultrasound and in plain radiographs.

Suggested Readings

Bancroft LW, Merinbaum DJ, Zaleski CG, Peterson JJ, Kransdorf MJ, Berquist TH. Hip ultrasound. *Semin Musculoskelet Radiol.* 2007;11(2):126-136.

Keller MS, Nijs EL. The role of radiographs and US in developmental dysplasia of the hip: how good are they? *Pediatr Radiol.* 2009;39(Suppl 2):S211-S215.

Paton RW. Developmental dysplasia of the hip: ultrasound screening and treatment. How are they related? *Hip Int.* 2009;19(Suppl 6):S3-S8.

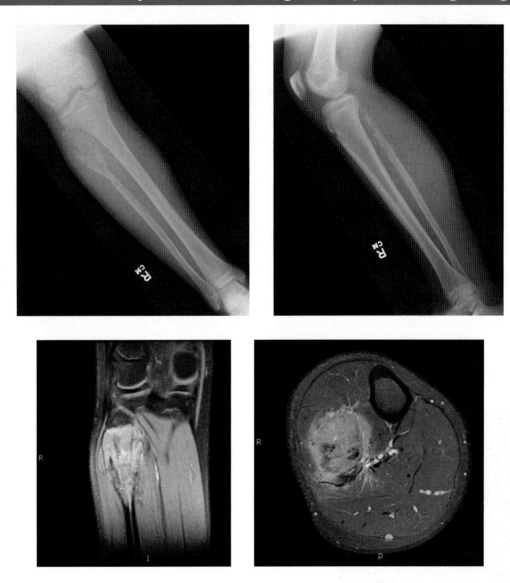

1. What are the findings?

2. In which portion of the bone does this lesion tend to occur?

3. In which bone is this lesion most prevalent?

4. What is the most common site of metastasis?

5. What are the clinical signs of this entity?

Case ranking/difficulty:

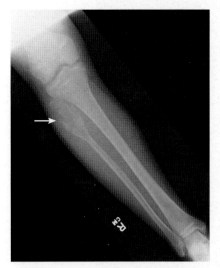

Frontal radiograph of the right leg demonstrates a permeative lytic lesion in the proximal fibula (*arrow*) with break of the periosteum. Irregular periosteal reaction noted extending to the surrounding soft tissue.

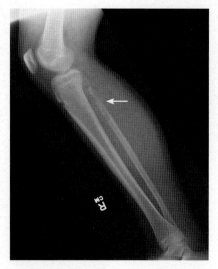

Lateral radiograph of the right leg demonstrates permeative lytic lesion in the proximal fibula (*arrow*) with break of the periosteum. Irregular periosteal reaction noted extending to the surrounding soft tissue.

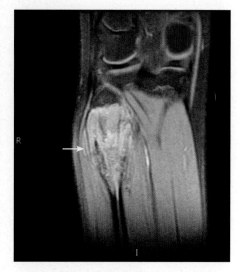

Coronal MRI-T2 of the proximal right fibula demonstrates irregular high signal lesion (*arrow*) with break of the periosteum. There is soft tissue edema in the proximal fibula around the lesion.

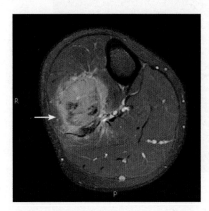

Axial contrast-enhanced MRI-T1 of the proximal right fibula demonstrates irregular enhancing lesion (*arrow*) with break of the periosteum. Ossification of the posterior aspect of the proximal fibula noted with surrounding enhancing edema.

Answers

1. An expansile lytic permeative lesion is seen in the proximal fibula with break of the periosteum. Irregular osteoid formation is seen in the surrounding with soft tissue edema. Vascular structures are not affected.

2. Osteosarcoma tends most commonly to affect the metaphysis of long bones.

3. Osteosarcoma is most prevalent in the distal femoral metaphysis (42%).

4. The most common site of metastasis is the lungs.

5. Clinical signs may include a palpable mass and pain. If the joint is involved, there might be a decrease in the range of motion. If lower extremity is involved, there may be a limp. Pathologic fractures are uncommon except in the telangiectatic type of osteosarcoma.

Pearls

- Osteosarcoma is an aggressive neoplasm producing malignant osteoid.
- Osteosarcoma is the most common form of bone cancer.
- The neoplasm has prevalence to originate from the metaphyseal region of long bones.
- High prevalence occurs in the distal femur.
- Metastasis to the lungs may occur. Metastases to other organs are rare.
- The imaging modality of choice for evaluation of the intramedullary region and soft tissue extension is MRI.

Suggested Readings

Campanacci M. Preface. *Bone and Soft Tissue Tumors: Clinical Features, Imaging, Pathology and Treatment.* 2nd ed. New York, NY: Springer-Verlag; 1999.

Hudson M, Jaffe MR, Jaffe N, et al. Pediatric osteosarcoma: therapeutic strategies, results, and prognostic factors derived from a 10-year experience. *J Clin Oncol.* 1990;8(12):1988-1997.

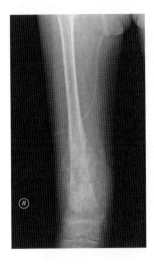 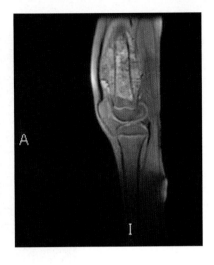 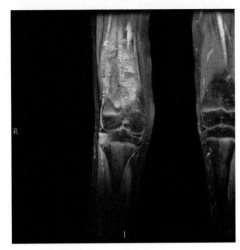

1. Describe the findings seen in the plain radiographs.

2. How this case may present clinically?

3. What is the anatomical site that this entity most commonly occurs?

4. What is the most common site that this lesion metastasizes?

5. What are the treatment options?

Case ranking/difficulty:

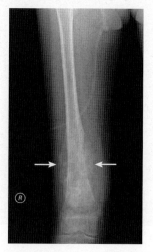

Frontal radiograph of the right femur reveals dense ossifications of the distal femoral diametaphyseal region. There are adjacent soft tissue ossifications (*arrows*).

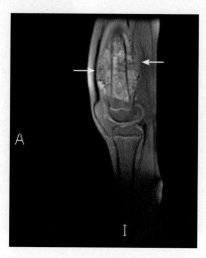

Sagittal MRI-T2 shows high signal of the distal right femur with adjacent soft tissue high signals (*arrows*).

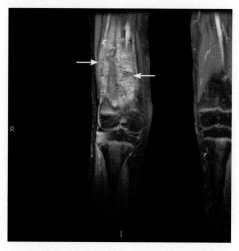

Coronal MRI-T1 with contrast shows high enhancement of the distal femur with enhanced soft tissue mass around the distal femur (*arrows*).

Pearls

- Osteosarcoma is the most common malignant bone tumor.
- Osteosarcoma is a deadly disease and most patients die from pulmonary metastatic disease.
- Most common site of occurrence is the distal femur.
- Imaging findings depend on the variant of the lesion. The classic osteoblastic type shows intramedullary ossification in the bone and in the adjacent soft tissue.

Suggested Readings

Campanacci M. Preface. *Bone and Soft Tissue Tumors: Clinical Features, Imaging, Pathology and Treatment.* 2nd ed. New York, NY: Springer-Verlag; 1999.

Ottaviani G, Jaffe N. The epidemiology of osteosarcoma. In: Jaffe N, et al., eds. *Pediatric and Adolescent Osteosarcoma.* New York, NY: Springer; 2009.

Answers

1. There is ossification of the distal right femur with adjacent soft tissue ossified mass.

2. This particular case may present with swelling, pain, and a decreased range of motion. If there are pulmonary metastatic lesions, then respiratory distress may occur.

3. The most common site of occurrence is the femur (42%, 75% of which are in the distal femur).

4. Pulmonary metastases are most common in osteosarcoma.

5. Treatment options include chemotherapy, radiation therapy, and surgery.

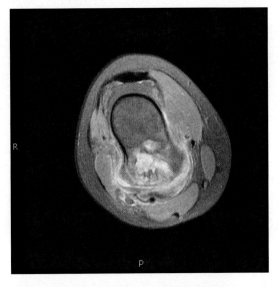
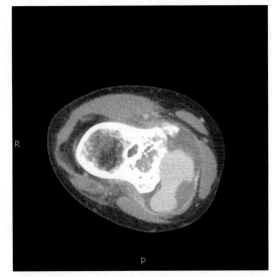
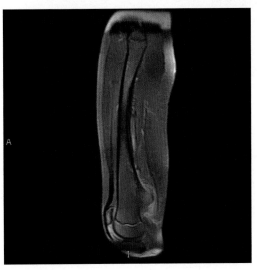
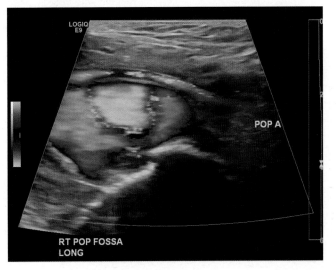

1. What is the diagnosis?

2. What is the differential diagnosis of the shown entity?

3. What are the sonographic findings of this entity?

4. What are the risk factors?

5. What are the treatment options?

Case ranking/difficulty: **Category:** Lower extremities

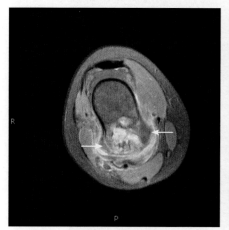

Axial MRI-T2 at the level above the right popliteal region demonstrates osteochondroma (*arrows*).

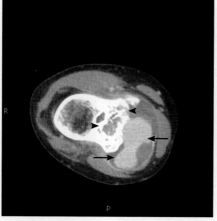

Axial-enhanced CT reveals an area in the popliteal region of the right femur that fills with blood (*arrows*) adjacent to osteochondroma (*arrowheads*).

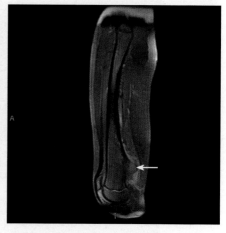

Sagittal MRI-T1 reveals osteochondroma above the right popliteal region (*arrow*).

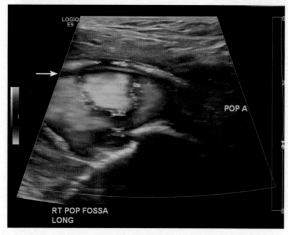

Color sonogram of the popliteal fossa demonstrates a mass filled with blood with swirling of the blood in to-and-fro direction (*arrow*). The mass connects to the popliteal artery and represents pseudoaneurysm.

Answers

1. The diagnosis is femoral osteochondroma causing pseudoaneurysm following irritation of the popliteal artery.

2. Differential diagnosis may include hematoma, abscess, arteriovenous fistula, lymphocele, and compartment syndrome.

3. The sonographic findings include in-color Doppler communication with an artery, swirling of blood, and to-and-fro direction of blood flow.

4. Risk factors may include endovascular procedure, gunshot wound, irritation of arterial wall, and catheterization.

5. Treatment options may include coiling, compression under ultrasound guidance, and surgery.

Pearls

- A pseudoaneurysm, or false aneurysm, is a hematoma that forms outside an arterial wall and communicates with the artery it surrounds.
- The communication with the artery is being created by a leaking arterial hole.
- Pseudoaneurysm can be caused by irritation and damage of the arterial wall, such as catheterization.
- During systole, blood enters the pseudoaneurysm and exists during diastole.

Suggested Readings

Belmir H, Azghari A, Mechchat A, et al. Rupture of a popliteal artery pseudo-aneurysm revealing a tibial osteochondroma: case report and review of the literature. *J Mal Vasc*. 2011;36(1):50-55.

Guder WK, Streitbürger A, Gosheger G, et al. Small sharp exostosis tip in solitary osteochondroma causing intermittent knee pain due to pseudoaneurysm. *BMC Res Notes*. 2013;6:142.

Oliveira FM, Fernandes Júnior N, Roberti T, Bolanho E, Costa Rde F. Popliteal artery pseudoaneurysm caused by a femoral osteochondroma: case report. *Rev Col Bras Cir*. 2012;39(6):558-559.

2-week-old male with sacral dimple

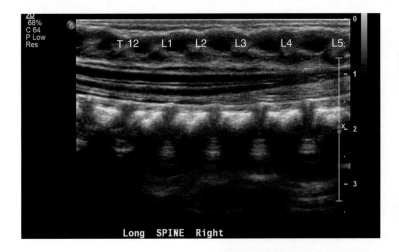

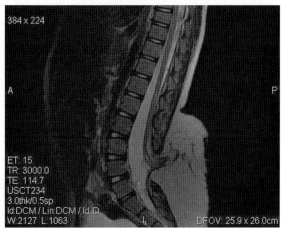

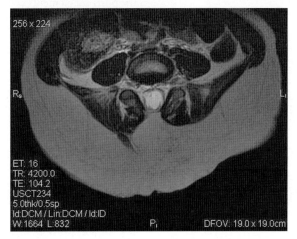

1. What are the findings?

2. What are the clinical presentations that may be seen in a newborn with this entity?

3. To which of the body system will you classify this disorder?

4. What is the level of the normal conus medullaris at birth?

5. What is the treatment?

Case ranking/difficulty:

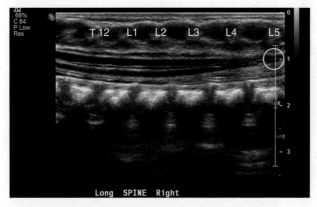

Longitudinal sonogram of the lumbosacral spine shows conus medullaris at the level of L5 (*circle*).

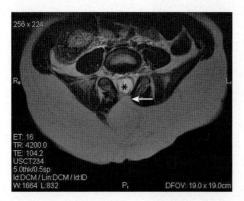

Axial MR-T2 image at the level of L5 shows failure of closure of the posterior elements of L5 (*arrow*). Lipomeningocele noted (*asterisk*).

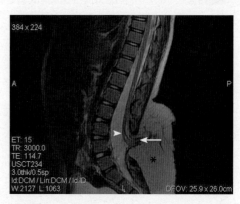

Sagittal midline MR-T2 image of the lumbosacral spine shows conus medullaris at the level of L5 (*arrowhead*). Failure of closure of the posterior elements of L5 is seen (*arrow*). A low back fatty mass is seen in continuity with the tethered conus medullaris (*asterisk*).

Answers

1. The diagnosis is tethered cord syndrome with lipomyelomeningocele. The conus medullaris is at the level of L5. There is failure of closure of the posterior elements of L5. There is herniation of the tethered cord and the meninges through the posterior elements of the lower lumbar spine, surrounded by a fatty mass.

2. Clinical presentation of a newborn with this entity may include dermal sinus tract, lipoma, sacral dimple, and hairy patches. The clinical presentation may also include paralysis and/or spasticity of the lower extremities, and later disturbances in bowel and urinary control.

3. This entity is a neurological disorder.

4. The normal conus medullaris at birth is at the level between L1 and L2.

5. Treatment of tethered cord may include physical therapy, analgesics, and surgery.

Pearls

- Tethered spinal cord syndrome consists of abnormal stretching of the cord due to tissue attachment that limits the movements of the spinal cord within the spinal column.
- Lipomyelomeningocele is associated anomaly that consists of herniation of the meninges and parts of the tethered cord through the posterior elements of the lower lumbar spine. A fatty mass surrounds the herniated sac.
- Symptoms may include lesions, hairy patches, dimples, or fatty tumors on the lower back, foot, and spinal deformities, weakness in the legs, lower back pain, scoliosis, and incontinence.
- Sonography and MR images demonstrate that the conus medullaris is low in position, below the level of L2. The filum terminale is usually thickened, more than 2 mm.
- Spina bifida is present with failure of closure of the posterior elements of L5 and sometimes S1.
- In children, early surgery is recommended to prevent further neurological deterioration. Pain medication is needed to relieve symptoms. Nerve roots can be cut if severe pain occurs.

Suggested Readings

Fitz CR, Harwood-Nash DC. The tethered conus. *AJR Am J Roentgenol.* 1975;125:515-523.

Hill CA, Gibson PJ. Ultrasound determination of the normal location of the conus medullaris in neonates. *AJNR Am J Neuroradiol.* 1995;16:469-472.

Korsvik HE, Keller MS. Sonography of occult spinal dysraphism in neonates and infants with MR imaging correlation. *Radiographics.* 1992;12:297-306.

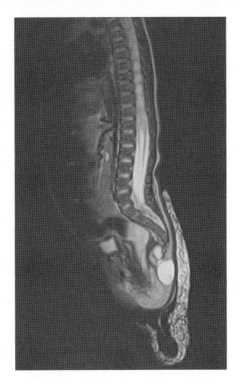
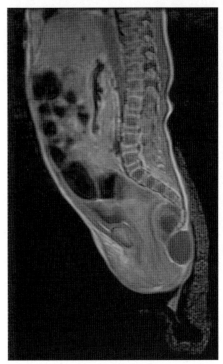

1. What are the findings?

2. What is the differential diagnosis?

3. What is the correct classification for this entity?

4. What are possible complications?

5. What is the survival rate in this entity?

Case ranking/difficulty:

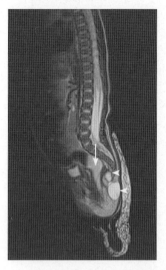

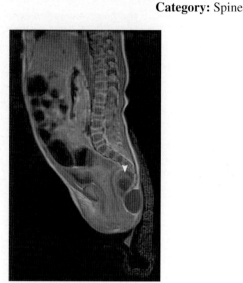

Polycystic lesion with minimal soft tissue component at the tip of the coccyx. There is an evident presacral extension, but without external posterior component (*arrowheads*). There is no infiltration of the spinal canal. The sacrum is intact. Fluid-filled rectum (*arrow*).

On T1WI, there is only minimal contrast enhancement at the periphery of the cysts (*arrowhead*), and no solid tumor component.

Answers

1. There is a polylobulated multicystic tumor mass behind the rectum, in front of the sacrum/coccyx, entirely within the pelvis. No anomaly of the sacrum/coccyx is seen. MRI is mandatory to evaluate for possible intraspinal infiltration.

2. Rhabdomyosarcoma may be located deep in the pelvis, but usually arises from the genitourinary tract, and therefore are rarely in presacral location. Neuroblastoma may be also considered, especially when originating from the organ of Zuckerkandl (chromaffin cells in para-aortal location from the renal arteries down to the aortic bifurcation). If the tumor is purely cystic, the teratoma is probably of benign nature.

3. The American Academy of Pediatric Surgical Section survey classified the teratoma according to its location. Type I is an extrafetal retrosacral teratoma, type II is an extrafetal teratoma with presacral infiltration of the pelvis, type III is an extrafetal teratoma with abdominopelvic infiltration, and type IV is an entirely intrapelvic presacral teratoma.

4. Surgery with complete resection is the treatment of choice but to avoid recurrence, resection of the coccyx where the tumor is attached is mandatory. Depending upon the volume of the tumor, chronic ventral compression of rectovesical structures during fetal life may lead to functional insufficiency. Intraspinal extension may produce spinal cord and radicular symptoms.

5. Ninety percent of benign teratoma will be cured after surgery and/or chemotherapy. In malignant teratoma, the cure rate is almost zero.

Pearls

- Commonest tumor in fetus and neonates.
- Solid and cystic components.
- Female predominance.
- Sixty percent mature/benign teratoma.
- Fifty percent are type I in extrafetal retrosacral location.

Suggested Readings

Marković I, Stamenović S, Radovanović Z, Bosnjàković P, Ilić D, Stojanov D. Ultrasound and magnetic resonance imaging in prenatal diagnosis of sacrococcygeal teratoma—case report. *Med Pregl*. 2013;66(5-6):254-257.

Shue E, Bolouri M, Jelin EB, et al. Tumor metrics and morphology predict poor prognosis in prenatally diagnosed sacrococcygeal teratoma: a 25-year experience at a single institution. *J Pediatr Surg*. 2013;48(6):1225-1231.

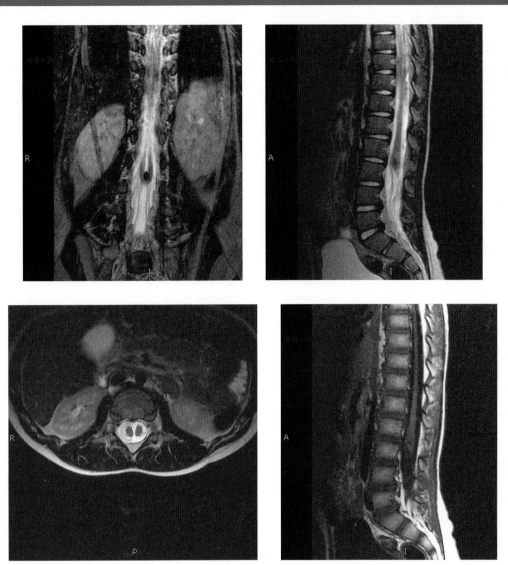

1. What are the findings?

2. Where is this abnormality most commonly located?

3. Which meningeal layer is common to the two hemicords in this case?

4. What can be the associated abnormalities?

5. What are the treatment options?

Case ranking/difficulty: 🌰🌰🌰   **Category:** Spine

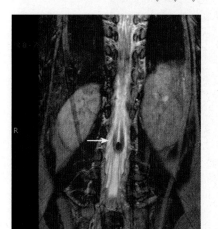 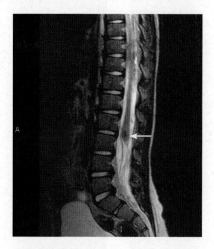 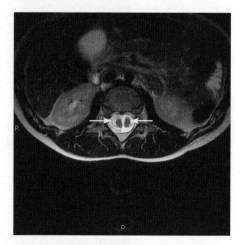

Coronal MRI-T2 demonstrates splitting of the cord at the level between L2 and L3. Bony septum separates the two hemicords (*arrow*).

Sagittal MRI-T2 demonstrates splitting of the cord at the level between L2 and L3. Bony septum separates the two hemicords (*arrow*).

Axial MRI-T2 demonstrates splitting of the cord at the level of L2, above the bony septum (*arrows*). CSF separates the two hemicords.

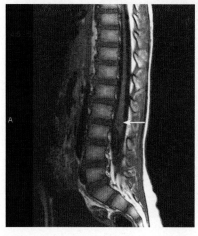

Sagittal MRI-T1 demonstrates splitting of the cord at the level between L2 and L3. Bony septum separates the two hemicords (*arrow*).

Answers

1. There is splitting of the cord. The cord is divided by a bony septum.

2. The cleft in diastematomyelia may be found at any level, but in most cases it is found at the lower thoracic or upper lumbar regions.

3. The hemicords usually have a distinct arachnoid membrane each with a common dura.

4. Associated anomalies may include open spina bifida, closed abnormalities of the vertebrae: scoliosis, kyphosis, hemivertebrae, butterfly vertebra; cutaneous manifestations on the dorsal midline consisting of telangiectasias, atrophic skin, hemangiomas, subcutaneous

lipomas, and cutaneous nevi. Among the cutaneous nevi, the most characteristic is the nevus pilosus, a large patch of long silky hair that is situated over the site of the cleft in the cord in 50 to 70% of the cases.

5. If the patient is symptomatic, then decompression of the hemicords is needed with removal of the bony or the cartilaginous elements producing the compression. Asymptomatic patients can just be observed.

Pearls

- Diastematomyelia occurs when the spinal cord is split into two columns.
- Diastematomyelia may occur with spina bifida or with a closed spine.
- Diastematomyelia may involve a single vertebra or extend to several vertebral segments.
- The cleft may be found at any level, but in most cases it is found in the lower thoracic or upper lumbar regions.
- Associated cutaneous and vertebral anomalies are often seen.
- If patient is symptomatic, decompression surgery may be required.

Suggested Readings

Cowie TN. Diastematomyelia with vertebral column defects; observations on its radiological diagnosis. *Br J Radiol.* 1951;24(279):156-160.

Dick EA, Patel K, Owens CM, De Bruyn R. Spinal ultrasound in infants. *Br J Radiol.* 2002;75(892):384-392.

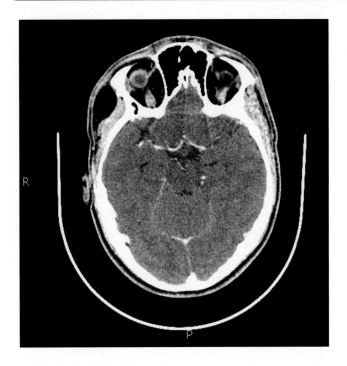
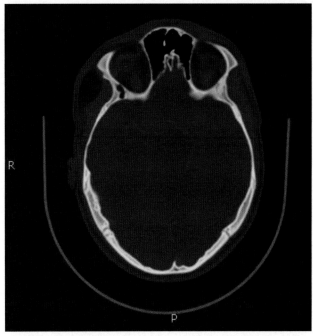

1. Describe the findings.

2. What is the cause of this entity?

3. Name few anatomical locations where such entity can be found.

4. What are the imaging modalities of choice for the diagnosis of this entity?

5. What are the treatment options?

Case ranking/difficulty:

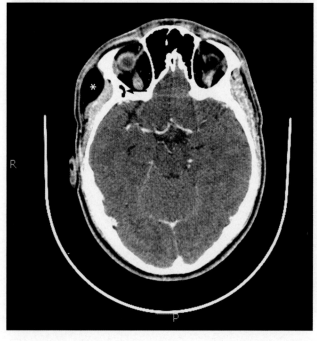

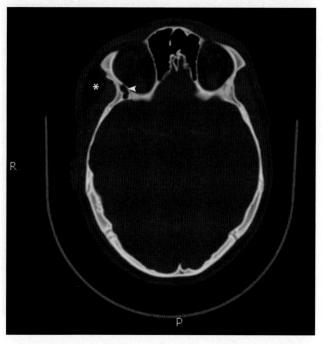

Axial CT of the head with contrast demonstrates subcutaneous fatty density cyst located lateral to the right orbit/suprazygomatic (*asterisk*) with extension into the right sphenoid buttress (*arrow*).

Axial CT of the head with contrast in bone window demonstrates subcutaneous fatty density cyst located lateral to the right orbit/suprazygomatic (*asterisk*) with extension into the right sphenoid buttress (*arrowhead*).

Answers

1. The CT of the head demonstrates subcutaneous fatty density cyst located lateral to the right orbit/suprazygomatic with extension into the right sphenoid buttress.

2. Dermoid cysts are caused by skin structures that become trapped during fetal development.

3. Dermoid cysts in the subcutaneous layer occur mostly in the face, neck, or in the scalp. They may also be seen intracranially, intra-abdominally, and in the pelvis as well.

4. CT and MRI are helpful in diagnosing dermoid cysts due to fatty dissemination. Calcification and teeth may also be assessed radiographically, mostly in ovarian cysts.

5. Surgical excision is the treatment of choice in any localization.

Pearls

- Dermoid cysts have walls that contain structures that are usually seen in the outer skin such as hair follicles and sweat glands.
- During fetal life these skin structures become trapped and a cyst is formed.
- MRI is helpful in planning surgical procedures and in assessing therapeutic success.

Suggested Readings

Chung EM, Murphey MD, Specht CS, Cube R, Smirniotopoulos JG. From the Archives of the AFIP. Pediatric orbit tumors and tumorlike lesions: osseous lesions of the orbit. *Radiographics*. 2009;28(4):1193-1214.

Pham NS, Dublin AB, Strong EB. Dermoid cyst of the orbit and frontal sinus: a case report. *Skull Base*. 2010;20(4):275-278.

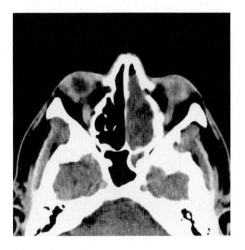
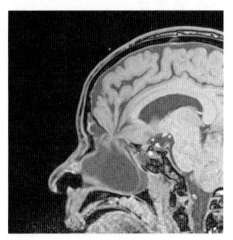
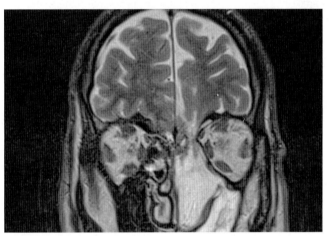
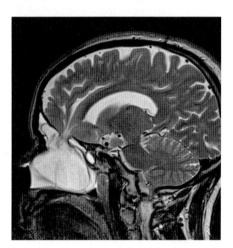

1. Which population has the highest prevalence of this entity?

2. How is the shown entity being formed during the fetal development?

3. Which part of the head is involved in the sincipital type of this entity?

4. In which part of the head this entity is most common?

5. What are the intracranial anomalies associated with this entity?

Case ranking/difficulty:

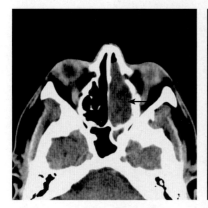

Non-contrast axial CT of the face demonstrates brain tissue inside the left ethmoidal sinus (*arrow*).

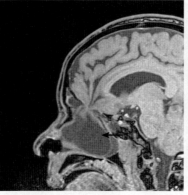

Sagittal MRI-T1 reveals a low signal inside the left ethmoidal sinus representing the cerebrospinal fluid (*arrow*).

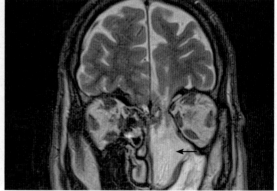

Coronal MRI-T2 reveals high signal inside the left ethmoidal sinus representing the cerebrospinal fluid (*arrow*).

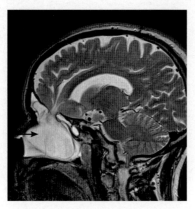

Sagittal MRI-T2 reveals high signal inside the left ethmoidal sinus representing the cerebrospinal fluid (*arrow*).

Pearls

- Encephalocele is a neural tube defect that consists of the brain protruding through an opening in the skull.
- Nasoethmoidal encephaloceles result from herniation of a dural diverticulum through the lamina cribrosa.
- Nasofrontal encephalocele is based on a persistence of the fonticulus nasofrontalis (which, when obliterated, becomes the foramen cecum).
- The imaging modalities of choice for the diagnosis are CT and MRI.

Suggested Readings

Goldstein RB, LaPidus AS, Filly RA. Fetal cephaloceles: diagnosis with US. *Radiology*. 1991;180(3):803-808.

Lowe LH, Booth TN, Joglar JM, Rollins NK. Midface anomalies in children. *Radiographics*. 2000;20:907-922.

Answers

1. Nasoethmoidal encephaloceles are more common in South and Southeast Asian population.

2. These defects are caused by failure of the neural tube to close completely during fetal development.

3. Sincipital encephaloceles involve the midface and occur about the dorsum of the nose, the orbits, and the forehead.

4. Occipital encephalocele is the most common.

5. Encephaloceles have a high prevalence of associated intracranial anomalies, including intracranial cysts, callosal agenesis, interhemispheric lipomas, facial clefts, and schizencephaly.

16-year-old male with seizures

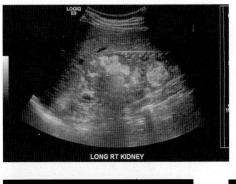
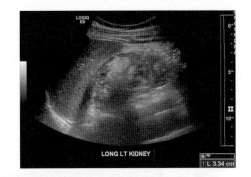
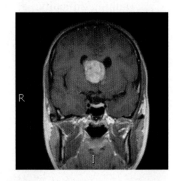
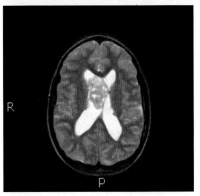
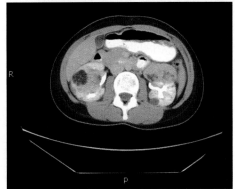
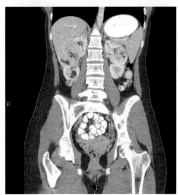

1. What are the findings in the ultrasound images?

2. What are clinical features of this case?

3. What is the tumor that most commonly develops in the heart in patients with this entity?

4. What is being represented by the echogenic foci in the kidneys?

5. What is the tumor that most commonly develops in the brain in patients with this entity?

Case ranking/difficulty: **Category:** Generalized diseases

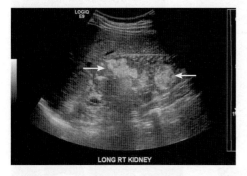

Longitudinal sonogram of the right kidney reveals two echogenic structures (*arrows*) representing angiomyolipomas.

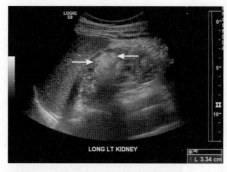

Longitudinal sonogram of the left kidney reveals echogenic structure (*arrows*) representing angiomyolipomas.

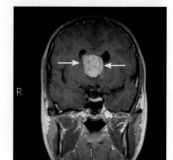

Contrast-enhanced MRI T1 of the head in coronal view reveals enhancing mass arising from the ependymal lining of the foramen of Monro (*arrows*) representing giant cell astrocytoma.

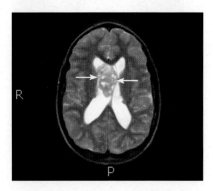

Axial MRI T2 of the head reveals a mass arising from the ependymal lining of the foramen of Monro (*arrows*) representing giant cell astrocytoma.

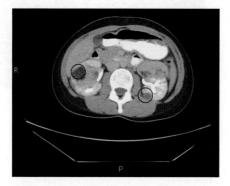

Axial contrast-enhanced CT of the abdomen reveals enlarged kidneys with numerous masses containing fat (*circles*) representing angiomyolipomas in a patient with tuberous sclerosis.

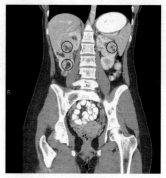

Coronal contrast-enhanced CT of the abdomen reveals enlarged kidneys with numerous masses containing fat (*circles*) representing angiomyolipomas in a patient with tuberous sclerosis.

Answers

1. There are bilateral echogenic foci in the kidneys.

2. Clinical features of the disease vary and may include seizures, mental retardation, skin lesions, and hematuria. The features depend on the organ being involved. The disease may affect any organ.

3. Patients with tuberous sclerosis tend to develop rhabdomyoma in the heart.

4. The echogenic structures represent the fat in angiomyolipomas. Patients with tuberous sclerosis tend to develop renal angiomyolipomas.

5. The mass is giant cell astrocytoma. Patients with tuberous sclerosis tend to develop giant cell astrocytoma that arises from the ependymal lining of the foramen of Monro.

Pearls

- Tuberous sclerosis is a genetic disease that affects many organs.
- Classically, the Vogt's classic triad was known as mental retardation, epilepsy, and cutaneous facial angiofibromas, but many other clinical features may be observed, depending on the affected organ.
- Patients tend to develop pneumothoraces if lungs are affected.
- Experimental treatment with Rapamycin (mTOR pathway inhibitor) shows reduction in size and number of angiofibromas.

Suggested Reading

Liu H, Cooke K, Frager D. Bilateral massive renal angiomyolipomatosis in tuberous sclerosis. *AJR Am J Roentgenol.* 2005;185(4):1085-1086.

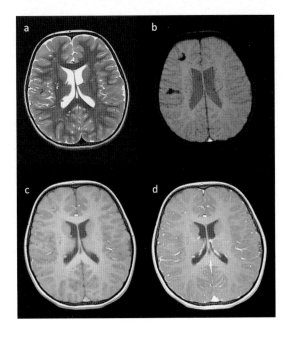

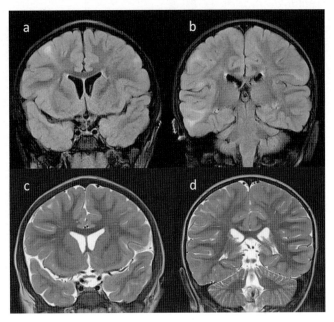

1. What are the three most important findings?

2. What is your diagnosis?

3. What is the other name for this entity?

4. What are the most common complications
   in this entity?

5. Where do calcifications occur in this entity?

Case ranking/difficulty:

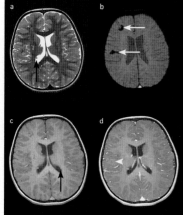

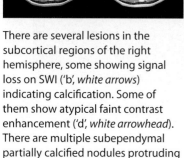

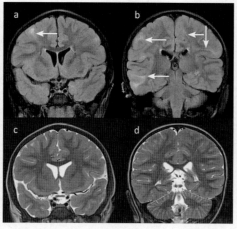

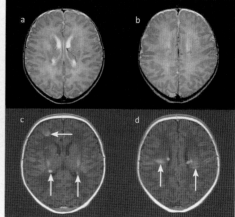

There are several lesions in the subcortical regions of the right hemisphere, some showing signal loss on SWI ('b', *white arrows*) indicating calcification. Some of them show atypical faint contrast enhancement ('d', *white arrowhead*). There are multiple subependymal partially calcified nodules protruding into the ventricles ('a', 'c', *black arrows*).

Multiple triangular-shaped signal hyperintensities best seen on FLAIR, which are typically cortex-based and pointing to the ventricle system ('a', 'b', *white arrows*). These represent dysmyelination along migration bands of abnormal giant cells and are barely seen on T2WI ('c', 'd').

In neonates, cortical tubers, white matter linear signal alterations, and subependymal nodules are all best seen on T1WI demonstrating highly T1 hyperintensities ('c', 'd', *white arrows*) and barely visible on T2WI ('a', 'b').

Answers

1. Neuroimaging findings in tuberous sclerosis complex are primarily driven by the presence of abnormal giant cells, which do not migrate normally. These cells accumulate at the subependymal level (producing subependymal nodules), induce myelination deficits along their migration pathway (leading to FLAIR hyperintense bands), and finally produce layering and myelination abnormalities in the cortical and subcortical regions (leading to cortical tubers).

2. The combination of subependymal nodules (which are accumulations of abnormal giant cells and do not show normal neuronal tissue and therefore are not to be confused with heterotopias), linear white matter signal alterations (which correspond to dysmyelination bands along migration of abnormal cells), and cortical tubers is characteristic for tuberous sclerosis complex.

3. Désirée-Magloire Bourneville was a French neurologist who was the first to perform autopsy and describe this entity. He was especially impressed by the many enlarged and protruding cerebral gyri (tuber is a bump or swelling in Latin). John James Pringle was an English dermatologist who described the facial skin rash called adenoma sebaceum and known nowadays as facial angiofibroma.

4. The number of cortical tubers is directly related with the mental cognitive abilities and the presence and severity of epilepsy. At the level of the foramen of Monro, growing subependymal nodules indicate their transformation into giant cell astrocytoma, which eventually will cause CSF flow obstruction and hydrocephalus.

5. Calcifications are characteristically present within the subependymal nodules, but cortical tubers may also calcify, whether they are located in the cerebral or cerebellar hemispheres.

Pearls

- Subependymal nodules consist of an accumulation of abnormal giant cells, which are progenitor cells for both neurons and astrocytes.
- Linear white matter signal alterations on FLAIR are myelination alterations along bands of migration anomalies showing scattered giant cells.
- Cortical tubers show evidence of layering disorder and dysmyelination.
- Subependymal nodules and cortical tubers may calcify.

Suggested Readings

Daghistani R, Widjaja E. Role of MRI in patient selection for surgical treatment of intractable epilepsy in infancy. *Brain Dev*. 2013;35(8):697-705.

Kalantari BN, Salamon N. Neuroimaging of tuberous sclerosis: spectrum of pathologic findings and frontiers in imaging. *AJR Am J Roentgenol*. 2008;190(5):W304-W309.

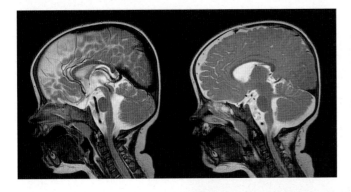
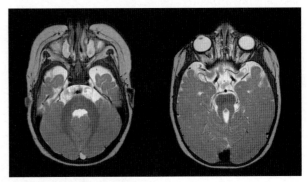

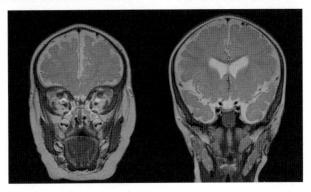

1. What are the characteristic findings of this entity?

2. Which white matter tracts have an aberrant course in this entity?

3. What are the clinical signs associated with this entity?

4. What is the red dot spot?

5. Which visceral organ may be involved in this entity?

Case ranking/difficulty: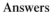

Category: Head

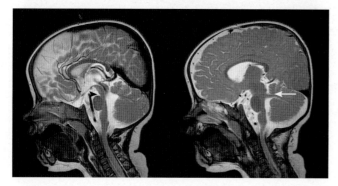

Absence of typical vermian lobules in the midline. Horizontally oriented superior cerebellar peduncles (*white arrow*). Brain stem is too small and the tegmentopontine sulcus is deepened (*black arrowhead*).

Answers

1. Vermis agenesis may be subtotal and small dysplasia elements can be found in the uppermost part. The absence of midline structure dictates the form of the fourth ventricle, which takes a batwing appearance. Cerebellar hemispheres are opposed but never fused (in contrary to rhombencephalosynapsis). There is also a deformity of the superior cerebellar peduncles, which take a molar tooth configuration in the axial plane and a horizontal direction in the parasagittal plane.

2. In Joubert syndrome, there is a failure of decussation of the corticospinal (pyramidal) tract at the level of the lower medulla, and also a lack of decussation of the dentatorubral and dentatothalamic tracts, both running parallel within the superior cerebellar peduncle.

3. In a neonate or young child with developmental delay, muscular hypotonia and abnormal eye movements related to ocular apraxia must trigger neuroimaging to exclude brain stem and cerebellar anomalies. These are obligate features of Jouberts syndrome, but can also be found in other entities as Cogan syndrome. Respiration anomaly is frequent.

4. Superior cerebellar peduncles and their dentorubral and dentospinal tracts decussate at the anterior tegmentum immediately above the pons. This right-left fiber decussation is readily identified as a "red spot" on DTI and is absent in Joubert syndrome. Absence of decussation may explain the hypoplasia at the mesencephalopontine sulcus seen on sagittal images. Hypoplasia of the brain stem has been associated with dyspnea/apnea symptoms that occur in many Joubert patients.

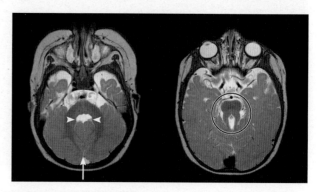

Absence of midline vermian structures with apposition of cerebellar hemispheres (*white arrow*) and abnormal batwing deformation of the fourth ventricle (*white arrowheads*). At the level of the superior cerebellar peduncles, the typical molar tooth sign is shown (*black circle*).

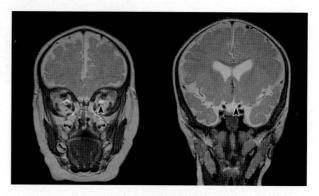

Absence of left optic nerve from retrobulbar up to the prechiasmatic region (*outlined black arrowheads*).

5. Especially in Joubert patients showing AHI1 mutation, there is a higher incidence of chronic kidney disease especially nephronophthisis and retinal dystrophy.

Pearls

- Vermian hypoplasia/aplasia.
- Horizontal superior cerebellar peduncles.
- Molar tooth aspect of the brainstem with posterior curvilinear pointing of the superior cerebellar peduncles.
- Optic nerve aplasia/hypoplasia is associated with retinal dystrophy.

Suggested Reading

Romani M, Micalizzi A, Valente EM. Joubert syndrome: congenital cerebellar ataxia with the molar tooth. *Lancet Neurol.* 2013;12(9):894-905.

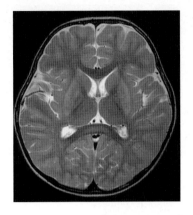
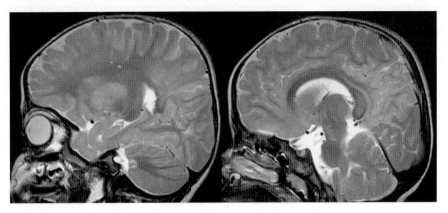

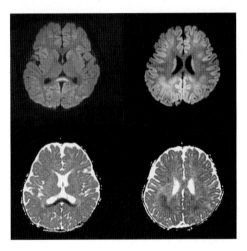
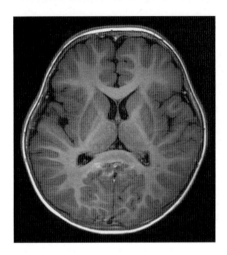

1. What are the findings?

2. What is the most probable diagnosis in the clinical context?

3. What is the differential diagnosis?

4. What are the treatment options?

5. What is the usual outcome after therapy is initiated?

Case ranking/difficulty: **Category:** Head

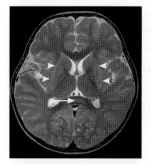

T2-hyperintensity in the splenium of the corpus callosum (*white arrow*) and the putamen bilaterally (*white arrowheads*).

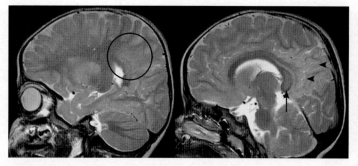

Diffuse T2-hyperintensity in the cortex of precuneus in the parietal lobe (*black arrowheads*), the deep parietal white matter (*black circle*), and the splenium of the corpus callosum (*black arrow*).

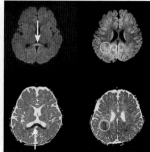

Upper row: DWI; Lower row: ADC maps diffusion restriction is seen in the deep white matter bilaterally, more on the right side (*white circle*) and within the splenium of the corpus callosum (*white arrow*).

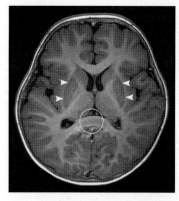

The demyelinated areas (*white arrowheads* and *white circle*) are slightly T1-hypointense without contrast enhancement.

Answers

1. Multifocal T2-hyperintensity in cortical regions (precuneus bilaterally), deep white matter areas (parietal lobe bilaterally and splenium of corpus callosum), and deep gray matter areas (putamen bilaterally). Diffusion restriction is limited to the white matter areas.

2. The combination of T2WI-FLAIR hyperintensity of cortex, white matter, and basal ganglia in the context of an acute encephalopathic child is highly suggestive of ADEM.

3. Viral encephalitis, especially of herpetic origin, cannot be excluded. The classic adult pattern of limbic system involvement and hemorrhagic component in herpetic encephalitis is not the rule in children. Some of the children diagnosed with ADEM may relapse a second or several times. In the setting of a multiple relapsing disease, the diagnosis may be revised and multiple sclerosis must be considered.

4. ADEM is treated primarily with steroidal therapy. Nevertheless, at presentation, as herpetic encephalitis cannot be excluded (neither clinically nor from neuroimaging), anti-herpetic treatment is always initiated until PCR-test from the CSF tapping returns negative.

5. After steroidal therapy, the outcome of ADEM is usually excellent.

Pearls

- ADEM is a multifocal demyelinating immune-mediated disease that may also involve the brainstem, cerebellum, and spinal cord.
- Demyelination involves not only white but also gray matter (cortex and basal ganglia may all be involved at the same time).
- Usually, some lesions may show DWI hyperintensity, but true restriction in the ADC maps is exceptional.
- Contrast enhancement is rare.

Suggested Readings

Leake JA, Albani S, Kao AS, et al. Acute disseminated encephalomyelitis in childhood: epidemiologic, clinical and laboratory features. *Pediatr Infect Dis J*. 2004;23(8):756-764.

Marin SE, Callen DJ. The magnetic resonance imaging appearance of monophasic acute disseminated encephalomyelitis: an update post application of the 2007 consensus criteria. *Neuroimaging Clin N Am*. 2013;23(2):245-266.

Tenembaum SN. Acute disseminated encephalomyelitis. *Handb Clin Neurol*. 2013;112:1253-1262.

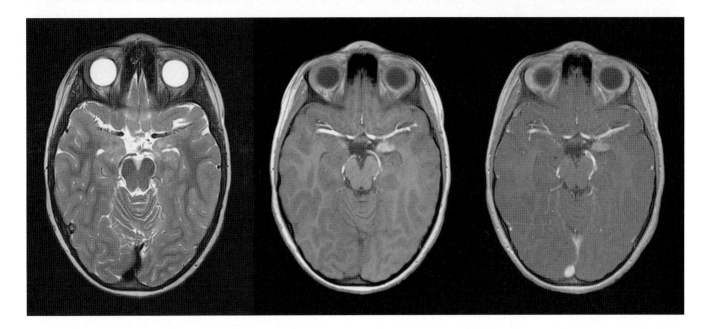

1. What are the findings?

2. What is your diagnosis?

3. Which other structure must be looked after?

4. Which malformation can be associated with this entity?

5. Which clinical signs may be associated with this entity?

Case ranking/difficulty:

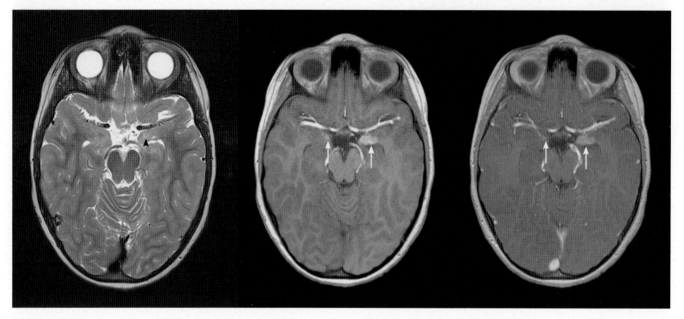

Predominantly left-sided T1-hyperintense lesions within the amygdala (*white arrows*) without contrast enhancement. The lesion is slightly T2-hyperintense (*black arrowhead*).

Answers

1. In the presence of pigmented/melanocytic cutaneous nevi, T1-hyperintense lesions most probably represent melanin deposition. These deposits may also show some T2-shortening (which is not the case here).

2. In the clinical context, and in the absence of malignant transformation of melanocytic nevi into a melanoma in which case metastasis could be considered, neurocutaneous melanosis is the most probable diagnosis.

3. In neurocutaneous melanosis, melanin deposition may occur within the leptomeninges of the brain and the spine, which can eventually obstruct CSF flow due to benign overgrowth.

4. In children affected by this phakomatosis, a Dandy-Walker malformation has been described in 8 to 10% of cases, and an association with Sturge-Weber has also been described.

5. Seizures are probably related to the superficial infiltration of the cortex by the leptomeningeal melanosis, which also leads to CSF flow obstruction and hydrocephalus. In the presence of spinal leptomeningeal infiltration, medullar compression with bladder control loss and cauda equina symptoms may occur.

Pearls

- Melanin is hyperintense on native T1WI.
- Melanin deposition occurs frequently in the amygdala and more rarely within the leptomeninges.
- Leptomeningeal overgrowth produces CSF obstruction and hydrocephalus.
- Spinal canal may be simultaneously involved.

Suggested Readings

Alikhan A, Ibrahimi OA, Eisen DB. Congenital melanocytic nevi: where are we now? Part I. Clinical presentation, epidemiology, pathogenesis, histology, malignant transformation, and neurocutaneous melanosis. *J Am Acad Dermatol.* 2012;67(4):495.e1-e17;quiz 512-514.

Ramaswamy V, Delaney H, Haque S, Marghoob A, Khakoo Y. Spectrum of central nervous system abnormalities in neurocutaneous melanocytosis. *Dev Med Child Neurol.* 2012;54(6):563-568.

Shah KN. The risk of melanoma and neurocutaneous melanosis associated with congenital melanocytic nevi. *Semin Cutan Med Surg.* 2010;29(3):159-164.

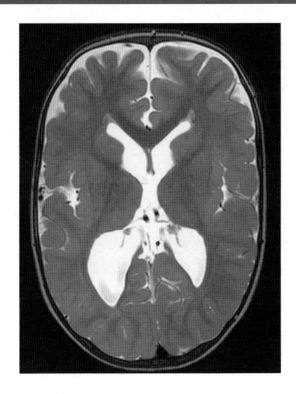 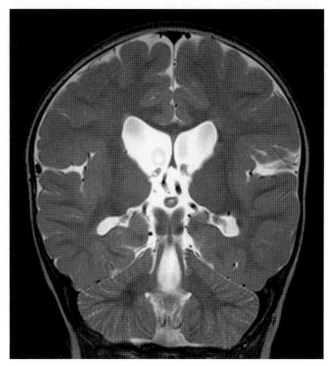

1. What are the findings?

2. What are the radiological characteristics of the affected area?

3. Which syndrome may present with similar malformation?

4. What is a common infectious etiology of this entity?

5. Which other cerebral anomaly may be associated?

Case ranking/difficulty:

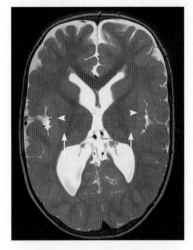

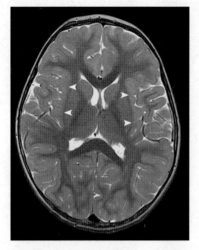

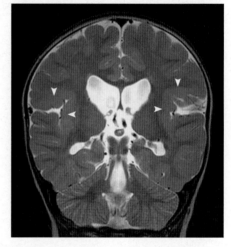

The cortex of the sylvian fissure is bilaterally thickened and shows too small gyri (*arrowheads*). The sylvian fissure itself is vertically oriented with typical T form and a shortened anteroposterior length. Ventricles are malformed and dilated. Putamen is moderately atrophic (*arrows*).

For comparison purposes, note the normal appearance of the sylvian fissure and gyrification of the insula in this normal control (*arrowheads*).

Polymicrogyria areas of the complete insular cortex with participation of the adjacent frontal areas (*arrowheads*).

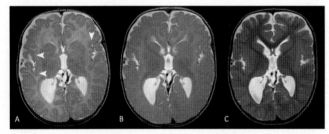

A: 4 months, B: 9 months, C: 19 months. This time series from the same patient illustrates the different appearances of polymicrogyria through age. Especially in neonates, thickening of the cortex is subtle but the blurring of the gray-white matter junction is more evident (*arrowheads*). It also demonstrates that due to ongoing myelination, imaging between 6 and 20 months should be avoided because of the intrinsic poor differentiation between cortex and white matter.

Answers

1. Bilateral polymicrogyria around the sylvian fissure and insula with atrophy of the basal ganglia (especially the putamen) and the corpus callosum (body and splenium on the coronal image) are present. The dilatation of the ventricle system is of malformative nature.

2. In polymicrogyria, the cortical ribbon demonstrates only four disorganized layers and is thinned (normal cortex has 6 layers). But due to the crowding of the many small gyri, there is a thickened appearance on MRI. Furthermore, the transition between cortex and white matter is blurred and wavy.

3. Zellweger disease (a peroxisomal disorder) presents with bilateral polymicrogyria especially located at the central region.

4. Cytomegalovirus infection, especially during the first trimester, may lead to disorganized cortical folding and polymicrogyria, which can be focal, unilateral or bilateral, and extensive.

5. In schizencephaly, there may be adjacent areas showing polymicrogyria. Microcephaly is more often present than macrocephaly. In extensive polymicrogyria, the deep white matter shows myelination deficiency or delay.

Pearls

- Cortical thickening due to polymicrogyria at the sylvian fissure on both sides.
- Sylvian fissure has an abnormal vertical orientation.
- There may be a variable extension in the adjacent cortical areas.
- Ventricles are often dilated and malformed.
- The appearance of polymicrogyria changes during the myelination process within the first 2 years of life.

Suggested Reading

Gropman AL, Barkovich AJ, Vezina LG, Conry JA, Dubovsky EC, Packer RJ. Pediatric congenital bilateral perisylvian syndrome: clinical and MRI features in 12 patients. *Neuropediatrics*. 1997;28(4):198-203.

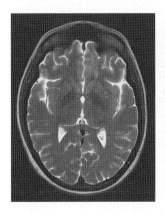 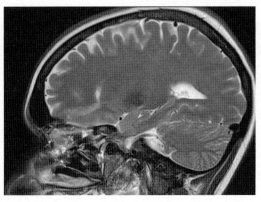 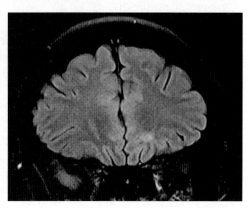

1. What are the findings?

2. Which complementary imaging can be done?

3. Which syndrome may be seen in association with this entity?

4. Which malformations can be associated with this entity?

5. What is the transmantle sign?

Case ranking/difficulty: **Category:** Head

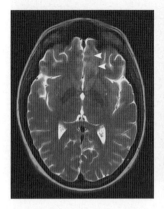 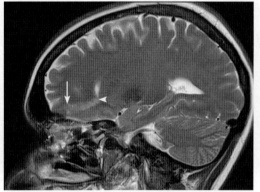 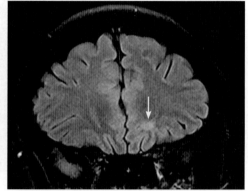

There is a band of abnormal tissue intensity frontopolar on the left side with blurring of the delineation between cortex and white matter (*arrowheads*).

The abnormal tissue has a triangular/conal form, based at the cortex (*arrow*) and pointing to the ventricular wall to which it abuts (*arrowhead*).

The lesion is most conspicuous on FLAIR with distinct signal hyperintensity (*arrow*).

Answers

1. Blurring of the corticomedullary junction and triangular cortex-based band of tissue hyperintensity is characteristic for focal cortical dysplasia.

2. Especially in intractable seizures with negative MRI findings, FDG PET may pick up the region of hypometabolism where the FCD is located.

3. In tuberous sclerosis complex (TSC), cytoarchitectonic anomalies may resemble focal cortical dysplasia, producing a similar neuroradiological appearance. Therefore, a formal clinical check-up to exclude TSC must be made.

4. Anomalies in cellular components and in cortical architecture can be found in the vicinity of tumors (especially ganglioglioma and DNET), but also at the periphery of vascular malformations.

5. The transmantle sign describes the fact that the malformation extends from the cortex to the ventricular wall, through the whole cerebral mantle (transmantle).

Pearls

- Cortex-based conical T2WI/FLAIR hyperintensity between cortex and side ventricle.
- T2WI and FLAIR hyperintensity is due to hypomyelination, different cellular constituents, and water content within the malformation.
- The transmantle conical form of the malformation indicates that a functional anomaly of the radial glial fibers is implicated during fetal neuronal migration.
- Highly epileptogenic focus often drug-resistant.
- Surgery may be considered.

Suggested Reading

Blümcke I, Thom M, Aronica E, et al. The clinicopathologic spectrum of focal cortical dysplasias: a consensus classification proposed by an ad hoc Task Force of the ILAE Diagnostic Methods Commission. *Epilepsia.* 2011;52(1):158-174.

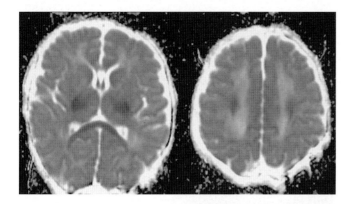
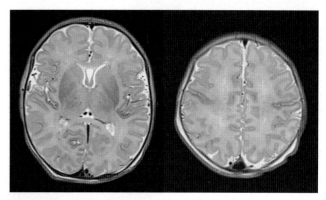
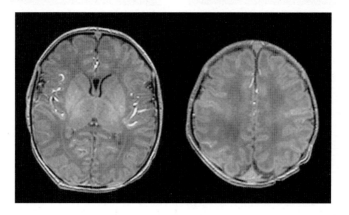

1. What are the findings?

2. What are possible causes of hypoxic-ischemic injury in term neonates?

3. What is the treatment of this condition?

4. What is the best timing for MR imaging of asphyctic neonates?

5. What is the aim of the cooling procedure?

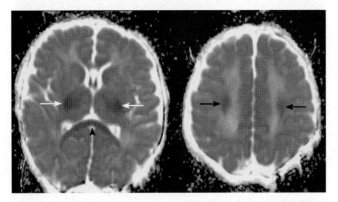

Diffusion restriction is seen at the PLIC, the ventrolateral thalamus and the posterolateral putamen (*white arrows*), the corona radiata (*black arrows*), and the splenium of corpus callosum (*arrowhead*).

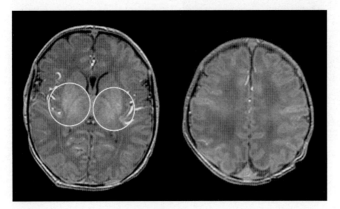

There is a characteristic T1-hyperintensity within the ventrolateral thalamus and dorsolateral putamina, and an absence of the myelinated part of corticospinal tracts within the posterior limb of the internal capsule (*large circles*).

Answers

1. Thalamus, putamen, and the corticospinal tracts are involved in this case. The gray matter at the central region appears spared, probably a consequence of the whole body cooling. Diffuse white matter edema and T2-hyperintensity are present (also in the splenium of the corpus callosum).

2. All of the listed conditions may result in impairment of circulation and pre-/perinatal asphyxia.

3. Placing the neonates at room temperature to reduce core temperature to 30°.

4. Immediately after birth, DWI may be negative, even in case of severe ischemia. Therefore, immediate cooling procedure is initiated first. Best time to detect diffusion restriction is between days 3 and 5. After that period, ADC values increase again, a phenomenon known as "pseudonormalization". Therefore, imaging after day 7 is not recommended.

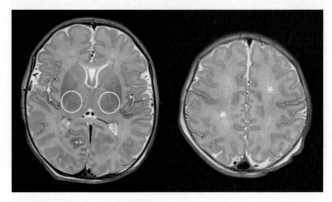

There is diffuse white matter T2-hyperintensity (*asterisks*) and inhomogeneity of the ventrolateral thalamus (*circles*).

5. Primary aim of whole body cooling is to protect the neurons in the cortex from the secondary energy failure, which results from the reperfusion of the ischemic areas. The white matter and the basal ganglia are less influenced by the procedure.

Pearls

- Neonatal asphyxia is due to interruption of normal blood supply during labor.
- The pattern of injury depends upon the length and the severity of ischemia.
- The severity of the clinical picture is mainly dependent on the amount of basal ganglia involved.
- Cooling is the treatment of choice.
- MRI is best to demonstrate the amount of ischemic injury immediately after the cooling procedure (generally at days 3 to 6).
- After day 7/8, there is a risk of missing the diffusion restriction on ADC maps because pseudonormalization of the diffusion values occurs around day 10.

Suggested Readings

Alderliesten T, de Vries LS, Benders MJ, Koopman C, Groenendaal F. MR imaging and outcome of term neonates with perinatal asphyxia: value of diffusion-weighted MR imaging and ¹H MR spectroscopy. *Radiology.* 2011;261(1):235-242.

Bednarek N, Mathur A, Inder T, Wilkinson J, Neil J, Shimony J. Impact of therapeutic hypothermia on MRI diffusion changes in neonatal encephalopathy. *Neurology.* 2012;78(18):1420-1427.

van Laerhoven H, de Haan TR, Offringa M, Post B, van der Lee JH. Prognostic tests in term neonates with hypoxic-ischemic encephalopathy: a systematic review. *Pediatrics.* 2013;131(1):88-98.

2-year-old female with leukocoria

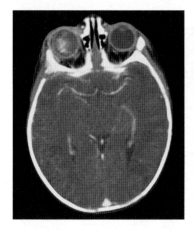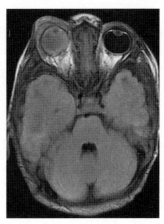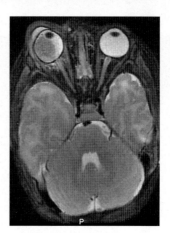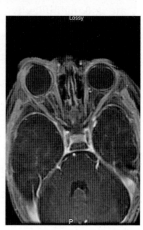

1. What are the findings?

2. What is the most likely diagnosis?

3. What is the differential diagnosis?

4. What is the peak age of the disease?

5. What is the treatment?

Case ranking/difficulty:

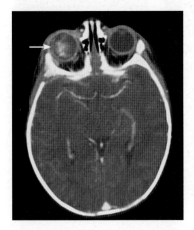

Contrast-enhanced axial CT of the orbits in soft tissue window reveals a calcified mass inside the right orbit (*arrow*).

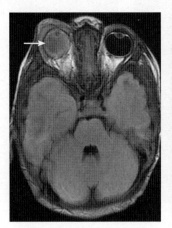

Axial MRI, FLAIR, of the orbits reveals a mass in the right orbit (*arrow*).

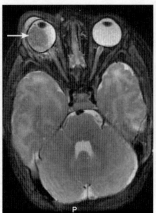

Axial T2 MRI of the orbits reveals a mass in the right orbit (*arrow*).

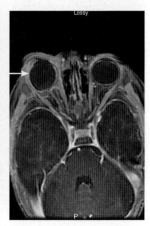

Axial T1 contrast MRI of the orbits reveals enhancing mass in the right orbit (*arrow*).

Answers

1. CT reveals a calcified mass in the right orbit. MRI reveals low signal of the mass in T1 and T2.

2. The most likely diagnosis is retinoblastoma.

3. Differential diagnosis may include retinopathy of prematurity, uveitis, retinal detachment, vitreous hemorrhage, and congenital cataract.

4. The peak age of the disease is 0 to 5 years.

5. Treatment of the disease includes chemotherapy, radiation, and, in extreme cases, enucleation.

Pearls

- Retinoblastoma is a malignancy of the retina.
- It is the most common eye tumor in children, usually occurring before the age of 5.
- The most common presenting clinical sign is leukocoria. Other visual disturbances may be present.
- Tumor can be calcified.
- In MRI, retinoblastoma has low signal in T1 and T2.

Suggested Readings

Abramson DH, Frank CM, Susman M, Whalen MP, Dunkel IJ, Boyd NW 3rd. Presenting signs of retinoblastoma. *J Pediatr.* 1998;132(3 Pt 1):505-508.

de Graaf P, Barkhof F, Moll AC, et al. Retinoblastoma: MR imaging parameters in detection of tumor extent. *Radiology.* 2005;235(1):197-207.

Ts'o MO, Zimmerman LE, Fine BS. The nature of retinoblastoma, I: photoreceptor differentiation: a clinical and histopathological study. *Am J Ophthalmol.* 1970;69:339-349.

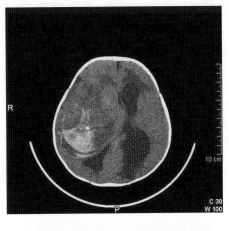
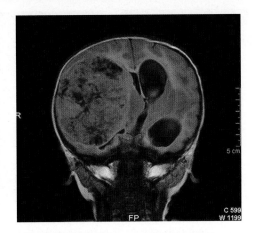
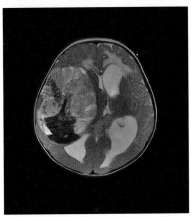
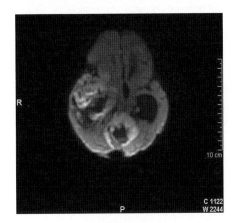

1. What are the findings?

2. What is the diagnosis?

3. Where does this entity most commonly occur?

4. What is the tumor that this entity is often misdiagnosed?

5. How is the definitive diagnosis made?

Case ranking/difficulty:

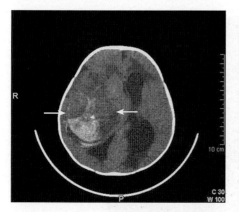

Axial CT of the head demonstrates a large heterogeneous mass in the right cerebral hemisphere with associated hemorrhage and calcification (*arrows*). Hydrocephalus seen with significant subfalcine herniation.

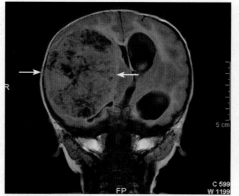

Coronal MRI FLAIR demonstrates a large supratentorial lesion in the right cerebral hemisphere, which has heterogeneous appearance and multiple areas of necrosis and hemorrhage (*arrows*). It is producing compression of the right lateral ventricle as well as right-to-left midline shift.

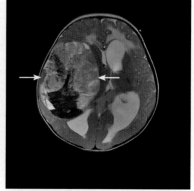

Axial MRI T2 demonstrates a large supratentorial lesion in the right cerebral hemisphere, which has heterogeneous appearance and multiple areas of necrosis and hemorrhage (*arrows*). It produces compression of the right lateral ventricle as well as right-to-left midline shift.

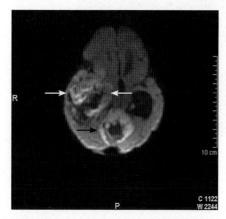

Axial MRI DWI demonstrates a large supratentorial lesion in the right cerebral hemisphere, which has heterogeneous appearance and multiple areas of necrosis and hemorrhage (*white arrows*). It produces compression of the right lateral ventricle as well as right-to-left midline shift. Increased diffusion restriction noted. The *black arrow* demonstrates increased diffusion restriction of the cerebellar vermis lesion.

Answers

1. Axial CT–A large heterogeneous mass in the right cerebral hemisphere with associated hemorrhage and calcification. Hydrocephalus seen with significant subfalcine herniation.

   MRI–A large supratentorial mass in the right cerebral hemisphere. It produces compression on the right lateral ventricle and right-to-left midline shift. A second mass seen in the upper and anterior portion of the cerebellar vermis.

2. The diagnosis is atypical teratoid rhabdoid tumor.

3. ATRT most commonly occurs in the cerebellopontine angle.

4. ATRTs are often misdiagnosed as primitive neuroectodermal tumors (PNET).

5. Definitive diagnosis of ATRT rests ultimately on immunohistochemical studies: the majority of these tumors are positive for epithelial membrane antigen, vimentin, and smooth-muscle actin, and negative for markers for germ-cell tumors, differentiating them from PNET.

Pearls

- ATRTs are rare childhood intracranial tumors that most commonly present before 2 years of age.
- Often misdiagnosed as PNET.
- Generally, patients present with classic symptoms of increased intracranial pressure, such as headache, vomiting, lethargy, and failure to thrive.
- The tumor classically appears as a bulky, heterogeneous, and solid cystic mass.
- Definitive diagnosis of ATRT rests ultimately on immunohistochemical studies.

Suggested Readings

Fenton LZ, Foreman NK. Atypical teratoid/rhabdoid tumor of the central nervous system in children: an atypical series and review. *Pediatr Radiol.* 2003;33(8):554-558.

Tang A, Franco A, Figueroa RE. Atypical Teratoid/Rhabdoid Tumor. Unknown case #30, SPR web site May 26-June 13, 2010. <http://mirc.childrensmemorial.org/storage/ss12/docs/20100526103632328/MIRCdocument.xml>.

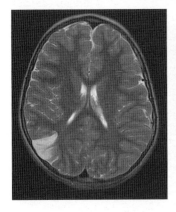
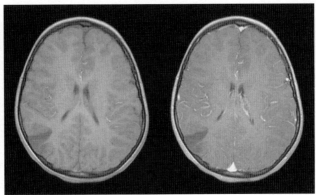
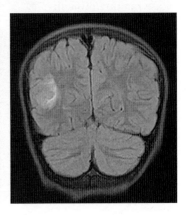

1. What are the findings?

2. What is the FLAIR ring sign?

3. What is the differential diagnosis?

4. Which are the predilection sites of this entity?

5. Which other anomaly may be associated with this entity?

Case ranking/difficulty: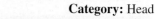

Category: Head

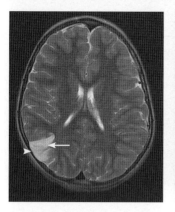

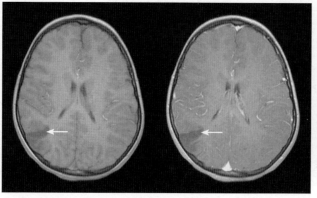

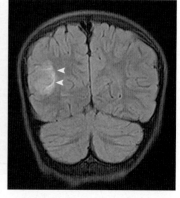

Cortical thickening of the right angular gyrus with very small intratumoral cysts (*arrow*). Vault scalloping is seen over the tumor (*arrowhead*).

The tumor is homogeneously T1-hypointense and does not show contrast enhancement (*arrows*).

The intracortical part of the tumor is isointense to normal cortex on FLAIR, but the periphery and white matter delimitation show a typical FLAIR-hyperintense ring (the "FLAIR ring sign", *arrowheads*).

Answers

1. The cortical thickening represents the tumor itself, infiltrating the cortical ribbon with displacement and blurring of the gray-white matter border. There are tiny intratumoral cysts, and contrast enhancement is usually absent (only 20% of cases). The overlying skull scalloping is due to the chronic pressure from the underlying tumor (which is a nonspecific but characteristic finding in slow-growing superficial tumors).

2. The "FLAIR ring sign" is demonstrated: this is a peripheral complete or incomplete FLAIR hyperintensity ring, whereas the cortical center of the tumor remains iso-, hypointense.

3. Dysembryoplastic neuroepithelial tumor (DNET) but also unspecific glioneuronal tumors or ganglioglioma arise within the cortical ribbon. In low-grade fibrillary astrocytoma, the tumor is primarily located within the white matter of the gyrus itself and tends only secondarily to invade the cortex. PNET must always be considered, but DNET is a low-grade slowly progressive tumor, whereas PNET is a high-grade rapidly progressive tumor that often metastasizes in the subarachnoideal space.

4. DNET and ganglioglioma have a predilection for cortex belonging to the limbic system (amygdala, hippocampus, temporal lobe, insula, and cingulate gyrus).

5. Classically, almost 80% of DNET have adjacent areas demonstrating foci of cortical dysplasia.

Pearls

- Low-grade tumor in cortical location.
- Mostly located at the limbic system.
- May present with small intratumoral cysts.
- FLAIR hyperintense ring (the "ring sign").
- Typically does not enhance.
- May produce scalloping of the skull.
- Surgery is curative.

Suggested Reading

Parmar HA, Hawkins C, Ozelame R, Chuang S, Rutka J, Blaser S. Fluid-attenuated inversion recovery ring sign as a marker of dysembryoplastic neuroepithelial tumors. *J Comput Assist Tomogr.* 2007;31(3):348-353.

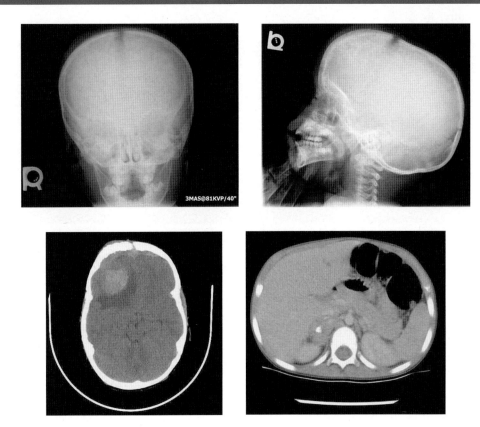

1. What are the findings in the plain skull radiographs?

2. What are the findings in the brain CT?

3. What are the findings in the abdominal CT?

4. What is included in the differential diagnosis of the brain CT image?

5. How is stage MS of the INRGSS staging system being treated?

Case ranking/difficulty:

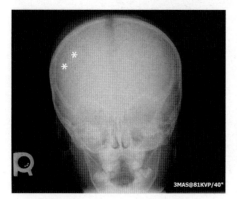

Frontal radiograph of the skull reveals mottle densities representing calcifications dispersed through the right side of the skull (*asterisks*).

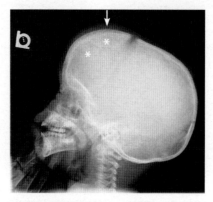

Lateral radiograph of the skull reveals mottle densities representing calcifications dispersed through the skull (*asterisks*). The periosteum is involved. Soft tissue swelling noted (*arrow*).

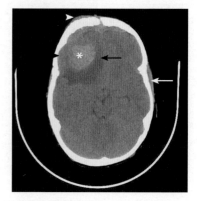

Axial CT of the head shows intraparenchymal bleed in the right frontal lobe (*asterisk*). Edema noted around the hemorrhage (*black arrows*). Subdural hematoma noted. There is bifrontal epidural collection with displacement of the superior sagittal sinus leftward. This is most probably due to subperiosteal metastasis and tumor infiltration of the epidural space. A subcutaneous soft tissue swelling noted on the side of the right frontal lobe (*arrowhead*). There is also subcutaneous soft tissue swelling on the opposite side (*white arrow*).

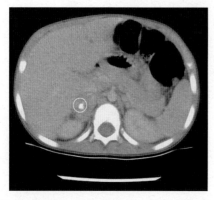

Axial CT of the abdomen reveals a mass in the right adrenal gland. Calcifications noted in the mass (*circle*).

Answers

1. There is thickening of the diploic space, calcifications, and soft tissue swelling.

2. CT reveals intraparenchymal hemorrhage, vasogenic edema around the bleed, soft tissue swelling, and subfalcine herniation.

3. The abdominal CT reveals a calcified mass in the region of the right adrenal gland.

4. The differential diagnosis may include astrocytoma, atypical teratoid rhabdoid tumor, relapse of acute lymphoblastic leukemia (ALL), and intracerebral hemorrhage.

5. Stage MS of the International Neuroblastoma Risk Group Staging System (INRGSS) is found in infants less than 1 year old. The tumor is already spread, but the malignant cells are less aggressive than in older children. Sometimes the tumor disappears without treatment. Low dose of radiation or low dose of chemotherapy may be used.

Pearls

- In children with solid tumors, brain metastasis is relatively uncommon.
- Brain metastasis occurs in 8% of cases of neuroblastoma.
- Neuroblastoma is the most common extracranial pediatric neoplasm and the third most common pediatric malignancy after leukemia and central nervous system tumors.
- Neuroblastomas can arise from anywhere along the sympathetic chain. About two-thirds of all neuroblastomas start in the abdomen, developing in the adrenal glands.
- Sometimes the neuroblastoma forms before birth, and in rare cases, a prenatal diagnosis can be made using ultrasound.

Suggested Readings

Monclair T, Brodeur GM, Ambros PF, et al. INRG Task Force. The International Neuroblastoma Risk Group (INRG) staging system: an INRG Task Force report. *J Clin Oncol.* 2009;27(2):298-303.

Posner J. Brain metastases: a clinician's view. In: Weiss L, Gilbert H, Posner J, eds. *Brain Metastases.* Boston: GK Hall; 1980:2-29.

Tasdemiroglu E, Patchell RA. Cerebral metastases in childhood malignancies. *Acta Neurochir.* 1997;139:182-187.

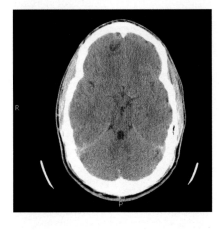 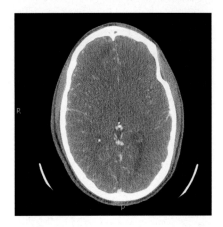 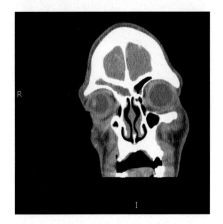

1. What are the findings?

2. What is the most likely etiology of this entity?

3. What are the clinical signs of this entity?

4. What is the most likely etiology for the lesion seen in the cerebrum?

5. What are the treatment options?

Case ranking/difficulty: **Category:** Head

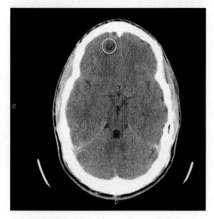

Noncontrast axial CT of the head demonstrates low attenuation in the right frontal lobe representing cerebritis (*circle*). The midline is slightly shifted to the left.

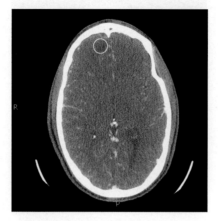

Contrast axial CT of the head demonstrates low attenuation in the right frontal lobe representing cerebritis (*circle*). The midline is slightly shifted to the left. Enhancement of the subdural space and the interhemispheric region adjacent to the area of cerebritis noted representing subdural empyema.

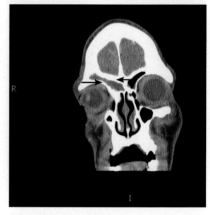

Coronal contrast CT of the head demonstrates opacification of the right frontal sinus (*arrows*). The right ethmoid and the right maxillary sinus are also partially opacified.

Answers

1. There is area of low attenuation in the right frontal lobe with midline shift to the left. Subdural empyema noted. The right frontal sinus is opacified.

2. The etiology is most likely bacterial infection. *Staphylococcus pneumoniae* and *Streptococcus pneumoniae* are the most likely community-acquired pathogens.

3. The clinical signs may include fever, headache, facial tenderness, and retro-orbital pain.

4. The most likely etiology for the lesion seen in the cerebrum is direct extension from the frontal sinus infection.

5. Treatment consists of neurology consultation and selection of appropriate antimicrobial therapy.

Pearls

- The frontal sinus develops at approximately the age of 10 years.
- Sinusitis is defined as an inflammation of the mucosal lining of one or more of the paranasal sinuses.
- Direct extension of infection can lead to cerebritis and the development of brain abscess.
- Risk factors include diseases that impair the muco-ciliary system.
- Cystic fibrosis is a risk factor.
- Imaging findings of sinusitis are mucosal thickenings, complete or partial opacification of the sinuses, and air-fluid levels in the acute phase.
- Imaging findings of cerebritis are low attenuation in CT with edema. If abscess develops, wall enhancement will be seen.

Suggested Readings

Benninger MS, Sedory Holzer SE, Lau J. Diagnosis and treatment of uncomplicated acute bacterial rhinosinusitis: summary of the Agency for Health Care Policy and Research evidence-based report. *Otolaryngol Head Neck Surg.* 2000;122(1):1-7.

Lusk RP, Stankiewicz JA. Pediatric rhinosinusitis. *Otolaryngol Head Neck Surg.* 1997;117(3 Pt 2):S53-S57.

6-year-old female with pain and tenderness in the neck anteriorly, above the level of the thyroid

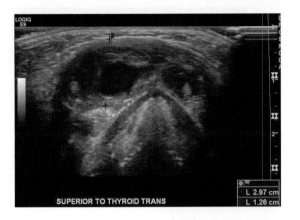

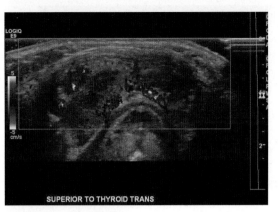

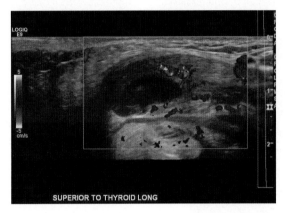

1. What is the most likely diagnosis?

2. What is the relevant embryology?

3. What are the clinical symptoms?

4. What is the most common location of this entity?

5. What are the treatment options?

Case ranking/difficulty:

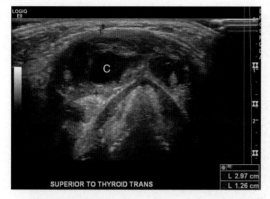

Transverse view sonography of the neck in the midline above the thyroid reveals a cystic structure (*C*) surrounded by inflammatory soft tissue.

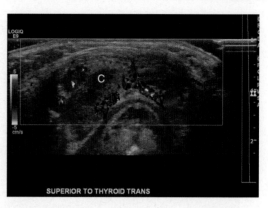

Transverse view sonography of the neck in the midline above the thyroid reveals a cystic structure (*C*) surrounded by inflammatory soft tissue. Increased blood flow seen.

5. Treatment of thyroglossal duct cyst is Sistrunk procedure that involves excision of the entire thyroglossal duct tract up to the foramen cecum and resection of hyoid bone. Simple aspiration of the cyst results in recurrence and is not recommended. Cyst aspiration with injection of OK-432 in the cyst as an alternative treatment has been tried and found to be effective by some researchers.

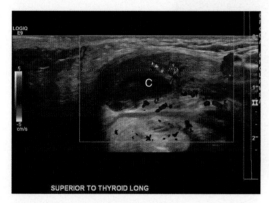

Longitudinal view sonography of the neck in the midline above the thyroid reveals a cystic structure (*C*) surrounded by inflammatory soft tissue. Increased blood flow seen.

Answers

1. The diagnosis is infected thyroglossal cyst.

2. Thyroid gland begins its development in the 4th gestational week as an endodermal swelling called tuberculum impar located on the floor of the pharynx between the 1st and the 2nd pharyngeal pouches. Tuberculum impar invaginates to form a diverticulum that descends in the midline through and around the hyoid bone to reach the normal location of thyroid in the neck. The thyroglossal duct involutes after 5th gestational week. Failure to involute results in persistence of a thyroglossal duct remnant or cyst.

3. Clinical symptoms may include palpable mass, neck pain, throat pain, and dysphagia. Patients can also be asymptomatic.

4. Thyroglossal duct cyst is commonly located at the infrahyoid or hyoid level. These cysts can also be seen in suprahyoid location. Rarely, they are seen in the tongue or in the mediastinum.

Pearls

- Site of the tuberculum impar becomes foramen cecum located at the dorsum of the tongue at the junction of anterior two-third and posterior one-third of the tongue.
- If the distal part of the thyroglossal duct fails to involute, pyramidal lobe of thyroid may form.
- Thyroglossal duct cyst may contain accessory thyroid tissue or it may be the only thyroid tissue in the patient.
- This thyroid tissue can rarely undergo malignant change with papillary carcinoma as the most common type.
- A mural nodule or calcification within the cyst may suggest malignancy.
- Enlarged lymph node may also suggest malignancy.
- Malignancy in the thyroglossal duct cyst may present with rapidly enlarging neck mass.
- Preferred treatment of thyroglossal duct cyst is Sistrunk procedure.

Suggested Readings

Acierno S, Waldhausen J. Congenital cervical cysts, sinuses and fistulae. *Otolaryngol Clin N Am.* 2007;40:161-176.

Deaver MJ, Silman EF, Lotfipour S. Infected thyroglossal duct cyst. *West J Emerg Med.* 2009;10(3):205.

Reede D, Bergeron R, Som P. CT of thyroglossal duct cysts. *Radiology.* 1985;157:121-125.

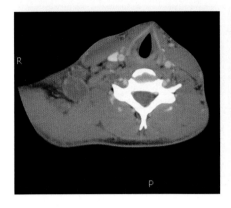 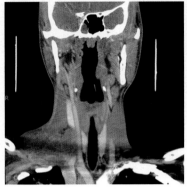 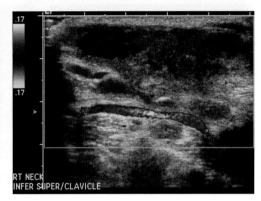

1. What are the findings?

2. What is the most likely diagnosis?

3. What is the common causative agent of this entity in children in the United States?

4. How does one make definitive diagnosis of this entity?

5. How does this entity present clinically?

Case ranking/difficulty: 🐞 🐞 🐞

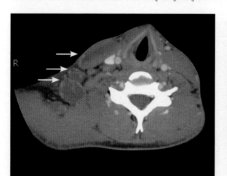

Axial contrast CT of the lower neck is remarkable for a cluster of low attenuation lymphadenopathy in the right supraclavicular cervical region (*arrows*).

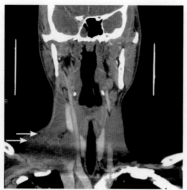

Coronal contrast CT of the neck is remarkable for a cluster of low attenuation lymphadenopathy in the right supraclavicular cervical region (*arrows*).

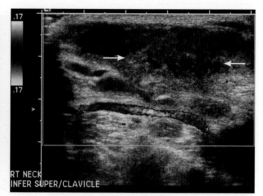

Ultrasound of the right supraclavicular cervical region shows a mixed cystic and solid fluid collection without increased peripheral flow (*arrows*). There are multiple fluid collections of mixed echogenicity adjacent to the larger fluid collection.

Answers

1. The CT and the ultrasound images demonstrate right supraclavicular cervical lymphadenopathy. The lymph nodes have low attenuation density in the CT and hypoechogenicity in ultrasound, consistent with necrotic lymphadenopathy.

2. Necrotic cervical lymph nodes with pulmonary opacities in a young patient are most likely due to tuberculosis. Tuberculous cervical lymphadenopathy is also known as scrofula.

3. The common causative agent of scrofula in children in the United States is *Mycobacterium scrofulaceum*.

4. The definitive diagnosis of scrofula is made by histology and culture of lymph node material.

5. Scrofula has an insidious onset and can be asymptomatic for a long duration. The cervical mass can be non-tender with or without induration of the overlying skin.

Pearls

- Cervical tuberculous lymphadenopathy is also called scrofula.
- Causative agent for scrofula in children in the United States is atypical mycobacteria *Mycobacterium scrofulaceum*.
- It is frequent in HIV-infected population.
- The onset is insidious.
- Cross-sectional images demonstrate enlarged cervical lymph nodes that may be necrotic.
- Surgical excision may be required as a definitive treatment.

Suggested Readings

Artenstein AW, Kim JH, Williams WJ, Chung RC. Isolated peripheral tuberculous lymphadenitis in adults: current clinical and diagnostic issues. *Clin Infect Dis*. 1995;20:876-882.

Dandapat MC, Mishra BM, Dash SP, Kar PK. Peripheral lymph node tuberculosis: a review of 80 cases. *Br J Surg*. 1990;77:911-912.

Kuhn L, Franco A. *Tuberculous Cervical Lymphadenitis*. Unknown case #28. SPR web site April 20-May 9, 2010. <http://mirc.childrensmemorial.org/storage/ss12/docs/20100420121950015/MIRCdocument.xml>.

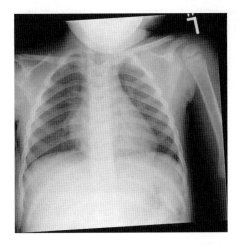
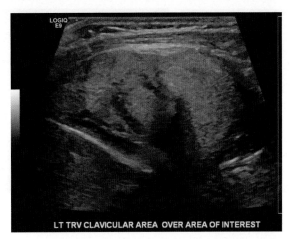

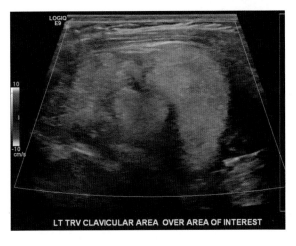
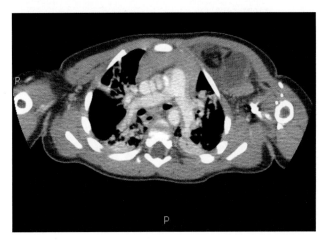

1. What are the findings?

2. What is included in the differential diagnosis?

3. Based on images, how will you differentiate between this entity and cystic hygroma?

4. What are the histologic features of this entity?

5. What is the most common age that this entity presents?

Case ranking/difficulty:

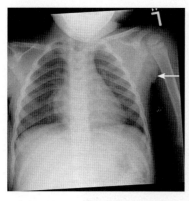

Frontal view of the chest demonstrates soft tissue swelling of the left axillary region with a lucent area (*arrow*) that represents fat.

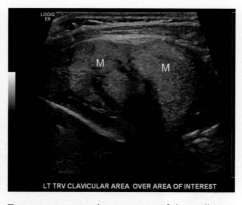

Transverse grayscale sonogram of the axillary region reveals a large echogenic mass (*M*).

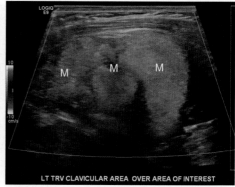

Transverse color sonogram of the axillary region reveals a large echogenic mass (*M*). The mass has no increased vascular supply.

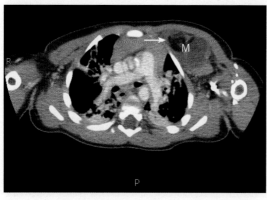

Axial CT of the upper chest reveals a mass in the left axillary region (*M*). The mass contains a region of low attenuation (*arrow*) representing fat. Note is made of airspace infiltrates in both lungs.

Pearls

- Lipoblastoma and lipoblastomatosis are uncommon benign mesenchymal lesions that predominantly occur in infancy and early childhood.
- It generally presents as asymptomatic mass that grows in size.
- Most commonly occur in the extremities, trunk, and abdomen.
- CT generally shows mostly fatty tissue with fibrous septae.
- Tumor composed of lipoblasts that abnormally proliferate during the postnatal period.
- Generally well circumscribed but can grow large enough to produce mass effects (a diffused form called lipoblastomatosis also exists).

Answers

1. Images reveal a left axillary mass containing fat.

2. Differential diagnosis includes lipoblastoma, liposarcoma, hematoma, teratoma, and cystic hygroma.

3. Cystic hygroma is mainly a cystic mass, while lipoblastoma is mainly solid. Both may contain septae. Cystic hygroma does not have fat, while lipoblastoma and teratoma contain fat elements.

4. Lipoblastoma is a benign tumor that develops from embryonic white fat. Histology shows immature and mature fat cells separated into lobules by fibrous septae containing vessels, collagen, and fibroblasts.

5. Ninety percent of the cases of lipoblastoma are diagnosed before the age of 3.

Suggested Readings

Chun YS, Kim WK, Park KW, et al. Lipoblastoma. *J Pediatr Surg*. 2001;36:905-907.

Coffin CM. Adipose and myxoid tumors. In: Coffin CM, Dehner LP, O'Shea PA, eds. *Pediatric Soft Tissue Tumors: A Clinical, Pathological, and Therapeutic Approach*. New Salt Lake City, Utah: JA Majors Company; 1997:254-276.

Moholkar S, Sebire NJ, Roebuck DJ. Radiological-pathological correlation in lipoblastoma and lipoblastomatosis. *Pediatr Radiol*. 2006;36:851-856.

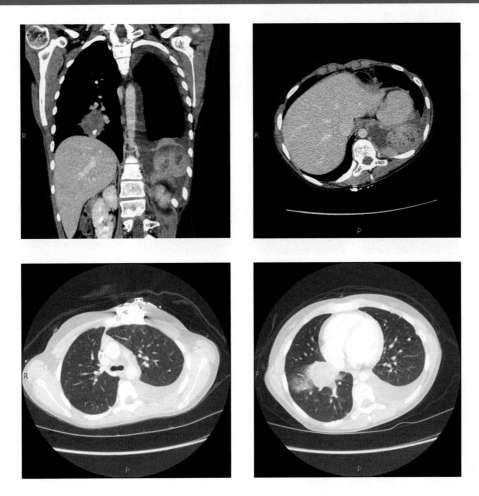

1. What are the findings?

2. What is the most common site of occurrence of primary osteosarcoma?

3. What is the most common site of metastasis from osteosarcoma?

4. What is the approximate percentage of lung metastases in patients with osteosarcoma?

5. What are the treatment options?

Case ranking/difficulty:

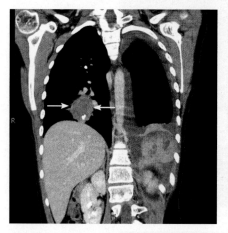

Coronal CT of the lungs. There is left-sided pleural effusion. There is round mass in the right lower lobe (*arrows*). Calcifications noted in the lower aspect of the mass. This represents metastasis from the patient's known osteosarcoma.

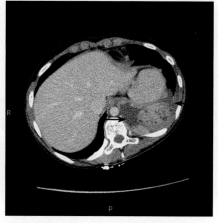

Axial CT of the lungs. There is left-sided pleural effusion. In the pleural cavity, there is a solid mass (*arrows*) with low attenuation foci inside. This represents pleural metastatic mass with areas of central necrosis.

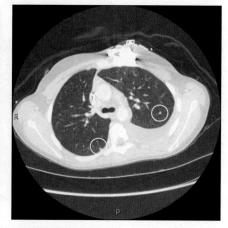

CT of the lungs in lung window demonstrates a nodule in the right upper lobe and a nodule in the left upper lobe (*circles*). The nodules represent metastatic lesions.

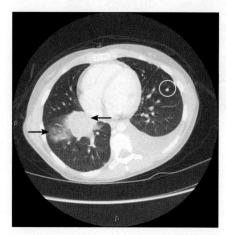

CT of the chest in lung window reveals a sub centimeter nodule in the left lower lobe (*circle*). The large mass seen in the coronal view is seen in the axial view (*arrows*) surrounding with density in its lateral aspect that represents compressive atelectasis.

4. Approximately 90% of patients with osteosarcoma will develop lung metastases.

5. In this particular case, surgery can be performed to remove the right lower lobe mass and the pleural cavity mass. However, if the disease is widespread, surgery is not an option and the treatment is mainly chemotherapy. Localized radiation can also be used.

Pearls

- Osteosarcoma is the third most common cancer in adolescence.
- Only lymphoma and brain tumors surpass osteosarcoma in frequency.
- Lung metastases are common occurrence in osteosarcoma and tend to calcify.
- Pleural metastases are less common.

Answers

1. There is a left-sided pleural effusion with a mass inside the pleural cavity. The mass has areas of low attenuation representing necrosis. There are multiple lung nodules with large mass in the right lower lobe. This represents metastatic disease from the patient's known osteosarcoma.

2. The most common site of occurrence of osteosarcoma is distal femur.

3. The lungs are the most common site of metastases from osteosarcoma.

Suggested Readings

Seo JB, Im JG, Goo JM, Chung MJ, Kim MY. Atypical pulmonary metastases: spectrum of radiologic findings. *Radiographics.* 2001;21(2):403-417.

Zwaga T, Bovée JV, Kroon HM. Osteosarcoma of the femur with skip, lymph node, and lung metastases. *Radiographics.* 2008;28(1):277-283.

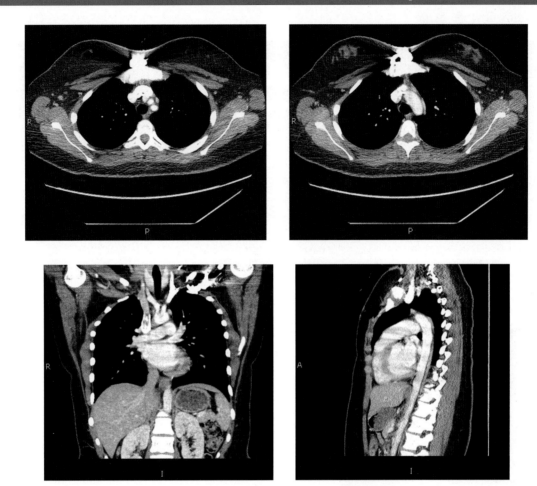

1. Which are the structures present in the images?

2. At what level does the hemiazygos vein join
   the azygos vein?

3. At what level does the accessory hemiazygos
   vein join the azygos vein?

4. What is the normal variant of the mediastinal
   vascularity seen in the images?

5. What is the second normal variant of the
   mediastinal vascularity seen in the images?

Case ranking/difficulty: **Category:** Thorax

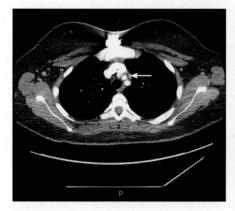

Axial CT of the chest reveals the accessory hemiazygos vein, seen in the left upper mediastinum anterior to the branching aortic vessels (*arrow*). It drains into the left brachiocephalic vein.

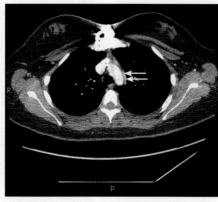

Axial CT of the chest reveals the accessory hemiazygos vein, seen in the mediastinum, left of the aortic arch (*arrows*).

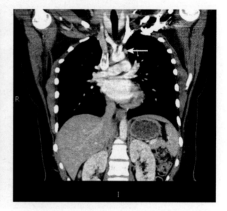

Coronal CT of the chest shows the accessory hemiazygos vein, seen in the mediastinum, left of the aortic arch (*arrow*).

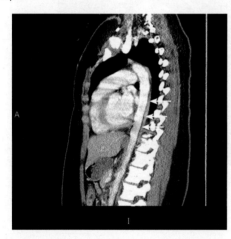

Sagittal CT of the chest shows the accessory hemiazygos, seen in the posterior mediastinum (*arrows*), posterior to the aorta, communicating with the hemiazygos.

Answers

1. The accessory hemiazygos vein is seen in the axial and coronal views. The sagittal view demonstrates that the accessory hemiazygos and hemiazygos form common channel posterior to the aorta.

2. The hemiazygos vein joins the azygos vein at the level of T8-T9.

3. The accessory hemiazygos joins the azygos at T7-T8 crossing posterior to the aorta.

4. The accessory hemiazygos that drains into the left brachiocephalic vein is a very rare normal variant.

5. The accessory hemiazygos vein that communicates with the hemiazygos vein posterior to the aorta is a rare normal variant.

Pearls

Two normal variants of the accessory hemiazygos vein are shown:
- Accessory hemiazygos that drains into the left brachiocephalic vein.
- The accessory hemiazygos communicates with the hemiazygos posterior to the aorta to form a common channel.

Suggested Readings

Blackmon JM, Franco A. Normal variants of the accessory hemiazygos vein. *Br J Radiol.* 2011;84:659-660.

Galwa RM, Prakash M, Khandelwal N. 16-MDCT depiction of the accessory hemiazygos vein draining into the left brachiocephalic vein. *Indian J Radiol Imaging.* 2007;17:50-51.

Lawler LP, Corl FM, Fishman EK. Multi-detector row and volume-rendered CT of the normal and accessory flow pathways of the thoracic systemic and pulmonary veins. *Radiographics.* 2002;22:S45-S60.

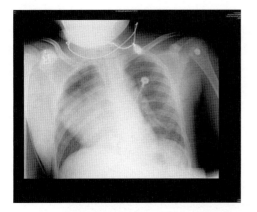
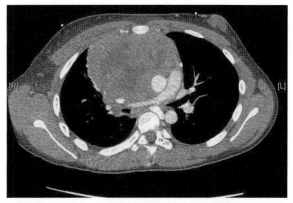
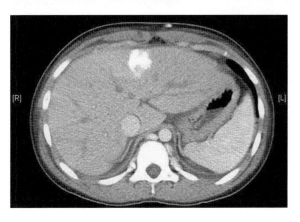
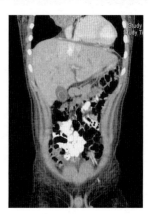

1. What is the etiology of this entity?

2. Describe the CT characteristics of the mass seen in the images.

3. What is the differential diagnosis?

4. What is the reason for the focal enhancement seen in the CT, in the left lobe of the liver?

5. What are the clinical symptoms of this entity?

Case ranking/difficulty: **Category:** Thorax

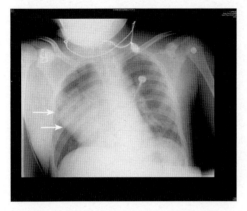

Frontal radiograph of the chest shows a mass occupying the right side of the chest (*arrows*).

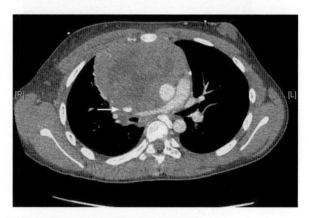

Axial CT of the same patient shows a large heterogeneous mass occupying the mediastinum and compressing the superior vena cava (*arrow*). The mass was diagnosed as lymphoma.

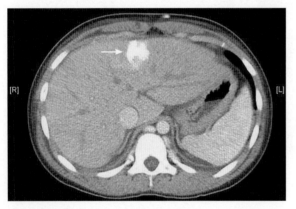

Axial CT of the abdomen shows focal enhancement of the medial segment of the left hepatic lobe (*arrow*).

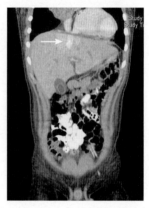

Coronal CT of the abdomen shows focal enhancement of the medial segment of the left hepatic lobe (*arrow*). Note is made of pericholecystic fluid.

Answers

1. The etiology is neoplastic.

2. The CT characteristic is a nonenhancing heterogeneous solid mass.

3. Differential diagnosis of anterior mediastinal mass includes teratoma, lymphoma, thyroid mass, and thymoma.

4. The focal enhancement seen in the CT, in the left lobe of the liver, is due to recanalization of the periumbilical veins.

5. Clinical symptoms may include wheezing, tachypnea, swollen face, and swollen right arm.

- Clinical manifestations include venous congestion of the face, neck, arms, and shortness of breath.
- The focal enhancement (hot spot) in the medial segment of the left lobe of the liver, seen in the images, is due to recanalization of collaterals of periumbilical veins.
- Management consists of treating the underline etiology. In the case of lymphoma (as is the case), it includes chemotherapy, radiation therapy, and surgery.

Suggested Readings

D'Angio GJ, Mitus A, Evans AE. The superior mediastinal syndrome in children with cancer. *Am J Roentgenol.* 1965;93:537-544.

O'Brien RT, Matlak ME, Condon VR, Johnson DG. Superior vena cava syndrome in children. *West J Med.* 1981;135(2):143-147.

Pearls

- Superior vena cava syndrome is due to obstruction of blood flow through the superior vena cava.

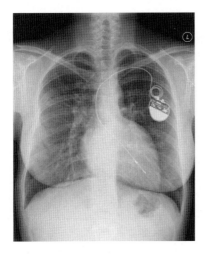
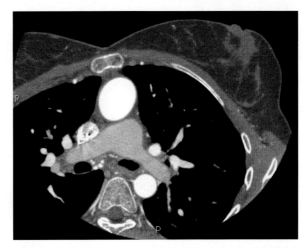
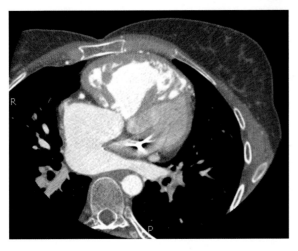
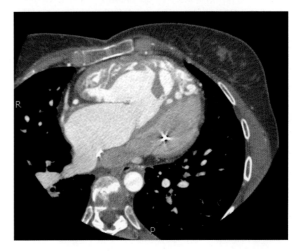

1. What is the normal position of the ascending aorta in relation to the main pulmonary artery?

2. Describe the relation of the ascending aorta in relation to the main pulmonary artery in this case.

3. What is the most likely diagnosis?

4. In this case where are the pulmonary veins draining?

5. What is the surgical procedure that was employed for treatment in this case?

Case ranking/difficulty: **Category:** Thorax

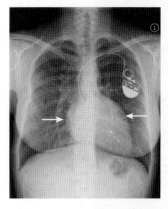

Frontal radiograph of the chest shows egg-shaped pattern of the cardiac silhouette (*arrows*). The patient has a pacemaker with the distal tip in the left ventricle.

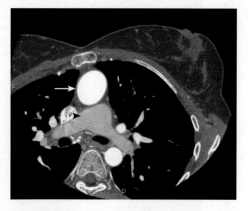

Axial CT of the chest reveals that the ascending aorta (*arrow*) is anterior and to the right in relation to the main pulmonary artery (*arrowhead*).

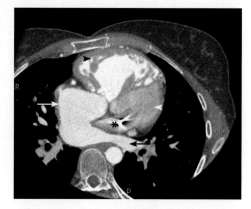

Axial CT of the chest reveals that the superior left pulmonary vein (*black arrow*) drains into the right atrium (*white arrow*). This is the status post Mustard procedure. *Black arrowhead* points to the right ventricle. *Black asterisk* points to the left atrium, and *white arrowhead* points to the left ventricle.

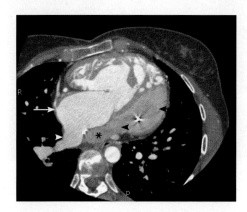

Axial chest CT reveals that the right superior pulmonary vein (*white arrowhead*) drains into the right atrium (*white arrow*). The inferior vena cava (*black asterisk*) drains into the left atrium (*black arrowhead*). This is status post Mustard procedure. The *black arrow* points to the left ventricle.

Answers

1. The ascending aorta is normally posterior and to the right of the main pulmonary artery.

2. In this case the ascending aorta is anterior and to the right of the main pulmonary artery.

3. This is corrected D-transposition of great arteries. Mustard procedure has been performed and the pulmonary veins drain into the right atrium through a baffle. The inferior vena cava drains into the left atrium.

4. The pulmonary veins drain into the right atrium.

5. Mustard procedure was employed. It consists of employing a baffle to direct oxygenated pulmonary venous return into the right atrium and then into the right ventricle, which is the pumping ventricle for the aorta and the systemic circulation. The inferior vena cava is directed to the left atrium.

Pearls

- Transposition of the great arteries is the most common cyanotic congenital heart lesion that presents in neonates.
- There is ventriculoarterial discordance.
- The aorta arises from the morphologic right ventricle, and the pulmonary artery arises from the morphologic left ventricle.
- There are two parallel circulations, leading to lack of tissue oxygen supply. This condition is incompatible with life.
- Surgical correction may be performed by arterial switch (Jatene procedure), to direct systemic venous blood to the left atrium and oxygenated blood to the right atrium (Mustard procedure), and to direct oxygenated blood from the left ventricle to the aorta (Rastelli procedure).

Suggested Readings

Neches WH, Park SC, Ettedgui JA. Transposition of the great arteries. In: *The Science and Practice of Pediatric Cardiology*. Vol 1. Baltimore: Williams & Wilkins; 1998:1463-1503.

Rao PS. Diagnosis and management of cyanotic congenital heart disease: part I. *Indian J Pediatr*. 2009;76(1):57-70.

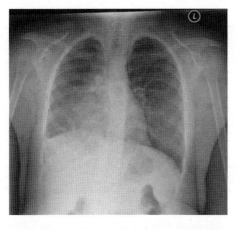
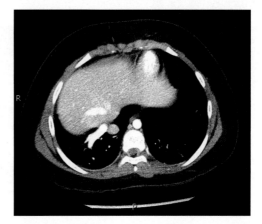
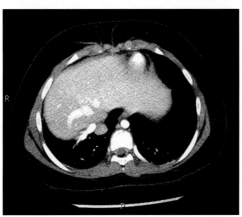
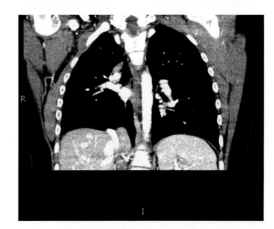

1. What is the diagnosis?

2. What kind of vascular shunt may appear with this entity?

3. What is the radiographic pattern of the lungs in this entity?

4. What are the associated anomalies that may be seen with this entity?

5. Why this syndrome has its name?

Case ranking/difficulty:

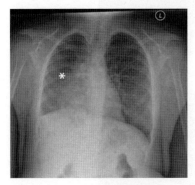

Frontal radiograph of the chest demonstrates small hypoplastic right lung (*asterisk*) with expansion of the left hemithorax.

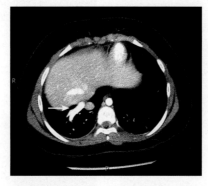
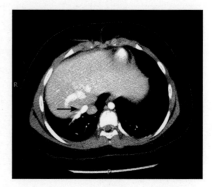

Chest CT in axial view reveals that the venous drainage in the right lower lung is abnormal. A right lower lung vein drains into the inferior vena cava at the level below the diaphragm (*arrow*).

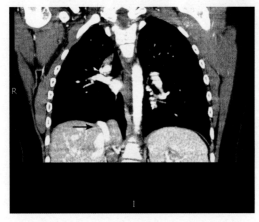

Chest CT in coronal view reveals that the venous drainage in the right lower lung is abnormal. A right lower lung vein drains into the inferior vena cava at the level below the diaphragm (*arrow*).

Pearls

- Venous drainage of the right lower lung is usually to the inferior vena cava below the level of the diaphragm.
- Scimitar syndrome is associated with small hypoplastic right lung.
- On chest radiograph, a curved shadow is seen near the right heart border that courses toward the diaphragm and coalesces with the inferior vena cava.

Suggested Readings

Gupta ML, Bagarhatta R, Sinha J. Scimitar syndrome: a rare disease with unusual presentation. *Lung India.* 2009;26:26-29.

Ho CB. Scimitar syndrome. *J Emerg Med.* 2001;21(3): 279-281.

Wang CC, Wu ET, Chen SJ, et al. Scimitar syndrome: incidence, treatment, and prognosis. *Eur J Pediatr.* 2008;167:155-160.

Answers

1. The diagnosis is Scimitar syndrome, which falls in the category of partial anomalous pulmonary venous return.

2. The vascular shunt that appears with Scimitar syndrome is left to right, which is acyanotic.

3. The pattern seen in the lungs is small and a hypoplastic right lung.

4. Associated anomalies that may be seen with Scimitar syndrome are lung sequestration, atrial septal defect, heart failure, accessory hemidiaphragm, and hypoplastic right pulmonary artery.

5. A "scimitar" appearance on chest x-ray has a resemblance to a Turkish sword for which the syndrome is named.

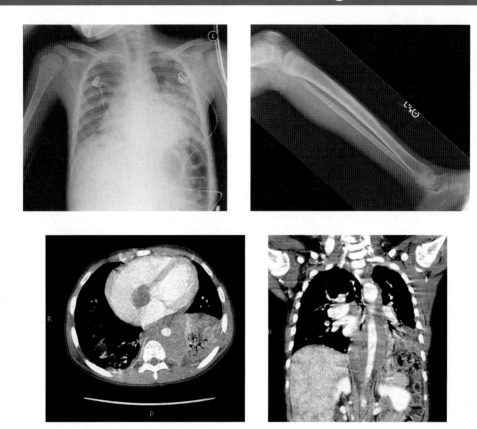

1. What are the findings?

2. What is the metabolic pattern of this entity as seen with PET/CT?

3. What kind of cells accumulate in lymph nodes in Rosai-Dorfman disease?

4. What is the disease that was described to be associated with Rosai-Dorfman disease?

5. What is the racial predilection of Rosai-Dorfman disease?

Case ranking/difficulty:

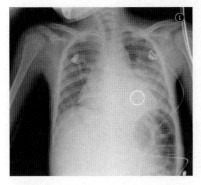

Frontal radiograph of the chest demonstrates opacity in the lower left mediastinum, in the retrocardiac region (*circle*). Initially, it is thought to represent left lower lobe airspace disease.

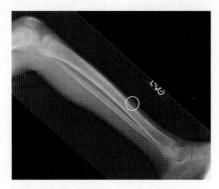

Lateral radiograph of the left leg reveals a subcutaneous nodule (*circle*).

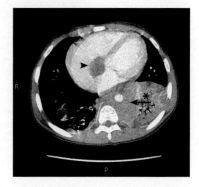

Axial contrast CT of the chest reveals a mass arising from the inter-atrial septum and expanding to both atria (*arrowhead*). A mass noted encasing the descending aorta (*arrow*). Compressive atelectasis of the left lower lobe noted (*asterisk*).

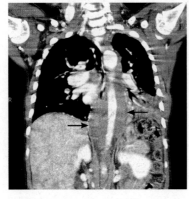

Coronal contrast CT of the chest reveals a mass noted encasing the descending aorta (*arrows*).

Pearls

- Rosai-Dorfman disease is a rare disorder characterized by over-production of histiocytes.
- Abnormal areas of accumulation appear almost anywhere in the body, including lymph nodes and central nervous system.
- The disease is more common in African-American children.
- Association with sickle cell disease was described.
- This case reveals that the mass that arises in the inter-atrial septa extends to the aortic root and encases the aorta. The mass is significantly hypermetabolic in PET/CT study.
- Some cases respond to chemotherapy.

Answers

1. There is a mass arising from the inter-atrial septum extending to both atria and contiguously encircling the aortic root, encasing the aortic arch and the descending aorta. The mass compresses the left lower lobe bronchus leading to atelectasis.

2. Rosai-Dorfman disease demonstrates a strongly hypermetabolic pattern in PET/CT study that is performed with F-18-FDG-fluorodeoxyglucose (18F).

3. Rosai-Dorfman disease is an uncommon histo-proliferative disease. It is a rare disorder characterized by over-production and accumulation of histiocytes in the lymph nodes of the body.

4. Sickle cell disease was described to be associated with Rosai-Dorfman disease.

5. The disease is more common in African-Americans.

Suggested Readings

Huang JY, Lu CC, Hsiao CH, Tzen KY. FDG PET/CT findings in purely cutaneous Rosai-Dorfman disease. *Clin Nucl Med*. 2011;36(4):e13-e15.

Santra G, Das BK, Mandal B, Kundu SS, Bandopadhyay A. Rosai-Dorfman disease. *Singapore Med J*. 2010;51(10):e173-e175.

Yontz L, Franco A, Sharma S, Lewis K, McDonough C. A case of Rosai-Dorfman Disease in a pediatric patient with cardiac involvement. *J Radiol Case Reports*. 2012;6(1):1-8.

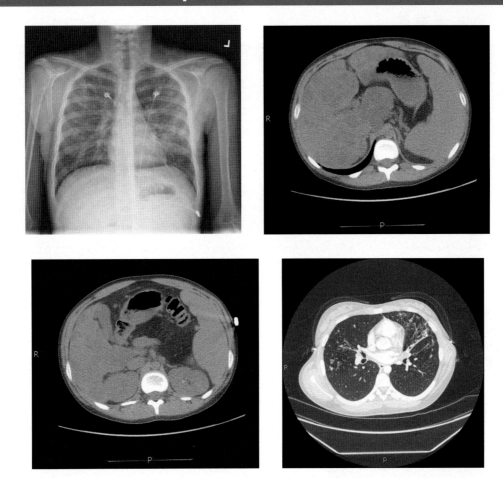

1. What are the findings?

2. Describe the pathophysiology of this entity.

3. In which racial group is the prevalence of this entity the highest?

4. What are the clinical features of newborns with this entity?

5. As this entity progresses, the pancreas undergoes . . . .

Case ranking/difficulty:

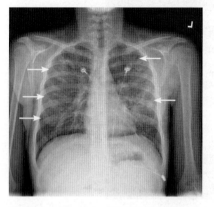

Frontal radiograph of the chest shows interstitial changes that are diffuse and bilateral (*arrows*).

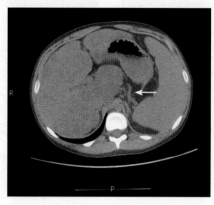

Axial non-contrast abdominal CT at the level of the liver shows fatty infiltration of the liver and hepatosplenomegaly. There is fatty transformation of the pancreas (*arrow*).

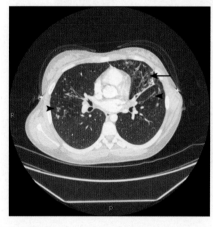

Axial cut of non-contrast high-resolution chest CT shows bronchiectatic changes (*arrowheads*). Interstitial architectural distortion and air space change noted in the lingula (*arrow*).

Answers

1. The chest radiograph demonstrates bilateral interstitial changes. The chest CT demonstrates bronchiectatic changes with tree-in-bud appearance consisting of small airways impacted by mucus. The abdominal CT demonstrates hepatosplenomegaly, fatty liver, and pancreatic fatty transformation.

2. Cystic fibrosis is caused by viscous secretions from the exocrine glands, which leads to bacterial overgrowth and recurrent infections.

3. Cystic fibrosis is more common in Caucasians.

4. Newborns may present with meconium peritonitis, meconium plug syndrome, or may present with microcolon, usually due to ileal atresia.

5. As the disease progresses, there is fatty transformation of the pancreas.

Pearls

- Cystic fibrosis is characterized by thick and viscous exocrine gland secretions, leading to infections mainly of the respiratory system.
- It is an inherited disease, most common in Caucasians with genetic traits.
- There is fatty transformation of the pancreas later in life.
- Fatty liver infiltration and cirrhosis may develop.
- Treatment is symptomatic and with antibiotics to treat recurrent infections.

Suggested Readings

Amorosa JK, Laraya-Cuasay LR, Sohn L, et al. Radiologic diagnosis of cystic fibrosis in adults and children. *Acad Radiol.* 1995;2(3):222-225.

Kliegman R, Kliegman RM. *Nelson Essentials of Pediatrics.* St. Louis, MO: Elsevier Saunders; 2006.

Ruzal-Shapiro C. Cystic fibrosis. An overview. *Radiol Clin North Am.* 1998;36(1):143-161.

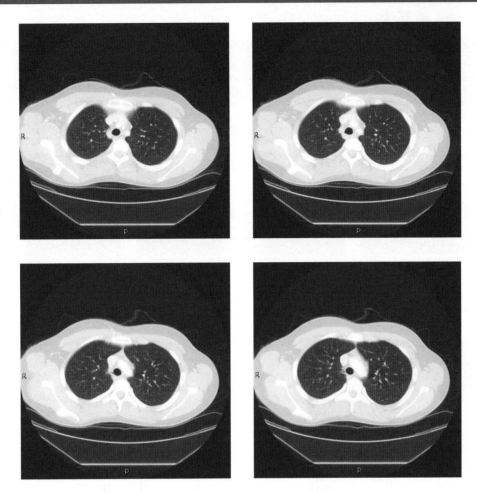

1. What is the diagnosis?

2. What is the best modality for diagnosing
   this entity?

3. What are the two types of this entity?

4. What happens when these patients are
   intubated?

5. What are the treatment options?

Case ranking/difficulty: **Category:** Thorax

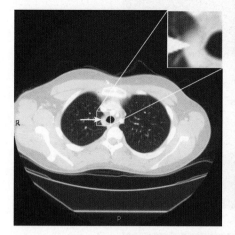

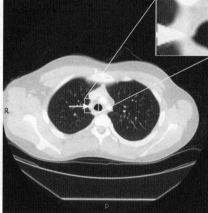

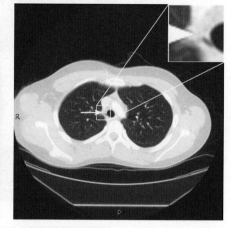

Axial CT of the upper chest above the carina demonstrates a lucent structure branching from the right tracheal wall (*arrow*).

Axial CT of the upper chest above the carina demonstrates a lucent structure branching from the right tracheal wall and coursing toward the right upper lobe (*arrow*).

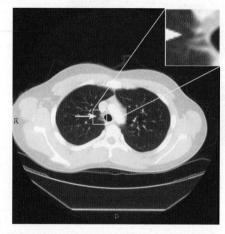

Axial CT of the upper chest above the carina demonstrates a lucent structure branching from the right tracheal wall and coursing toward the right upper lobe (*arrow*).

Answers

1. The diagnosis is tracheal bronchus.

2. CT scan is the best modality. Surface rendered images with 3D reconstructions and coronal reconstructions clearly demonstrate this anomaly.

3. Tracheal bronchus may be supernumerary (23%) or displaced (77%). Supernumerary bronchus is an additional bronchus coexisting with a normally originating right upper lobe bronchus. Displaced bronchus is a tracheal bronchus with associated absence of a normally branching upper lobe bronchus.

4. Right upper lobe collapse can be seen when an endotracheal tube is advanced beyond the origin of

tracheal bronchus and it expands when endotracheal tube is retracted above the origin of tracheal bronchus.

5. Treatment depends on the severity of symptoms. No treatment is required if the patient is asymptomatic. Treatment may include antibiotics, respiratory therapy, intubation, and lobectomy.

Pearls

- A tracheal bronchus is an aberrant bronchus that arises from the tracheal wall above the carina. It commonly arises from the right wall of the trachea and supplies the right upper lobe. It is also known as pig bronchus.
- Tracheal bronchus may be asymptomatic. Symptomatic tracheal bronchus presents with recurrent pneumonia, chronic bronchitis, or bronchiectasis.
- Right tracheal bronchus is much more common than left tracheal bronchus.
- Left tracheal bronchus arises from the distal part of left main bronchus and supplies apicoposterior segment of left upper lobe.
- Bridging bronchus arises from left main bronchus and crosses the midline to supply right lower lobe.

Suggested Readings

Barat M, Konrad HR. Tracheal bronchus. *Am J Otolaryngol.* 1987;8(2):118-122.

Franquet T. Anomalous bronchi. Dx. Statdx Premier. Amirsys Inc. 2005-2012.

Ghaye B, Szapiro D, Fanchamps J-M, Dondelinger RF. Congenital bronchial abnormalities revisited. *Radiographics.* 2001;21(1):105-119.

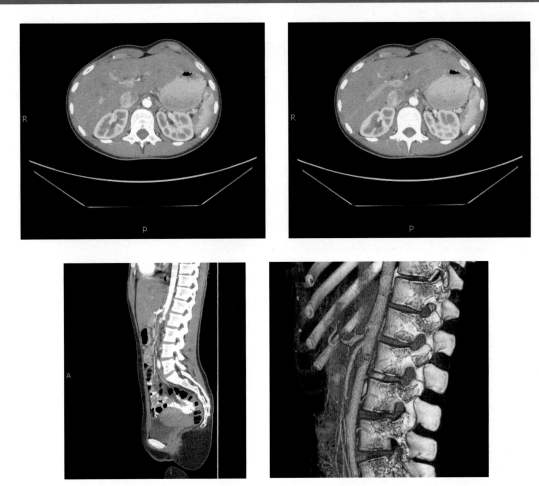

1. Describe the findings.

2. What is the pathophysiology of the case?

3. What are the clinical symptoms?

4. Ten to twenty-four percent of the population has the anatomic variant that contributes to the case. Most are asymptomatic. What is the percentage of these individuals that are symptomatic?

5. What are the treatment options?

Case ranking/difficulty: **Category:** Abdomen

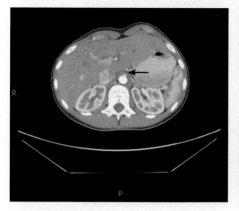

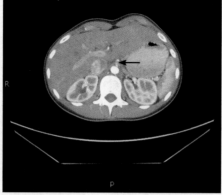

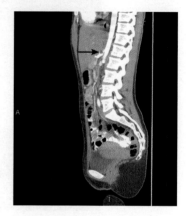

Axial CT of the abdomen at the level of the celiac artery shows narrowing of the proximal portion of the artery (*arrow*).

Sagittal CT of the abdomen at the level of the celiac artery shows narrowing of the proximal portion of the artery (*arrow*).

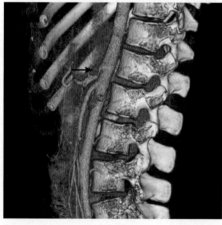

3D CT reconstruction in sagittal view of the abdomen at the level of the celiac artery shows narrowing of the proximal portion of the artery (*arrow*).

Answers

1. The images demonstrate stenosis of the proximal celiac artery.

2. The median arcuate ligament usually passes superior to the origin of the celiac axis. In 10 to 24% of people, the ligament may cross anterior to the artery; in some of these individuals, the ligament may actually compress the celiac axis, compromising blood flow and causing clinical symptoms.

3. Patients present with epigastric pain and weight loss. The abdominal pain may be associated with eating, but not always. At physical examination, an abdominal bruit that varies with respiration may be audible in the midepigastric region.

4. In 1% of the individuals in which the median arcuate ligament crosses anterior to the celiac axis, the ligament may actually compress the celiac axis, compromising blood flow and causing symptoms.

5. Treatment of the median arcuate ligament syndrome is surgical resection of the ligament's fibers around the celiac axis. In patients with continued stenosis after the ligation of the ligament, it is advisable to place a stent to prevent fibrotic stenosis.

Pearls

- The median arcuate ligament is a fibrous arch that unites the diaphragmatic crura on either side of the aortic hiatus.
- The ligament usually passes superior to the origin of the celiac axis.
- In 10 to 24% of people, the ligament may cross anterior to the celiac axis.
- In some of these individuals, the ligament may compress the celiac axis, compromising blood flow and causing symptoms.

Suggested Readings

Horton KM, Talamini MA, Fishman EK. Median arcuate ligament syndrome: evaluation with CT angiography. *Radiographics*. 2008;25(5):1177-1182.

Lindner HH, Kemprud E. A clinicoanatomic study of the arcuate ligament of the diaphragm. *Arch Surg*. 1971;103:600-605.

Manghat NE, Mitchell G, Hay CS, Wells IP. The median arcuate ligament syndrome revisited by CT angiography and the use of ECG gating-a single centre case series and literature review. *Br J Radiol*. 2008;81(969):735-742.

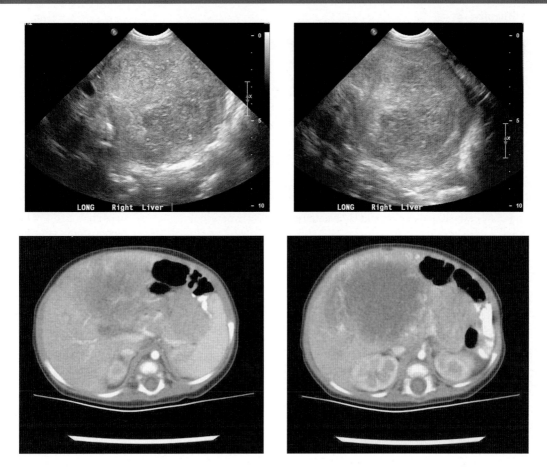

1. What are the findings?

2. What is the most common presentation
   of the disease?

3. What are complications of this case?

4. What are other congenital anomalies that
   the case may be associated with?

5. What are the treatment options?

Case ranking/difficulty:

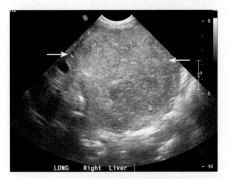 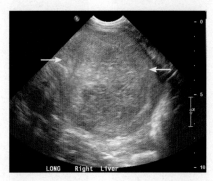

Longitudinal sonography of the liver demonstrates large heterogeneously hyperechoic hepatic mass (*arrows*).

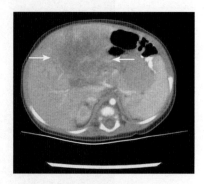

Axial contrast CT of the liver demonstrates large hepatic mass with peripheral enhancement and low attenuation centrally (*arrows*).

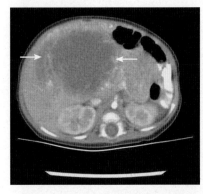

Axial contrast CT of the liver demonstrates large hepatic mass with peripheral enhancement and low attenuation centrally (*arrows*).

Answers

1. The sonogram demonstrates heterogeneously echogenic mass. In the CT, the mass is enhancing in the periphery; however, the center has low attenuation.

2. The most common presentation of infantile hemangioendothelioma is abdominal mass. Most patients are asymptomatic.

3. In up to 50% of the patients with infantile hemangioendothelioma, there is high-output cardiac failure as a result of A-V shunting of the tumor. Platelet sequestration within the tumor may lead to thrombocytopenia and bleeding, known as Kasabach-Merritt syndrome.

4. Infantile hemangioendothelioma may be associated with other congenital anomalies, such as bilateral renal agenesis, Beckwith-Wiedemann syndrome, and meningomyelocele. In 10% of the cases, cutaneous hemangiomas are present.

5. Hemangioendothelioma may regress, and if the patient is asymptomatic, no treatment is necessary. Symptomatic patients may undergo resection and embolization. Corticosteroids and supportive care including diuretics and blood product replacement have been employed.

Pearls

- Infantile hemangioendotheliomas are liver lesions composed of large endothelial-lined vascular channels. They are histologically distinct from hemangiomas.
- Typical presentation of infantile hemangioendothelioma includes an abdominal mass and 10% have cutaneous hemangiomas.
- In up to 50% of patients, there is high-output cardiac failure as a result of A-V shunting of the tumor.
- Platelet sequestration within the tumor may lead to thrombocytopenia and bleeding, known as Kasabach-Merritt syndrome.
- Serum alpha fetoprotein levels are usually within the normal range.

Suggested Readings

Bruegel M, Muenzel D, Waldt S, Specht K, Rummeny EJ. Hepatic epithelioid hemangioendothelioma: findings at CT and MRI including preliminary observations at diffusion-weighted echo-planar imaging. *Abdom Imaging.* 2011;36(4):415-424.

Chung EM, Cube R, Lewis RB, Conran RM. From the archives of the AFIP: pediatric liver masses: radiologic-pathologic correlation part 1. Benign tumors. *Radiographics.* 2010;30(3):801-826.

Feng ST, Chan T, Ching AS, et al. CT and MR imaging characteristics of infantile hepatic hemangioendothelioma. *Eur J Radiol.* 2010;76(2):e24-e29.

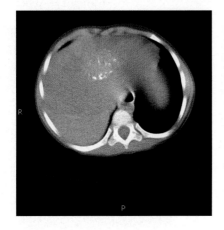
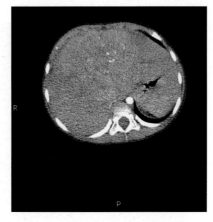
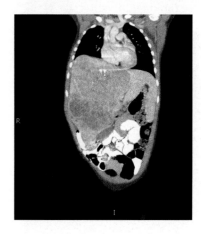

1. What are the findings?

2. What are the diseases associated with this case?

3. What is the differential diagnosis?

4. Which tumor marker is elevated in this case?

5. What is the peak age of presentation of this case?

Case ranking/difficulty:

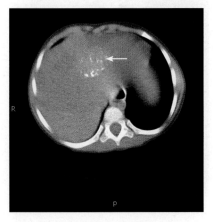

Non-contrast axial CT of the upper abdomen demonstrates large infiltrating hepatic mass with chunky calcifications (*arrow*).

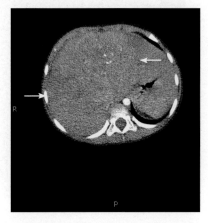

Contrast axial CT of the upper abdomen in arterial phase demonstrates large minimally enhancing heterogeneous hepatic mass (*arrows*) with chunky calcifications.

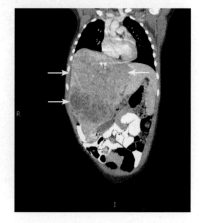

Contrast coronal CT of the abdomen in portal venous phase demonstrates large heterogeneously enhancing hepatic mass (*arrows*) with chunky calcifications.

Answers

1. Large infiltrating hepatic mass. The enhancement is heterogeneous. Calcification is seen. The enhancement is more intense in the portal venous phase. There are foci of low attenuation that represent necrosis. Most of the liver surface is involved.

2. Hepatoblastoma is associated with hemihypertrophy and Beckwith-Wiedemann syndrome, bilateral polycystic kidneys, polyposis coli, very low birth weight, and maternal exposure to metals.

3. Differential diagnosis includes hemangioendothelioma, metastatic disease, mesenchymal hamartoma, and hepatoblastoma. Hepatocellular carcinoma is very unlikely before the age of 5 years.

4. Serum alpha-fetoprotein (AFP) is elevated in most patients with hepatoblastoma.

5. Most cases of hepatoblastoma present between 1 and 2 years of age.

Pearls

- Hepatoblastoma is the most common liver cancer in children.
- The disease is usually diagnosed as an asymptomatic abdominal mass.
- In most of the patients, the serum level of alpha-fetoprotein is found to be elevated.
- In cross-sectional images, the tumor usually demonstrates heterogeneous enhancement, seen in the portal phase.

Suggested Readings

Berdon WE. Hepatoblastoma. *Pediatr Radiol.* 2001;31(4):306.

Chung EM, Lattin GE Jr, Cube R, et al. From the archives of the AFIP: pediatric liver masses: radiologic-pathologic correlation. Part 2. Malignant tumors. *Radiographics.* 2007;31(2):483-507.

Roebuck DJ, Aronson D, Clapuyt P, et al. 2005 PRETEXT: a revised staging system for primary malignant liver tumours of childhood developed by the SIOPEL group. *Pediatr Radiol.* 2007;37(2):123-132.

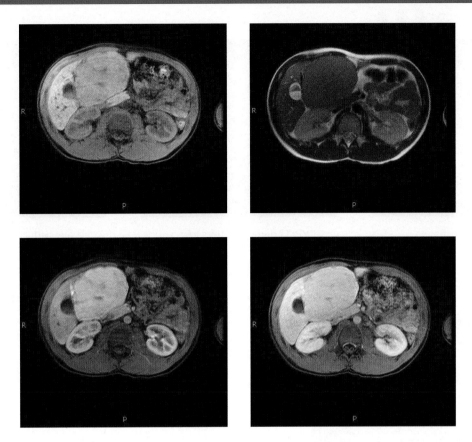

1. What are the findings?

2. What is the differential diagnosis?

3. What is the percentage of calcification seen in this entity?

4. What is the pathophysiology of the case?

5. What are the treatment options?

Case ranking/difficulty:

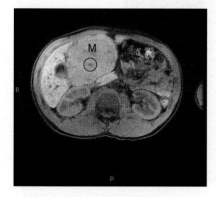

LAVA pre-contrast axial image demonstrates a liver mass (*M*) that is slightly of lower signal than the liver. It has low-signal central scar (*circle*) with radiating fibrous septae.

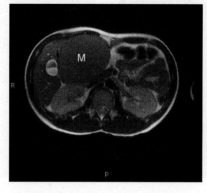

Axial MRI T2 demonstrates a low-signal liver mass (*M*) with same signal attenuation as the liver.

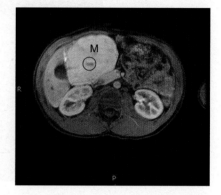

Axial LAVA with arterial phase contrast demonstrates a liver mass (*M*) that has higher signal than the liver parenchyma. A non-enhancing low-signal central scar seen (*circle*) with radiating septae.

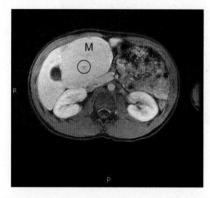

Axial LAVA with portal venous phase contrast demonstrates a liver mass (*M*) that has the same signal as the liver parenchyma. A non-enhancing low-signal central scar seen (*circle*) with radiating septae.

Answers

1. Discrete and well-defined hepatic mass is seen. The lesion has the higher signal than liver parenchyma in the arterial phase of contrast-enhanced MRI T1 and has the same signal as liver parenchyma in the portal venous phase of contrast-enhanced MRI T1.

2. Differential diagnosis includes focal nodular hyperplasia, hepatic adenoma, and fibrolamellar hepatocellular carcinoma.

3. The presence of calcification in a liver lesion suggests a diagnosis other than focal nodular hyperplasia because only 1% of patients with focal nodular hyperplasia have calcification.

4. Focal nodular hyperplasia is a benign hyperplastic process in which all the normal constituents of the liver are present but in an abnormally organized pattern.

5. Treatment is not mandatory unless large size, compression symptoms, or fear of traumatic hemorrhage

indicates otherwise. Ethanol embolotherapy offers a safe and effective alternative to surgery. FNH lends itself particularly well to embolotherapy because it is usually fed by a single end-artery with no intratumoral arteriovenous shunting or parasitic blood supply.

Pearls

- Focal nodular hyperplasia is the second most common tumor of the liver.
- May be associated with oral contraceptives.
- Cross-sectional images demonstrate well-defined mass with central scar and radiating fibrous septae.
- Variable intensity in T1-weighted MRI images.
- On T2-weighted images, the lesion is slightly hyperintense to isointense.
- The central scar of FNH is hypointense on T1-weighted images, but on T2-weighted images, the central scar shows a pattern of variable signal intensity.
- Following administration of a gadolinium-based contrast agent, the enhancement pattern parallels that of contrast-enhanced CT.

Suggested Readings

Chung EM, Cube R, Lewis RB, Conran RM. From the archives of the AFIP: pediatric liver masses: radiologic-pathologic correlation part 1. Benign tumors. *Radiographics*. 2010;30(3):801-826.

Do RK, Shaylor SD, Shia J, et al. Variable MR imaging appearances of focal nodular hyperplasia in pediatric cancer patients. *Pediatr Radiol*. 2011;41(3):335-340.

Hussain SM, Terkivatan T, Zondervan PE, et al. Focal nodular hyperplasia: findings at state-of-the-art MR imaging, US, CT, and pathologic analysis. *Radiographics*. 2004;24(1):3-17;discussion 18-19.

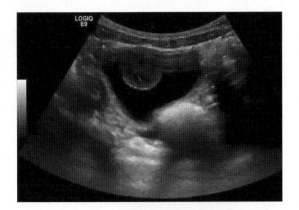
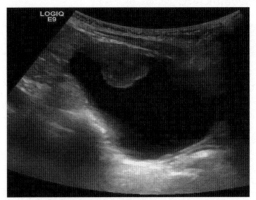

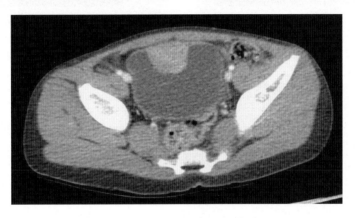

1. What are the findings?

2. What is the differential diagnosis?

3. What is the most common bladder tumor in children?

4. What is the most common presenting clinical sign of this entity?

5. How a definite diagnosis of this case can be made?

Case ranking/difficulty:

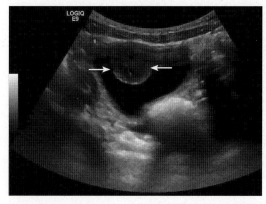

Sonogram of the bladder in transverse view demonstrates a solid heterogeneous mass (*arrows*) extending from the anterior-superior wall of the bladder and projecting into the lumen.

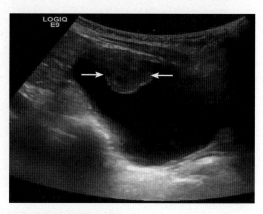

Sonogram of the bladder in longitudinal view demonstrates a solid heterogeneous mass (*arrows*) extending from the anterior-superior wall of the bladder projecting into the lumen.

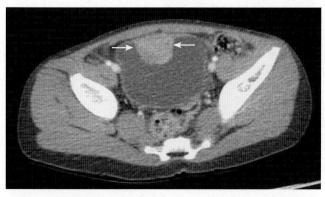

A CT of the pelvis of the patient, later diagnosed with a rhabdoid tumor of the bladder, demonstrates a solid, heterogeneous, well-circumscribed mass (*arrows*) arising from the anterior-superior wall of the bladder.

Answers

1. There is a solid heterogeneous mass, well circumscribed extending from the anterior-superior wall of the bladder projecting into the lumen.

2. Primitive neuroectodermal tumor, rhabdoid tumor, rhabdomyosarcoma, and sarcoma botryoides (which is a subtype of rhabdomyosarcoma) are in the differential diagnosis. Wilms' tumor is not in the differential diagnosis and appears in the kidneys.

3. Rhabdomyosarcoma is the most common bladder tumor in children.

4. Hematuria is the most common presenting clinical sign of this case (rhabdoid tumor of the bladder). Hematuria is also the most common presenting clinical sign of other bladder tumors including the most common tumor, rhabdomyosarcoma.

5. Imaging is part of a wide range of tools that can be used for diagnosis. However, there are no specific imaging findings for the diagnosis of rhabdoid tumor of the bladder. Therefore, cytological and molecular evaluations are used to complement imaging in making the diagnosis.

Pearls

- Rhabdoid tumor is a very uncommon bladder neoplasm.
- Differential diagnosis includes rhabdomyosarcoma and primitive neuroectodermal tumors.
- Rhabdoid tumors are notorious for aggressive metastases, especially pulmonary, with high mortality rate.
- No specific imaging findings can direct to a definite diagnosis.
- Diagnosis is made by cytological and molecular evaluations.

Suggested Readings

Duvdevani M, Mass D, Neumann Y, Leibovitch I, Ramon J, Mor Y. Pure rhabdoid tumor of the bladder. *J Urol.* 2001;166:2337.

Roebuck D. The role of imaging in renal and extra-renal rhabdoid tumors. *Australas Radiol.* 1996;40:310-318.

Savage N, Linn D, McDonough C, et al. Molecularly confirmed primary malignant rhabdoid tumor of the urinary bladder: implications of accurate diagnosis. *Ann Diagn Pathol.* 2012;16(6):504-507.

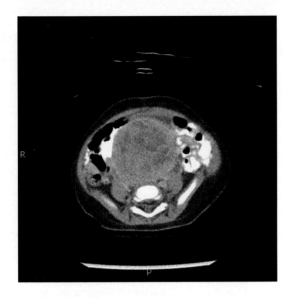 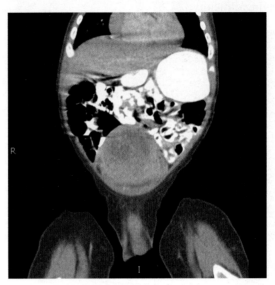

1. What are the findings?

2. What are the two most common forms/
   subtypes of this entity?

3. What is the incidence of this entity?

4. What is the most common anatomic system
   that this entity most commonly occurs in
   young children?

5. What are the treatment options?

Case ranking/difficulty:

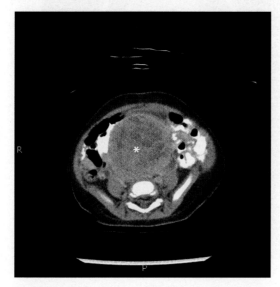

Axial contrast CT of the abdomen. There is large lower abdominal mass (*asterisk*) with areas of low attenuation noted to be necrotic. The mass was diagnosed as rhabdomyosarcoma.

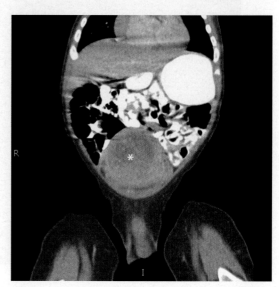

Coronal contrast CT of the abdomen. There is large lower abdominal mass (*asterisk*) with areas of low attenuation noted to be necrotic. The mass was diagnosed as rhabdomyosarcoma.

Answers

1. CT of the lower abdomen in axial and coronal views demonstrates a large mass with areas of low attenuation, representing necrosis. This mass was diagnosed as rhabdomyosarcoma.

2. The two most common forms/subtypes are embryonal rhabdomyosarcoma and alveolar rhabdomyosarcoma.

3. The incidence of rhabdomyosarcoma is 6 cases per 1,000,000 population per year in children and adolescents younger than 15 years.

4. In young children, rhabdomyosarcoma most commonly occurs in the lower genitourinary system. Bladder and prostate are common sites of occurrence.

5. Rhabdomyosarcoma is treated with a combination of chemotherapy, radiation therapy, and surgery.

Pearls

- Rhabdomyosarcoma is the most common soft tissue sarcoma in children.
- Alveolar rhabdomyosarcoma has poor prognosis. The prognosis of embryonal rhabdomyosarcoma is more favorable.
- With adequate treatment children with localized disease have 70% chance of long-term survival.
- Imaging modality of choice for the diagnosis are CT and MRI; however, pathologic diagnosis is needed for confirmation.

Suggested Readings

Franco A, Henderson PR, McDonough CH. Unusual concentration of Tc-99m methylendiphosphonate in rhabdomyosarcoma. *J Radiol Case Rep*. 2012;6(9):29-34.

Grimsby GM, Ritchey ML. Pediatric urologic oncology. *Pediatr Clin North Am*. 2012;59(4):947-959.

Prabhakaran P, Sanjayan R, Somanathan T, Narayanan G. Rhabdomyosarcoma of prostate presenting as bladder outlet obstruction in a young adult. *Ecancermedicalscience*. 2013;7:360.

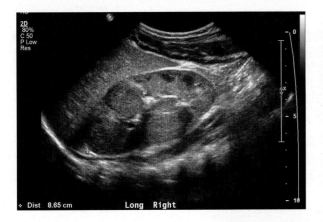

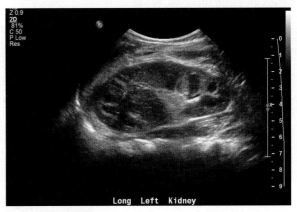

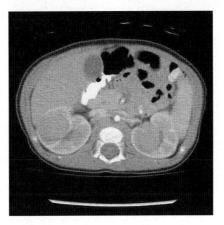

1. What are the findings?

2. What is the most likely diagnosis?

3. What is the most common natural history of this entity?

4. What are the types of this entity?

5. What is the treatment?

Case ranking/difficulty: **Category:** Genitourinary

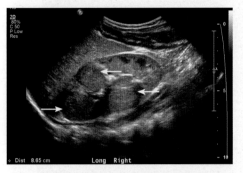

Longitudinal sonogram of the right kidney demonstrates multiple homogeneous echogenic masses (*arrows*).

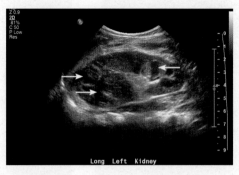

Longitudinal sonogram of the left kidney demonstrates multiple homogeneous echogenic masses (*arrows*).

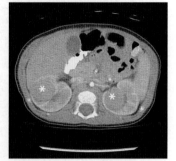

Axial CT at the level of the kidneys demonstrates masses in both kidneys. The masses are hypodense, homogenous, and are not enhancing with contrast material (*asterisks*).

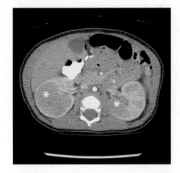

Axial CT at the level of the kidneys demonstrates masses in both kidneys. The masses are hypodense, homogenous, and are not enhancing with contrast material (*asterisks*).

Answers

1. The sonogram demonstrates bilateral multiple renal masses that are homogeneous and echogenic. The contrast CT demonstrates that the masses are nonenhancing and of low attenuation.

2. Nephroblastomatosis.

3. The majority of nephroblastomatosis regress. Some may develop Wilms' tumor. Nephrogenic rests are seen in up to 40% of patients with unilateral Wilms' tumor and in more than 90% of patients with synchronous or metachronous bilateral Wilms' tumor.

4. Perilobar and intralobar. Perilobar rests are more common (90% of all nephrogenic rests), located at cortex or corticomedullary junction, and have less risk (2%) for Wilms' tumor than intralobar rest (5%).

5. Chemotherapy may be used. Close follow-up is necessary because of the risk of transformation to Wilms' tumor.

Pearls

- A nephrogenic rest is an abnormal persistence of metanephric blastema after 36 weeks of gestation.
- Nephroblastomatosis is defined as the persistence of multifocal or diffuse nephrogenic rests.
- During development, the blastema differentiates into nephrons.
- The peripheral portion of the kidney is formed last and is more likely to contain persistent nephrogenic rests.
- Nephroblastomatosis is considered to be a precursor to Wilms' tumor.
- It is also associated with entities that are associated with Wilms' tumor, such as Beckwith-Wiedemann syndrome, Denys-Drash syndrome, sporadic aniridia, and hemihypertrophy.
- CT or MR scanning typically demonstrates multifocal or diffuse subcapsular layer of abnormal, homogenous non-enhancing tissue. Nephroblastomatosis is hypodense on CT and homogeneously echogenic on ultrasound.
- Hemorrhage and necrosis within these lesions usually indicate transformation to Wilms' tumor.

Suggested Readings

Donnelly LF, Jones BV, O'hara SM, et al. *Diagnostic Imaging: Pediatrics*. Salt Lake City, UT: Amirsys; 2005.

Lonergan GJ, Martínez-León MI, Agrons GA, Montemarano H, Suarez ES. Nephrogenic rests, nephroblastomatosis, and associated lesions of the kidney. *Radiographics*. 1998;18:947-968.

Lowe LH, Isuani BH, Heller RM, et al. Pediatric renal masses: Wilms' tumor and beyond. *Radiographics*. 2000;20:1585-1603.

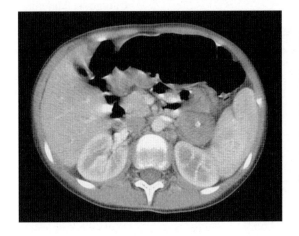 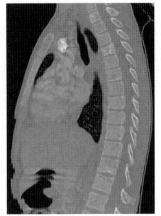 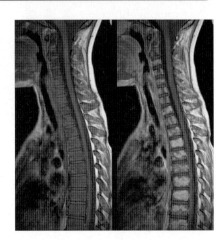

1. What is the differential diagnosis in this patient?

2. What is the stage of this disease?

3. What is the risk of this patient in terms of disease relapse?

4. What is the characteristic age at presentation?

5. What is the most specific imaging method for this entity?

Case ranking/difficulty:

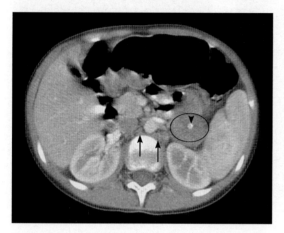

There is a soft tissue mass in the suprarenal left region (*black circle*) with central calcification (*black arrowhead*). Note interaortocaval and left paraaortic lymph node (*black arrows*).

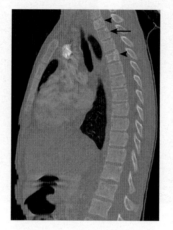

Sagittal reconstruction with bone algorithm shows diffuse osteopenia of the spine with lack of trabeculations (especially at the level of the *black arrow*). At the same time, several vertebral bodies demonstrate increased density and height loss, compatible with insufficiency fractures (*black arrowheads*).

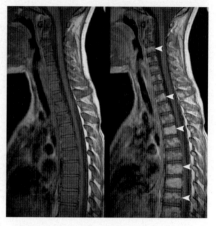

Left without, right with contrast enhancement T1WI demonstrates the severity and dissemination of the metastatic process within the whole spine (including the lower part, not shown) involving virtually all vertebral bodies (intensive contrast enhancement, *white arrowheads*).

Answers

1. Neuroblastoma and malignant ganglioneuroblastoma originate from the sympathetic nervous system. Both may show calcifications and distant metastasis to bone and bone marrow. Rhabdomyosarcoma may mimic these tumors. Only nephroblastoma (Wilms' tumor) exceptionally metastasizes to bones, and such a diffuse infiltration as seen in this patient would be atypical. Langerhan's cell histiocytosis may present with a diffuse osseous infiltration, but without an intra-abdominal mass.

2. An abdominal neuroblastoma in a 10-year-old child with distant metastasis (bone, bone marrow) is classified as a Stage 4. Stage 4S is only applicable in infants under 1 year of age.

3. A 10-year-old child with the diagnosis of metastatic neuroblastoma is always a high-risk patient. Spontaneous tumor regression is seen in up to 40% of neonates and these children are assigned to the low-risk group. This low-risk group is primarily followed up by imaging (or curative surgery may be considered as an alternative), and has an overall survival rate of 90%.

4. Typical age at presentation is within the first year of life. Two percent of neuroblastoma may occur in adulthood.

5. Ultrasound as a screening method may demonstrate the abdominal mass with calcifications (salt and pepper appearance). MRI/CT is the best to demonstrate locoregional tumor and distant metastasis (eg, liver, bone). MIBG scintigraphy is very specific to diagnose neuroblastomas and will be positive in >90% hormone-producing tumors, showing primary tumor sites and metastases as well.

Pearls

- Neuroblastomas are mainly localized in the region of the adrenal gland.
- Neonatal neuroblastoma has a very good prognosis and often regresses spontaneously.
- MIBG scintigraphy is specific and positive in >90% of cases.
- Staging of the tumor is done according to the clinic and image-defined risk factors depending upon tumor location and extension.

Suggested Readings

Charron M. Contemporary approach to diagnosis and treatment of neuroblastoma. *Q J Nucl Med Mol Imaging*. 2013;57(1):40-52.

Liu W, Zheng J, Li Q. Application of imaging modalities for evaluating neuroblastoma. *J Pediatr Endocrinol Metab*. 2013:1-6.

Nour-Eldin NE, Abdelmonem O, Tawfik AM, et al. Pediatric primary and metastatic neuroblastoma: MRI findings: pictorial review. *Magn Reson Imaging*. 2012;30(7):893-906.

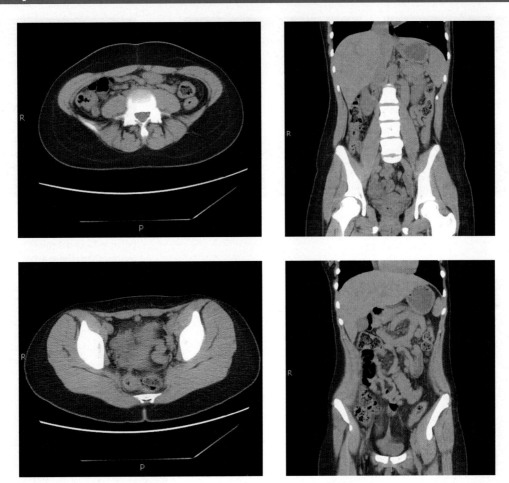

1. What are the findings?

2. What are the sonographic findings of this case?

3. What are the anatomic structures that the urachus connects during the fetal life?

4. What is the anatomical space of the urachus?

5. Why is it essential to remove asymptomatic urachal remnants?

Case ranking/difficulty:

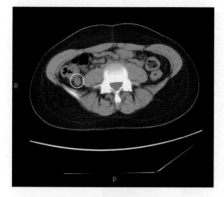

Axial CT at the level of the appendix reveals thickened wall and dilated appendix (*circle*).

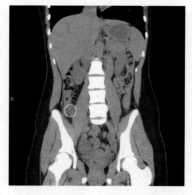

Coronal CT reveals thickened wall and dilated appendix (*circle*).

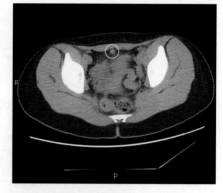

Axial CT at the level of the pelvis reveals small nodule adjacent to the anterior pelvic wall, in the midline space of Retzius, representing the urachal diverticulum (*circle*).

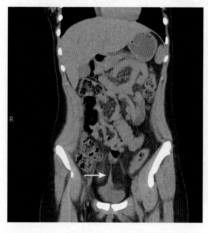

Coronal CT reveals a density branching from the dome of the bladder (*arrow*) representing urachal diverticulum.

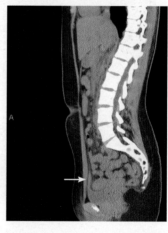

Sagittal CT reveals a density branching from the anterior aspect of the dome of the bladder (*arrow*) representing urachal diverticulum.

Answers

1. The images demonstrate dilated and thickened appendix. Incidentally, urachal diverticulum is noted.

2. The sonographic findings of acute appendicitis include increased flow to the appendix, noncompressible appendix, diameter of the appendix more than 6 mm, and appendicolith that may be seen.

3. During the fetal life, the urachus connects the anterior superior aspect of the bladder to the umbilicus.

4. The urachus is located in the space of Retzius.

5. Urachal remnants are associated with increased risk for the development of adenocarcinoma during adulthood.

Pearls

- This case demonstrates acute appendicitis in a non-contrast CT.
- Urachal diverticulum noted as an incidental finding.

Suggested Readings

Strouse PJ. Pediatric appendicitis: an argument for US. *Radiology*. 2010;255(1):8-13.

Yu JS, Kim KW, Lee HJ, Lee YJ, Yoon CS, Kim MJ. Urachal remnant diseases: spectrum of CT and US findings. *Radiographics*. 2002;21(2):451-461.

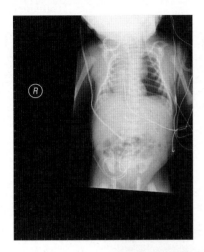
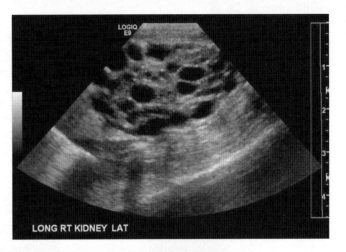
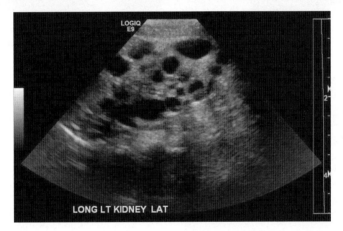

1. What is the diagnosis?

2. Which organ during fetal life produces the amniotic fluid?

3. What are the facial characteristics of the shown entity?

4. Which organ needs the amniotic fluid during the fetal life for normal development?

5. What are the other associated abnormalities of this entity?

Case ranking/difficulty: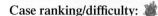

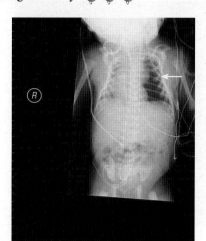

Frontal radiograph of the chest reveals left-sided pneumothorax (*arrow*).

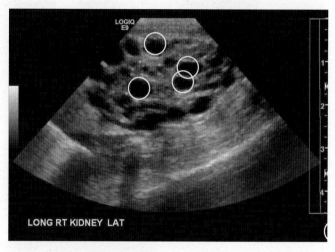

Sonogram of the right kidney reveals multiple cysts (*circles*). The cortex is thinned. This is consistent with multicystic dysplastic kidney.

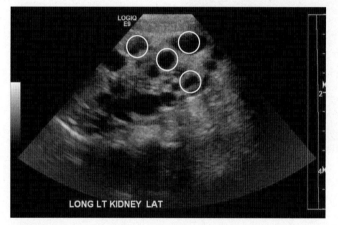

Sonogram of the left kidney reveals multiple cysts (*circles*). The cortex is thinned. This is consistent with multicystic dysplastic kidney.

5. This disease may be associated with hemivertebrae, sacral agenesis, and limb anomalies. Pulmonary hypoplasia and pneumothoraces are often seen.

Pearls

- Potter's syndrome is a direct result of oligohydramnios.
- Amniotic fluid is produced by the kidneys. It is composed of the urine produced during the fetal life.
- Normal amount of amniotic fluid is necessary for a normal lung development.
- Oligohydramnios may cause abnormalities in the development of the lungs. Pulmonary hypoplasia and pneumothoraces may occur at birth.
- Renal abnormalities such as obstructive uropathies, polycystic kidney disease, and multicystic dysplastic kidneys are all causes for decreased urine output during the fetal life and oligohydramnios.
- Newborns with Potter's syndrome have characteristic facies, and multiple other anomalies may be present.

Answers

1. The diagnosis is Potter's syndrome.

2. The amniotic fluid is the urine that the fetus produces by his kidneys. Any renal abnormality with decreased urine output may cause oligohydramnios.

3. Affected infants have characteristic facies: a flattened nose, recessed chin, prominent epicanthal folds, and low-set abnormal ears.

4. The mechanism of lung hypoplasia in Potter's syndrome is not clear. It is believed that adequate space in the fetal thorax and the movement of amniotic fluid into the fetal lungs are required for the normal development of lungs.

Suggested Reading

Dhundiraj KM, Madhukar DN, Ambadasrao PG, Wamanrao KS, Prem ZM. Potter's syndrome: a report of 5 cases. *Indian J Pathol Microbiol.* 2006;49(2):254-257.

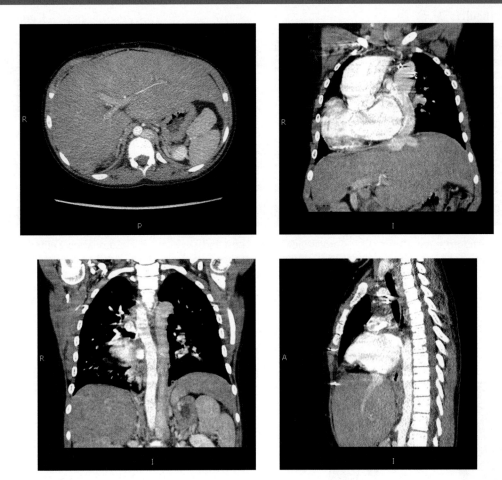

1. What is the diagnosis?

2. What are associated abnormalities of this entity?

3. How many lobes are there in both lungs in a case of polysplenia?

4. What kind of situs anomaly is seen in this entity?

5. What are the treatment options?

Case ranking/difficulty: 🦴 🦴 🦴

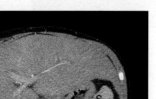

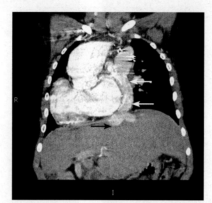

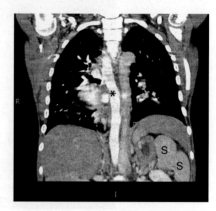

Axial CT of the upper abdomen reveals polysplenia (*S*). The aorta is on the right (*white arrow*) and the *black arrow* points to the dilated hemiazygos vein. Inferior vena cava is not visualized.

Coronal view of the chest and abdomen reveals that the liver tends to be in midline position (situs ambiguous). The hepatic veins (*black arrow*) drain into the inferior vena cava (*white arrows*) that in turn drains into the heart. The patient has complex congenital heart disease.

Coronal view of the chest reveals right-sided aorta (*black asterisk*). Dilated hemiazygos continuation (*white asterisk*) noted. Polysplenia is seen (*S*).

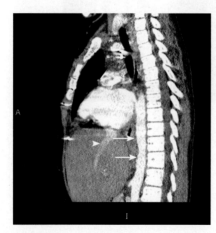

Sagittal view of the chest demonstrates the right-sided aorta (*arrows*). Hepatic vein is seen (*arrowhead*).

Answers

1. Diagnosis is Heterotaxy syndrome which includes in our case polysplenia, azygos continuation, congenital heart disease, and dextrocardia.

2. Associated abnormalities include congenital heart disease with situs ambiguous, asplenia or polysplenia, midgut malrotation, and biliary atresia.

3. With polysplenia, both lungs have 2 lobes (left-sided lungs). With asplenia, both lungs have 3 lobes (right-sided lungs).

4. The type of situs anomaly seen is situs ambiguous.

5. Treatment options are surgical repair of congenital heart disease; Ladd's procedure if the syndrome is associated with midgut malrotation; Kasai procedure if the syndrome is associated with biliary atresia; and antibiotics if associated with asplenia, or with non-functioning spleen.

Pearls

- Heterotaxy syndrome is associated with situs ambiguous and midline liver.
- There is presence of asplenia or polysplenia.
- With asplenia, the morphology of both the lungs is the same as that of right-sided lung (3 lobes bilaterally).
- With polysplenia, the morphology of both lungs is the same as that of left-sided lung (2 lobes bilaterally).
- Bilateral eparterial bronchi are associated with asplenia.
- Bilateral hyparterial bronchi are associated with polysplenia.
- Associated anomalies may include cardiac abnormalities, midgut malrotation, and biliary atresia.

Suggested Readings

Applegate KE, Goske MJ, Pierce G, Murphy D. Situs revisited: imaging of the heterotaxy syndrome. *Radiographics*. 1999;19(4):837-852; discussion 853-854.

Yoo SJ, Kim YM, Choe YH. Magnetic resonance imaging of complex congenital heart disease. *Int J Card Imaging*. 1999;15(2):151-160.

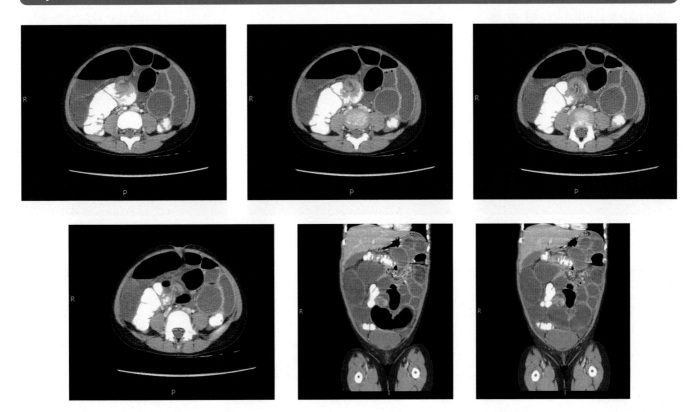

1. What is the diagnosis?

2. What may be the risk factors for the development of this entity?

3. What are the cross-sectional imaging findings of this entity?

4. What is the major complication of this entity?

5. What are the treatment options?

Case ranking/difficulty:

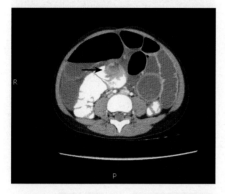 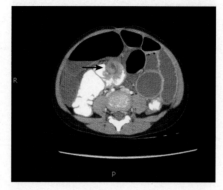 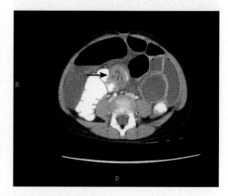

Axial CT of the abdomen with rectal contrast reveals swirling of the ileum representing a volvulus (*arrow*). Fluid-filled bowel loops noted representing an ileus.

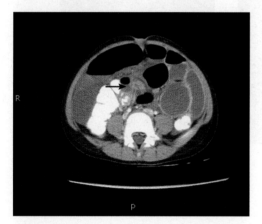 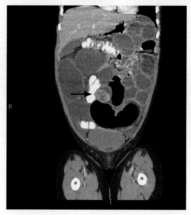

Axial CT of the abdomen with rectal contrast reveals swirling of the ileum representing a volvulus (*arrow*). Fluid-filled bowel loops noted representing an ileus.

Coronal CT of the abdomen with rectal contrast reveals swirling of the ileum representing a volvulus (*arrow*). Fluid-filled bowel loops noted representing an ileus.

Answers

1. The diagnosis is ileal volvulus.

2. Among the risk factors for the development of ileal volvulus are Henoch-Schönlein purpura, Meckel's diverticulum, intestinal lymphoma, and intestinal lipoma.

3. On CT and MR, the characteristic findings include the "whirl" sign of the rotated vessel and "peacock's tail" sign (due to torsion of the bowel around the vessel axis). Small bowel ischemia or infarction is suggested on CT by the presence of bowel wall thickening, intra-mucosal air, and intra-peritoneal fluid.

4. The major complication is ischemia and bowel necrosis.

5. Treatment is emergent surgery to untwist bowel loop, avoid vascular compromise, and prevent ischemia and bowel necrosis. If there is necrosis, the affected segment should be resected.

Pearls

- Henoch-Schönlein purpura is a small-vessel vasculitis characterized by purpura, abdominal pain, hematuria, and arthritis.
- The common complication is small bowel intussusception, but rarely ileal volvulus may occur as in this case of Henoch-Schönlein purpura.
- Volvulus is an intestinal obstruction, in which a loop of bowel has abnormally twisted on itself.

Suggested Readings

Chen Y, Tseng SH, Lai HS, Chen WJ. Primary volvulus of the ileum in a preterm infant. *J Formos Med Assoc.* 2003;102(12):896-898.

Sheen AJ, Drake I, George PP. A small bowel volvulus caused by a mesenteric lipoma: report of a case. *Surg Today.* 2003;33(8):617-619.

23-month-old male with midgut volvulus. There was no midgut malrotation

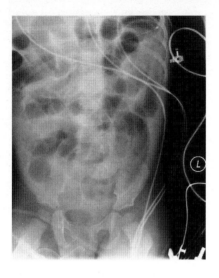 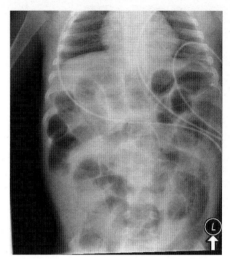

1. What should be your impression of the abdominal radiographs?

2. What is the differential diagnosis of intestinal obstruction in this patient's age group?

3. What are the signs of free intraperitoneal air in supine frontal radiograph of the abdomen?

4. Following review of the abdominal radiographs, what should be the next step?

5. What is the most common risk factor for midgut volvulus in infants?

Case ranking/difficulty:

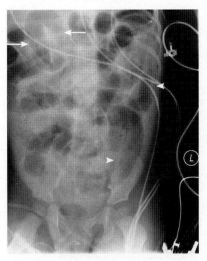

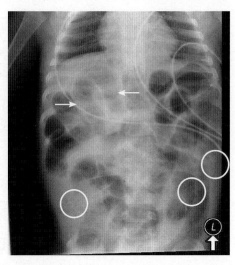

Frontal radiograph of the abdomen reveals a loop of small bowel (*arrows*) that has coffee-grain appearance that represents the midgut volvulus. The bowel loops are dilated and tubular. Bubbly appearance noted with intramural air (*arrowheads*).

Frontal radiograph of the abdomen reveals a loop of small bowel (*arrows*) that has coffee-grain appearance that represents the midgut volvulus. The bowel loops are dilated and tubular. Bubbly appearance is seen that represents submucosal intramural air (*circles*).

Answers

1. The images should raise suspicion for possible bowel obstruction and ischemia.

2. Differential diagnosis may include the different etiologies for obstruction such as midgut volvulus, post-surgical adhesions, acute appendicitis, incarcerated inguinal hernia, and Meckel's diverticulum.

3. Signs of intraperitoneal free air in supine frontal radiograph include visualization of the falciform ligament, Rigler's sign, and the right upper quadrant of the abdomen being more lucent than the chest retrocardiac region.

4. There is no right answer. Each of the answers may be the right one. The best answer is that clinical correlation is essential. In this particular case, the patient was very sick and the best thing was to take him immediately to the operating room.

5. The most common risk factor for midgut volvulus in infants is malrotation.

Pearls

- The abdominal image is very nonspecific; however, a loop of bowel in the right upper quadrant that has coffee-grain appearance may suggest the possibility of midgut volvulus.
- There are in the abdominal radiographs findings that are suggestive of ischemic bowel, such as bubbly appearance and linear lucencies in the margins of few bowel loops. The loops of bowel are extremely dilated and tubular with loss of the normal bowel mosaic appearance.
- Midgut volvulus without malrotation is a very rare occurrence.
- Midgut volvulus is an extreme emergency. There is a risk of necrotic bowel due to occlusion of blood supply.

Suggested Readings

Andrassy RJ, Mahour GH. Malrotation of the midgut in infants and children: a 25-year review. *Arch Surg.* 1981;116(2):158-160.

Kealey WD, McCallion WA, Brown S, Potts SR, Boston VE. Midgut volvulus in children. *Br J Surg.* 1996;83(1): 105-106.

Seashore JH, Touloukian RJ. Midgut volvulus. An ever-present threat. *Arch Pediatr Adolesc Med.* 1994;148(1):43-46.

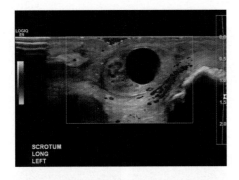
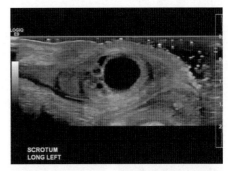
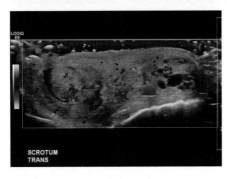
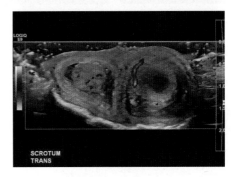

1. What is the differential diagnosis?

2. What is the serum marker of the shown entity?

3. What are the clinical findings at presentation?

4. What is the percentage of metastatic spread at presentation?

5. What is the most common testicular neoplasm in pre-pubertal children?

Case ranking/difficulty:

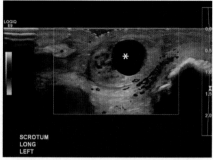

Longitudinal sonogram of the left testicle reveals a large cyst in the left testicle (*asterisk*). The large cyst is surrounded by smaller cysts. The left testicle has heterogeneous echo texture.

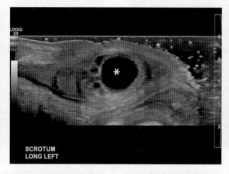

Longitudinal sonogram of the left testicle reveals a large cyst in the left testicle (*asterisk*). The large cyst is surrounded by smaller cysts. The left testicle has heterogeneous echo texture.

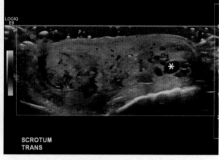

Transverse sonogram of the testicles reveals a large cyst in the left testicle (*asterisk*). The large cyst is surrounded by smaller cysts. The left testicle has heterogeneous echo texture.

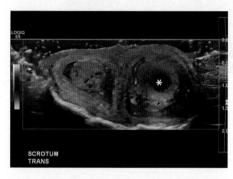

Transverse sonogram of the testicles reveals a large cyst in the left testicle (*asterisk*). The left testicle has heterogeneous echo texture.

Pearls

- Yolk sac tumor, also known as endodermal sinus tumor, is part of the germ cell tumor group.
- These cells secrete alpha-fetoprotein, which can be detected in the tumor, cerebrospinal fluid, serum, urine, and the amniotic fluid.
- Children present with painless testicular mass. Metastasis at presentation occurs in less than 10% of cases.
- Images may demonstrate the elements of teratoma: bone, hair, or cartilage. Calcifications may be seen.

Answers

1. Differential diagnosis includes teratoma, choriocarcinoma, seminoma, embryonal carcinoma, and testicular torsion.

2. The cells of yolk sac tumor secrete alpha-fetoprotein, which can be detected in the tumor, cerebrospinal fluid, serum, urine, and the amniotic fluid.

3. Children present with painless testicular mass.

4. Metastasis at presentation occurs in less than 10% of cases.

5. Yolk sac tumor is the most common testicular neoplasm in pre-pubertal children.

Suggested Readings

Barth RA, Teele RL, Colodny A, Retik A, Bauer S. Asymptomatic scrotal masses in children. *Radiology.* 1984;152(1):65-68.

Luker GD, Siegel MJ. Pediatric testicular tumors: evaluation with gray-scale and color Doppler US. *Radiology.* 1994;191(2):561-564.

Thava V, Cooper N, Egginton JA. Yolk sac tumour of the testis in childhood. *Br J Radiol.* 1992;65(780):1142-1144.

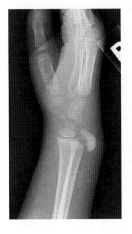 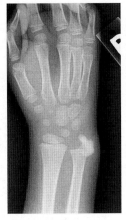 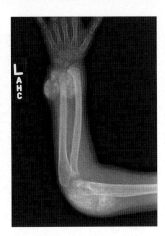 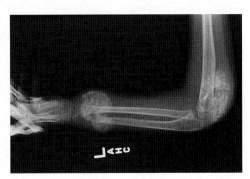

1. Describe the findings.

2. What are the entities included in the differential diagnosis?

3. What are the complications of this case?

4. What are the serum findings of the case?

5. What are the treatment options?

Case ranking/difficulty:

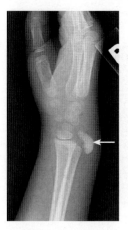

Lateral radiograph of the wrist demonstrates amorphous calcifications in the soft tissue adjacent to the joint (*arrow*).

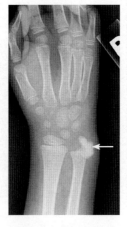

Oblique radiograph of the wrist demonstrates amorphous calcifications in the soft tissue adjacent to the joint (*arrow*).

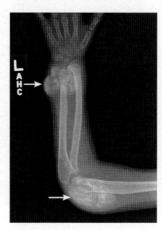

Oblique radiograph of the wrist of another 4-year-old female demonstrates amorphous calcifications in the soft tissue adjacent to the wrist and elbow (*arrows*). Ulnar minus variance noted.

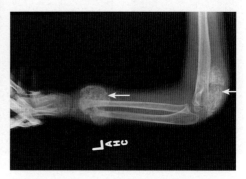

Lateral radiograph of the wrist of another 4-year-old female demonstrates amorphous calcifications in the soft tissue adjacent to the wrist and elbow (*arrows*). Ulnar minus variance noted.

Answers

1. Plain radiograph of the wrist demonstrates amorphous calcifications in the soft tissue adjacent to the joints. In images on the left, the calcifications are seen adjacent to the wrist. Images on the right, of another patient, demonstrate calcifications adjacent to the wrist and the elbow. Ulnar minus variance is seen on the two right images.

2. Entities that may be included in the differential diagnosis are hyperparathyroidism, heterotopic ossification, hypervitaminosis D, dermatomyositis, and renal osteodystrophy.

3. Complications may include compression of peripheral nerves, rare bone erosion, erosion through skin and drainage of chalky material through sinus tract, and development of amyloidosis.

4. There is normal renal and parathyroid function. There is normal or slightly elevated serum calcium, phosphorus, uric acid, and alkaline phosphatase.

5. The masses of calcification can be removed surgically, but recurrence is common if the masses are incompletely excised.

Pearls

- Tumoral calcinosis is not specific for a particular disease entity, but simply refers to the mass-like calcific deposits seen in the soft tissue adjacent to joints.
- Onset is usually during childhood or adolescence, and there may be an increased prevalence in patients of African descent.

Suggested Readings

Fernbach SK, Gore MD, Poznanski AK. Pediatric case of the day. Tumoral calcinosis. *Radiographics*. 1989;9(4):774-776.

Olsen KM, Chew FS. Tumoral calcinosis: pearls, polemics, and alternative possibilities. *Radiographics*. 2011;26(3):871-885.

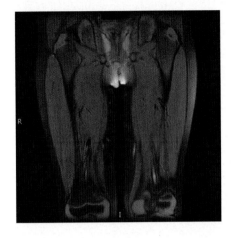 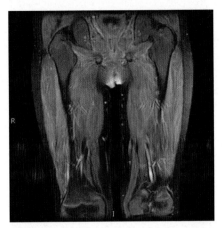 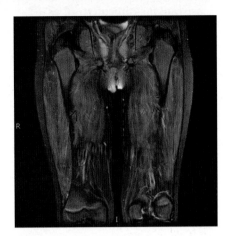

1. Describe the findings.

2. What are the clinical symptoms?

3. What are the medications that the shown case can be a side effect?

4. Which blood marker is elevated in this case?

5. What is the most common etiology of the case?

Case ranking/difficulty:

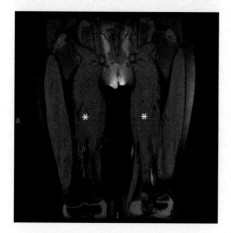

Coronal MRI-T1 of the lower extremities demonstrates intermediate signal of the musculature of the lower extremities (*asterisks*).

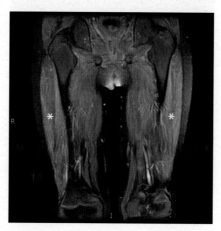

Coronal MRI-T1 of the lower extremities following contrast administration demonstrates enhancement of the musculature of the lower extremities (*asterisks*).

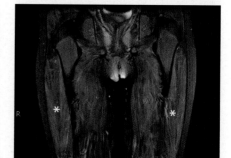

Coronal MRI-T2 of the lower extremities demonstrates high signal of the musculature of the lower extremities (*asterisks*).

Answers

1. MRI-T1 demonstrates intermediate signal of the muscles of both thighs. There is diffuse enhancement in post contrast T1 bilaterally. MRI-T2 demonstrates diffuse high signal of the muscles bilaterally.

2. Clinical symptoms of myositis include weakness, fatigue, and muscle pain.

3. Myositis is a documented side effect of the lipid-lowering drugs statins and fibrates.

4. Elevation of creatine kinase in blood is indicative of myositis.

5. Myositis is a general term for inflammation of the muscles. Many such conditions are considered to be caused by autoimmune process.

Pearls

- Myositis is defined as inflammation of the muscles.
- Dermatomyositis is defined as inflammation of the muscles and the skin.
- Usually bilateral.
- Most children with myositis are between 5 and 15 years old.
- MRI findings are muscular low or intermediate signal in T1 and high signal in T2.
- Treatment includes corticosteroids and immunosuppressants.

Suggested Readings

Peetrons P. Ultrasound of muscles. *Eur Radiol.* 2002;12(1):35-43.

Soler R, Rodríguez E, Aguilera C, Fernández R. Magnetic resonance imaging of pyomyositis in 43 cases. *Eur J Radiol.* 2000;35(1):59-64.

Trusen A, Beissert M, Schultz G, Chittka B, Darge K. Ultrasound and MRI features of pyomyositis in children. *Eur Radiol.* 2003;13(5):1050-1055.

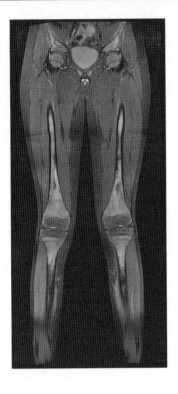 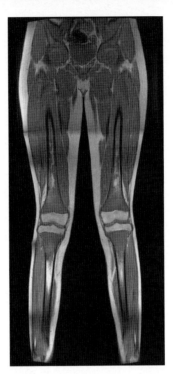 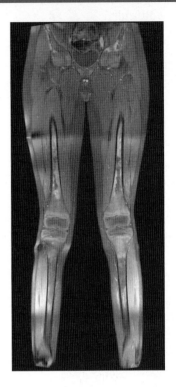

1. What are the findings?

2. What is the differential diagnosis?

3. What are known risk factors?

4. What are the different types of cells that may be involved?

5. What is the expected overall outcome of this entity?

Case ranking/difficulty: **Category:** Lower extremities

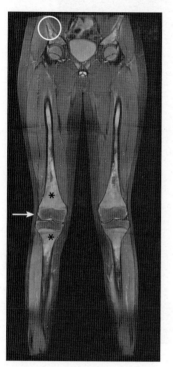

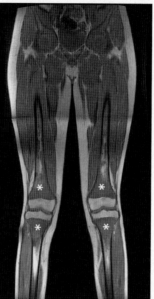

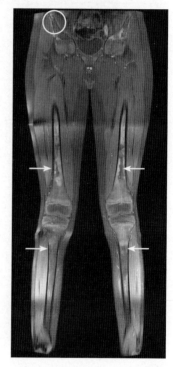

Diffuse STIR-hyperintense infiltration of the bone marrow of the femora and tibiae (*asterisks*). Note the sparing of the epiphysis (*arrow*). At the pelvic level (*circle*), there is a subperiosteal infiltration on both sides of the ilium.

The infiltrated areas demonstrate a classical T1-hypointensity (*asterisks*).

All infiltrated areas demonstrate intense contrast enhancement with a serpiginous aspect (*arrows*) in the metadiaphysis of the long tubular bones, but also in the subperiosteal region at the pelvis (*circle*).

Answers

1. Bone marrow infiltration is localized at the metadiaphysis of the long tubular bones. Subperiosteal infiltration is mostly seen in the flat bones, eg, the pelvic girdle. Epiphysis is spared.

2. Burkitt lymphoma may involve the bones, but this is mainly in the head and neck region (especially the mandibule), and usually presents as a soft tissue mass. Main differential diagnoses are bone metastasis in neuroblastoma and Langerhan's cell histiocytosis (LCH). In LCH, bone involvement demonstrates a typical geographic osteolysis, whereas the infiltration is diffuse without edges in leukemia.

3. Especially Down syndrome predisposes to ALL and AML, but has a benign course than non-Down syndrome associated leukemia.

4. Germ stem cells differentiate into myeloid or lymphoid stem cells. The latter differentiates further into lymphoblasts, and eventually either B or T or natural killer lymphocytes are produced. All of these cells have been involved in leukemia.

5. Remission can be achieved with chemotherapy in over 95% of children and 80% of children with newly diagnosed ALL will be long-term survivors.

Pearls

- Diffuse infiltration of the bone marrow.
- Characteristic T1-hypointensity/T2-hyperintensity and contrast enhancement.
- On x-rays metaphyseal band lucencies can be observed.
- Absence of a tumorous mass (in contrast to Burkitt leukemia/lymphoma).

Suggested Readings

Dugan LO, Meyer SJ, Chua GT. General case of the day. Acute lymphoblastic leukemia. *Radiographics*. 1993;13(1):221-223.

Vázquez E, Lucaya J, Castellote A, et al. Neuroimaging in pediatric leukemia and lymphoma: differential diagnosis. *Radiographics*. 2002;22(6):1411-1428.

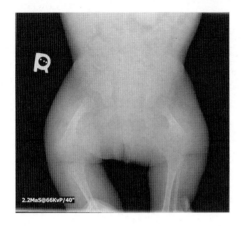 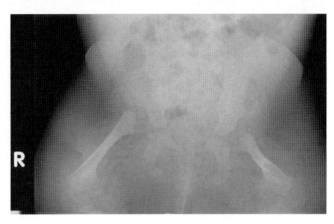

1. What are the findings?

2. What is the relevant anatomy of this entity?

3. How newborn with this entity presents?

4. What is the histopathology of this entity?

5. What are the associated anomalies?

Case ranking/difficulty:

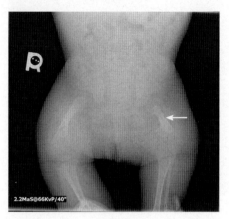

Frontal view of the pelvis and both femora demonstrates shortening of the left femur (*arrow*) in comparison to the right femur. In addition, both femora do not align with the acetabula suggestive of bilateral developmental hip dysplasia.

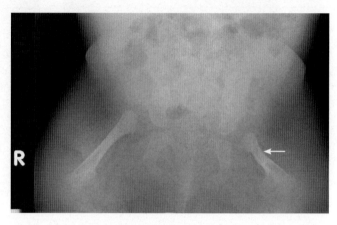

Frontal view of the pelvis and both femora in abduction view demonstrates shortening of the left femur (*arrow*) in comparison to the right femur. In addition, both the femora do not align with the acetabula suggestive of bilateral developmental hip dysplasia.

Answers

1. There is short left femur. Both hips are dysplastic. Both proximal femora do not align with the acetabula.

2. In proximal femoral focal deficiency, the proximal femur is partially absent, and the entire limb is overall shortened.

3. The appearance of proximal focal femoral deficiency is not subtle, so it is easily recognized. The femur is shortened, flexed, abducted, and externally rotated.

4. A defect in proliferation and maturation of chondrocytes in the proximal growth plate.

5. The knee is uniformly unstable in an anteroposterior plane secondary to absent cruciate ligaments. Generalized knee hypoplasia has been reported. Fibular deficiencies are found in as many as 70 to 80% of persons with PFFD. Approximately 50% of patients with PFFD have other limb anomalies.

Pearls

- Proximal femoral focal deficiency (PFFD) is an uncommon disorder.
- The modality of choice for the diagnosis is plain radiograph.

Suggested Readings

Epps CH. Proximal femoral focal deficiency. *J Bone Joint Surg Am.* 1983;65(6):867-870.

Gillespie R, Torode IP. Classification and management of congenital abnormalities of the femur. *J Bone Joint Surg Br.* 1983;65(5):557-568.

Panting AL, Williams PF. Proximal femoral focal deficiency. *J Bone Joint Surg Br.* 1978;60(1):46-52.

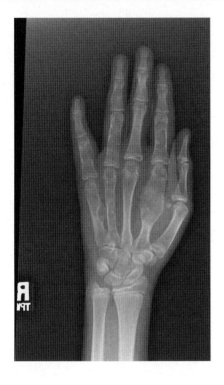 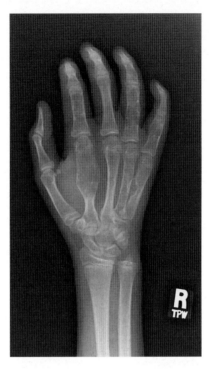 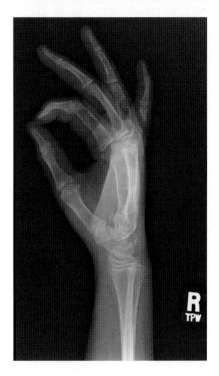

1. What are the findings?

2. What is the major complication of the case?

3. What are pathologic characteristics of the lytic lesions in the right hand?

4. What is Maffucci syndrome?

5. What are the treatment options?

Case ranking/difficulty: **Category:** Generalized diseases

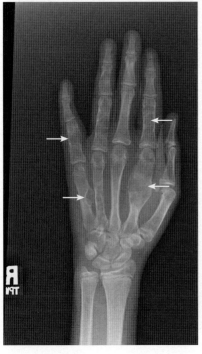

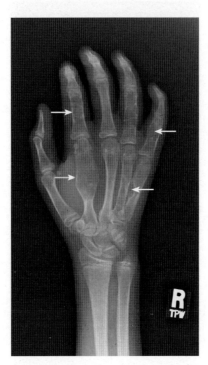

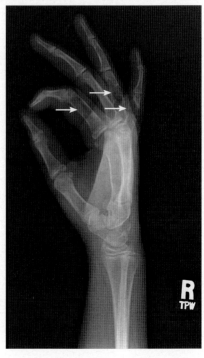

Radiograph of the right hand in frontal view reveals multiple lytic lesions through all metacarpals and phalanges (*arrows*). The larger lesions show cartilage calcification in a typical rings-and-arcs pattern.

Radiograph of the right hand in oblique view reveals multiple lytic lesions through all metacarpals and phalanges (*arrows*). The larger lesions show cartilage calcification in a typical rings-and-arcs pattern.

Radiograph of the right hand in lateral view reveals multiple lytic lesions through all metacarpals and phalanges (*arrows*). The larger lesions show cartilage calcification in a typical rings-and-arcs pattern.

Answers

1. The right hand reveals multiple lytic lesions through all metacarpals and phalanges. The larger lesions show cartilage calcification in a typical rings-and-arcs pattern.

2. There is an increased risk of chondrosarcoma occurring later in life. The risk has been reported to be up to 25 to 30% at 40 years.

3. The lytic lesions are enchondromas with cartilaginous matrix.

4. Ollier disease or multiple enchondromatosis associated with multiple angiomas is called Maffucci syndrome.

5. There is no medical treatment for Ollier disease. Surgery is indicated in case of complications (pathological fractures, growth defect, malignant transformation).

Pearls

- Ollier disease is a skeletal disorder characterized by cartilaginous tumors.

- The disease consists of multiple enchondromas which usually develop in childhood.
- Most patients have bilateral involvement, with predominance on one side. Enchondromas most frequently involve the short tubular bones of hands and feet.
- Plain radiographs reveal the classic appearance of multiple lytic lesions through the metacarpals and phalanges. Lesions may demonstrate cartilage calcification in a typical rings-and-arcs pattern.
- Patients with Ollier disease have increased risk of a secondary chondrosarcoma developing later in life.

Suggested Readings

Mainzer F, Minagi H, Steinbach HL. The variable manifestations of multiple enchondromatosis. *Radiology*. 1971;99(2):377-388.

Vázquez-García B, Valverde M, San-Julián M. Ollier disease: benign tumours with risk of malignant transformation. A review of 17 cases. *An Pediatr (Barc)*. 2011;74(3):168-173.

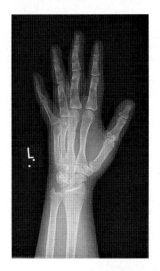 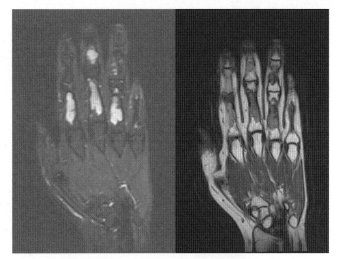

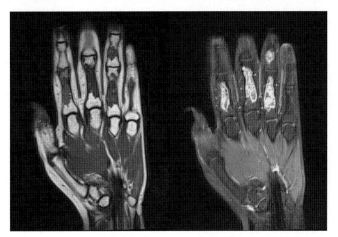

1. What is the diagnosis?

2. What are the possible complications?

3. What are the treatment options?

4. Which syndromes may be associated?

5. What are the possible complementary examinations?

Case ranking/difficulty: **Category:** Syndromes

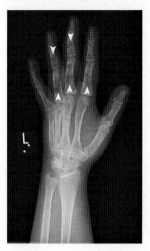

Hyperlucent areas in the proximal and middle phalanges of digits 2/3/4 (*arrowheads*). The cortex is thinned and shows signs of scalloping.

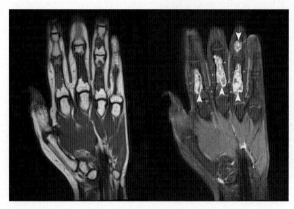

Serpiginous contrast enhancement of all lesions (right image, *arrowheads*).

Answers

1. Multiple cartilaginous tumors with T2WI hyperintensity and typical serpiginous enhancement pattern. The meta-diaphyseal but not epiphyseal location is typical for enchondroma.

2. Pathological fracture is always a possibility especially when enchondroma are getting larger. More centrally located lesions (femur, humerus) have a higher rate of malignant transformation into chondrosarcoma.

3. If tumor resection due to concerns about malignant transformation is needed, a primary complete R0 resection is advocated. Biopsy alone should not be performed to avoid spilling of tumor cells into the soft tissues (higher recurrence rates). In enchondroma larger than 5 cm, the risk of malignant degeneration is markedly elevated. Resection is not advised in asymptomatic non-syndromic patients.

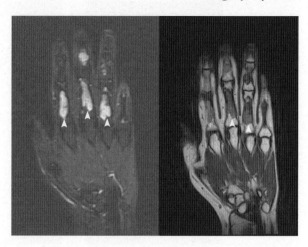

The tumors appear T2-hyperintense (STIR image on the left side) and of intermediate signal on proton density (PD right side), similar to cartilage (*arrowheads*). No extra osseous component is noted.

4. In case of multiple enchondromas, a syndromic enchondromatosis must be suspected. In Ollier disease, enchondromas are often all located on one body-side (eg, left leg and left arm). In Maffucci syndrome, multiple hemangioma of the skin and other visceral organs (including bones) are present. In these syndromic patients, there is a higher incidence of malignant transformation.

5. Scintigraphy is the method of choice to screen for multiple enchondromas in case a syndromic condition is suspected. Whole body MRI can be used as an alternative.

Pearls

- Enchondromas are benign cartilaginous tumors mainly occurring in tubular bones of the hand.
- They appear T2WI-hyperintense and take up contrast on MR in a serpiginous pattern.
- They may have a columnar appearance and are based at the epiphyseal growth plate.
- Enchondromatosis must be suspected in case of multiple enchondroma.

Suggested Readings

Choi BB, Jee WH, Sunwoo HJ, et al. MR differentiation of low-grade chondrosarcoma from enchondroma. *Clin Imaging*. 2012;37(3):542-547.

Douis H, Saifuddin A. The imaging of cartilaginous bone tumours. I. Benign lesions. *Skeletal Radiol*. 2012;41(10):1195-1212.

Larbi A, Viala P, Omoumi P, Lecouvet F, et al. Cartilaginous tumours and calcified lesions of the hand: a pictorial review. *Diagn Interv Imaging*. 2013;94(4):395-409.

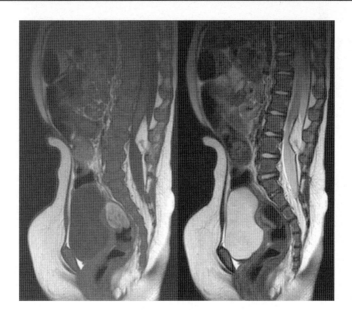

1. What are the findings?

2. What is the diagnosis?

3. What is the embryologic origin of this entity?

4. What are the clinical complications of this entity?

5. What is the etiology of non-congenital variant of this entity?

Case ranking/difficulty:

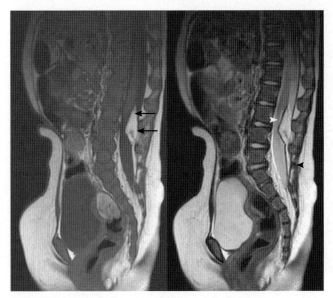

Left: T1WI, Right: T2WI. There is a sacralization of L5 and a posterior arch anomaly with atrophy of the spinal process of L5 (*black arrowhead*). There is a large fatty but slightly heterogeneous mass (*black arrows*), posteriorly attached to the conus which is too low (L3/L4), and tethered (*white arrowhead*).

Answers

1. The T1WI and T2WI hyperintense but slightly heterogeneous mass represents mostly fat which is always dorsal of the conus medullaris. It is an intraspinal extramedullary located but can also have an intramedullary component in cases where the spinal cord is splayed. As this mass arises during the fetal period when the conus is normally low at the lumbosacral region, it will impede its normal ascension due to spinal vertebral development, and produce a tethered cord.

2. Spinal dermoid/epidermoid mass is a slow growing benign tumor that contains mainly fat but also possibly cystic-appearing elements of dermal and/or epidermal origin. Growth is not due to cellular proliferation but desquamation and normal cellular turnover from the dermal/epidermal inclusions. Hence, neurological complications will appear after some time, mainly due to compression of adjacent neuronal elements.

3. The precocious separation of epithelial and neuronal layers during neurulation induces exposure of the infolding central neural canal to peripheral mesenchymal cells which will transform into fat. Therefore, fatty tissue will always be located at the dorsal part of the conus. Furthermore, dermal and epidermal elements may also be scattered within the infolding neural tube before its normal closure, inducing the presence of dermal/epidermal cysts.

4. Only 1 to 2% of the cystic dermoids/epidermoids may rupture (especially during surgery, rarely spontaneously), and produce an irritative meningitis. Rupture also produces a spilling of the fatty contents within the subarachnoid space and fat embolism.

5. Lumbar puncture has been proven to possibly push some epithelial cells during skin puncture for lumbar puncture into the subarachnoid space of the spinal canal. These cells may eventually lead to epidermoid cysts.

Pearls

- Dermoid/epidermoid cyst is a congenital malformation due to focal incomplete closure of the primitive neural placode.
- Fatty mass is located posteriorly to the medulla.
- Dermoid cysts occur most frequently at the level of the conus or distal medulla.
- Associated vertebral anomaly is frequent.
- Rupture of the dermoid cyst may occur in 1 to 2% of cases and may induce irritative chemical meningitis.

Suggested Readings

Alexiou GA, Prodromou N. Spinal dermal sinus tract. *Childs Nerv Syst.* 2010 May;26(5):597.

De Vloo P, Lagae L, Sciot R, Demaerel P, van Loon J, Van Calenbergh F. Spinal dermal sinuses and dermal sinus-like stalks analysis of 14 cases with suggestions for embryologic mechanisms resulting in dermal sinus-like stalks. *Eur J Paediatr Neurol.* 2013 Nov;17(6):575-584.

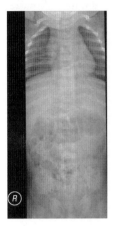 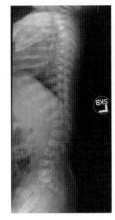 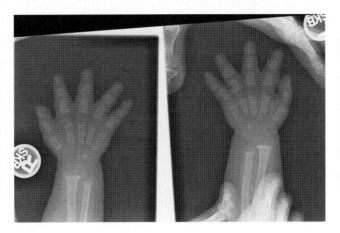 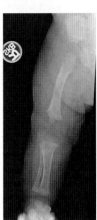

1. Describe the findings seen in both hands.

2. What is the finding that is usually seen in the spine of this entity?

3. What is the characteristic appearance of the pelvis in this entity?

4. What is the pathophysiology of this entity?

5. What are the treatment options?

Case ranking/difficulty: Category: Generalized diseases

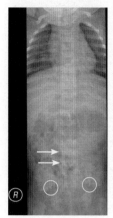 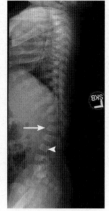 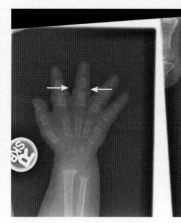 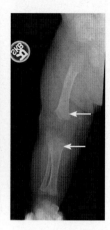

Frontal radiograph of the thoracolumbar spine and the pelvis demonstrates narrowing of the interpediculate space of vertebral bodies in the caudal direction (*arrows*). The pelvis has squared iliac wings (champagne-glass appearance) with bilateral sacroiliac notch (*circles*). Horizontal acetabular roof noted. The ribs are short.

Lateral radiograph of the thoracic spine demonstrates loss of the normal lumbar lordosis and the normal thoracic kyphosis. Vertebral bodies may have bullet-shape appearance with anterior beaking (*arrow*). Posterior scalloping of the vetebral bodies is seen (*arrowhead*).

Frontal radiograph of the hands shows trident hands–the second, third, and fourth fingers appearing separated and similar in length (*arrows*).

Frontal radiograph of the right femur demonstrates short limbs with widening and flaring of the metaphyses (*arrows*).

Pearls

- Achondroplasia is the most common short-limbed dwarfism.
- The disease is characterized as being rhizomelic dwarfism.
- Primary defect is abnormal endochondral ossification.
- There is decrease in the interpediculate distance of the vertebral bodies in the caudal direction.
- The pelvis has champagne-glass appearance.
- The hands have trident appearance.

Answers

1. The frontal view of the hands reveals trident hands–the second, third, and fourth fingers appearing separated and similar in length. There is undertubulation of the bones–broad phalanges. There is no osteopenia and the interphalangeal joints are not narrowed.

2. There is decrease in the interpediculate distance of the vertebral bodies in the caudal direction, which may lead to spinal stenosis.

3. In achondroplasia, the pelvis is squared and has champagne-glass appearance.

4. The primary defect found in patients with achondroplasia is abnormal endochondral ossification.

5. Growth hormone is currently being used to augment the height of patients with achondroplasia. The greatest acceleration in growth velocity is seen during the first year of treatment and in those with the lowest growth velocities before treatment.

Suggested Readings

Cheema JI, Grissom LE, Harcke HT. Radiographic characteristics of lower-extremity bowing in children. *Radiographics*. 2003;23(4):871-880.

Dighe M, Fligner C, Cheng E, et-al. Fetal skeletal dysplasia: an approach to diagnosis with illustrative cases. *Radiographics*. 2008;28(4):1061-1077.

Reeder MM, Felson B. *Reeder and Felson's Gamuts in Radiology, Comprehensive Lists of Roentgen Differential Diagnosis*. Springer Verlag; 2003. ISBN:0387955887.

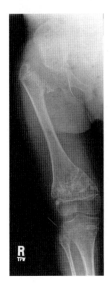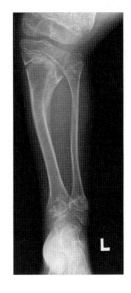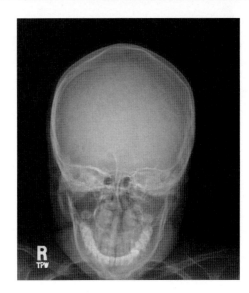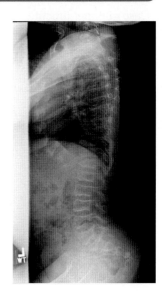

1. What are the findings?

2. What are the spinal changes?

3. What are the skull changes?

4. What is the pattern of the femoral heads?

5. What is the metabolic disorder of this case?

Case ranking/difficulty:

Category: Syndromes

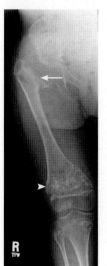

Frontal radiograph of the right femur demonstrates coxa vara. The femoral heads are not visualized (*arrow*). There is widening and sclerosis of the distal femoral metaphysis (*arrowhead*).

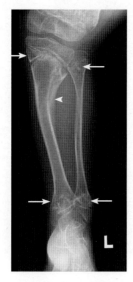

Frontal radiograph of the left tibia and fibula demonstrates widening and sclerosis of the metaphysis (*arrows*). There is mild bowing of the tibia (*arrowhead*).

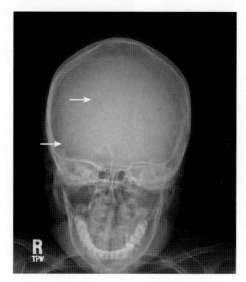

Frontal radiograph of the skull demonstrates wormian bones (*arrows*).

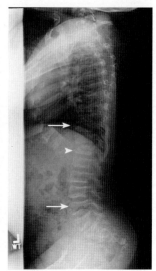

Lateral view of the thoracolumbar spine shows decrease in height of few of the vertebral bodies (*arrows*), beaking, and deformities (*arrowhead*).

Answers

1. Lower extremities bones are bowed. There is widening and sclerosis of the epiphyses. Femoral heads are unformed. There is bilateral coxa vara.

2. Changes in the spine include sclerosis and platyspondyly.

3. Wormian bones are seen.

4. Coxa vara is frequently seen.

5. Abnormal collagen prevents bones and other connective tissues from developing properly, which leads to the signs and symptoms of spondyloepimetaphyseal dysplasia, Strudwick type.

- The disorder affects mainly the spine, epiphyses, and metaphyses of long bones.
- The characteristic changes are short-stature, short trunk, and limbs.
- The hands and feet are usually average-sized.
- Platyspondyly, pectus carinatum, coxa vara, and clubfoot are seen.
- There is scoliosis and lumbar lordosis that may lead to respiratory difficulties.
- Visual disturbances are also part of the syndrome.
- The changes in the vertebral bodies may lead to spinal cord damage.

Suggested Readings

Bieganski T, Lipczyk Z, Kozlowski K. Rhizomelic spondyloepimetaphyseal dysplasia. *Clin Dysmorphol.* 2001;10(4):285-288.

Shebib SM, Chudley AE, Reed MH. Spondylometepiphyseal dysplasia congenita, Strudwick type. *Pediatr Radiol.* 1991;21(4):298-300.

Pearls

- Spondyloepimetaphyseal dysplasia, Strudwick type is an inherited disorder that results in bone deformities and dwarfism.
- The disorder interferes with the assembly of type II collagen molecule that prevents bone from proper development.

14-year-old male with chronic bone disease

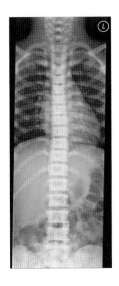
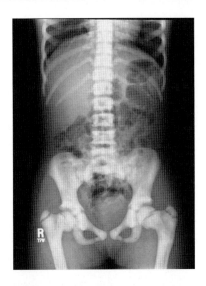
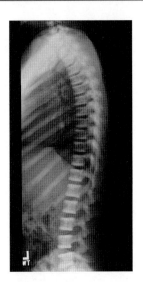

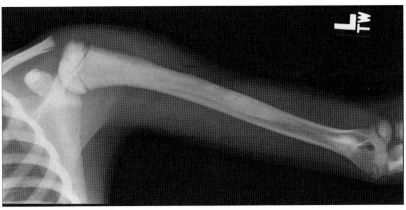
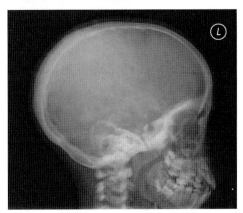

1. Which cell function is impaired in this case?

2. What is the differential diagnosis?

3. What is the radiographic pattern of the bones?

4. How will you characterize the pattern of the femoral heads?

5. What are the treatment options?

Case ranking/difficulty: 🐾 🐾 🐾

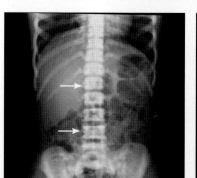
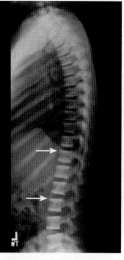
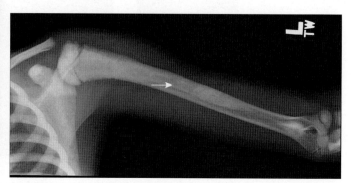

Frontal radiograph of the thoracic lumbar spine reveals high density of the cortex of all the vertebral bodies (*arrows*). Ribs are sclerotic. The pelvis is extremely sclerotic and the femurs are sclerotic. Bilateral coxa vara noted.

Lateral radiograph of the thoracic lumbar spine reveals high density of the cortex of all the vertebral bodies (*arrows*). Ribs are sclerotic.

Frontal radiograph of the left humerus demonstrates sclerotic medullary region. The cortex extends to the medullary portion of the bone (*arrow*).

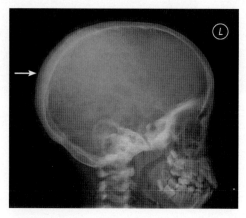

Lateral radiograph of the skull shows thickened cortex (*arrow*).

Answers

1. In osteopetrosis, there is impaired function of the osteoclasts. Bone resorption is impaired.

2. Differential diagnosis includes hypoparathyroidism, pseudohypoparathyroidism, and lead toxicity.

   Paget disease is the differential diagnosis of adult type osteopetrosis, not the infantile type. Our case is a child.

3. There is severe osteosclerosis. The pattern of osteopetrosis is characterized as bone within a bone.

Vertebral bodies have the appearance of a picture frame. Vertebrae are extremely radiodense. They may show alternating bands, known as the Rugger-Jersey spine sign.

4. The pattern of the femoral head is coxa vara. The angle between the femoral neck and the femoral diaphysis is decreased. This pattern is not specific for osteopetrosis.

5. Treatment includes vitamin D that stimulates osteoclasts, gamma interferon to improve white blood cells function, erythropoietin to correct anemia, and corticosteroids to stimulate bone resorption and treat anemia.

Pearls

- The disease has two major types: adult type, which is autosomal dominant with good prognosis; and infantile type, which is autosomal recessive with poor prognosis.

Suggested Readings

Gelman MI. Autosomal dominant osteosclerosis. *Radiology*. 1977;125(2):289-296.

Kelley CH, Lawlah JW. Albers-Schönberg disease: a family survey. *Radiology*. 1946;47(5):507-513.

Troeger J, Seidensticker P. Osteopetrosis. *Paediatric Imaging Manual*. Springer; 2008:137-138.

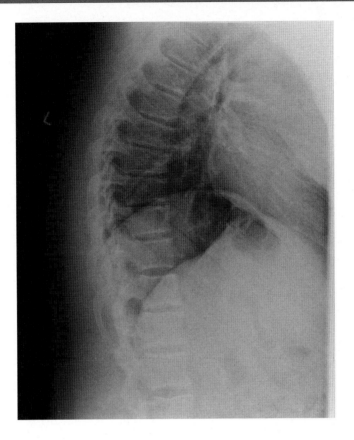

1. What are the findings?

2. What age group is affected by this entity?

3. What are the presumptive causative factors for this entity?

4. What are the radiographic signs of this disease?

5. What are the treatment options?

Case ranking/difficulty: **Category:** Spine

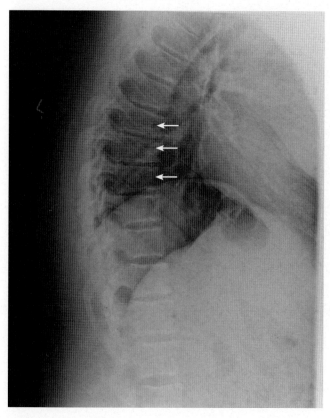

Lateral radiograph of the thoracic spine reveals anterior wedging of T8 and to a lesser degrees of T6, T7, and T9 (*arrows*). Kyphosis is present.

Answers

1. There is kyphosis. Anterior wedging of T6, T7, T8, and T9 noted. Schmorl's nodes of the inferior anterior end plate of T9 noted.

2. Patients with Scheuermann's disease generally are affected at age 13 to 16 years.

3. There is osteochondrosis of the secondary ossification centers of the vertebral bodies. Osteochondritis of the upper and lower cartilaginous vertebral plates and trauma seem to be the causative factors.

4. Wedge-shaped vertebral bodies are the changes described in the lateral radiographs of the thoracic spine. These changes are usually seen in at least three consecutive vertebral bodies. Kyphosis is seen. Vertebral plates that are poorly formed and multiple herniations of the nucleus pulposus (Schmorl's nodes) are being developed. The intervertebral disk spaces are narrowed.

5. Scheuermann's disease is self-limited after growth is complete; however, deformity will be maintained. Surgical treatment includes spinal fusion and orthopedic hardware instrumentation. Physical therapy is performed to relieve or decrease the deformity, and analgesics can be prescribed to relieve pain.

Pearls

- Patients with Scheuermann's disease have an increased kyphosis in the thoracic or thoracolumbar spine with associated backache and localized changes in the vertebral bodies.
- In lateral radiograph, anterior wedging of at least three consecutive vertebral bodies is seen.
- Vertebral plates are poorly formed and there is development of multiple herniations of the nucleus pulposus (Schmorl's nodes).
- The kyphosis angle should be more than 50 degrees for the diagnosis to be made.
- Patients with Scheuermann's disease generally are affected at age 13 to 16 years.
- This is a self-limited disease. Changes cease to develop after growth is complete.

Suggested Readings

Ali RM, Green DW, Patel TC. Scheuermann's kyphosis. *Curr Opin Pediatr*. 1999;11(1):70-75.

Lowe TG. Scheuermann's disease. *J Bone Joint Surg Am*. 1990;72(6):940-945.

Summers BN, Singh JP, Manns RA. The radiological reporting of lumbar Scheuermann's disease: an unnecessary source of confusion amongst clinicians and patients. *Br J Radiol*. 2008;81(965):383-385.

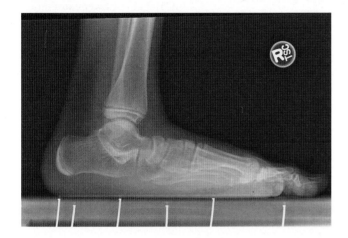
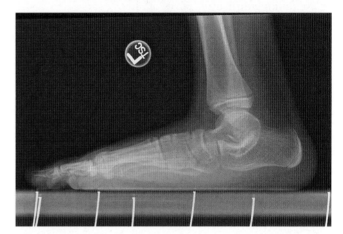
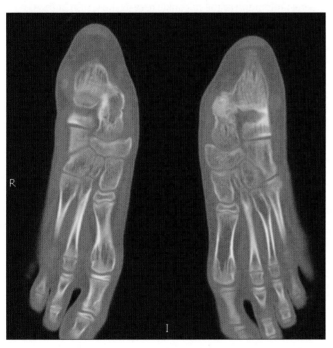
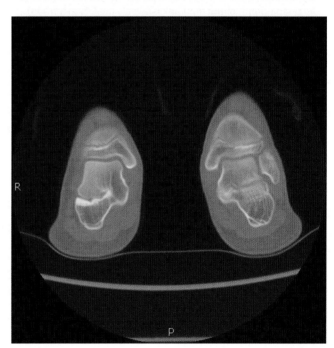

1. What is the sign that is shown in the lateral foot radiographs?

2. What part of the joint is most commonly involved?

3. At what age group does this entity become symptomatic?

4. In which side of the sub-talar joint is this entity characteristically seen?

5. What other sign may be seen in a lateral foot radiograph of this entity?

Case ranking/difficulty: **Category:** Lower extremities

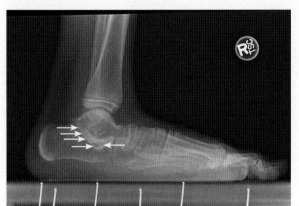

Lateral radiograph of the right ankle reveals the C sign (*arrows*) consistent with talocalcaneal middle facet coalition.

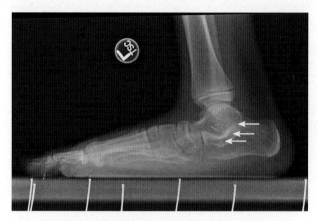

Lateral radiograph of the left ankle reveals the C sign (*arrows*) consistent with talocalcaneal middle facet coalition.

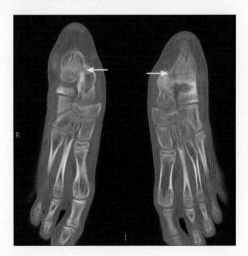

Axial CT of both ankles demonstrates the middle facet with talocalcaneal coalition (*arrows*).

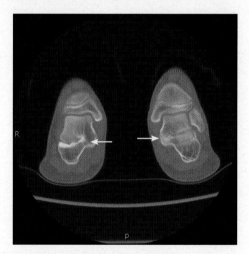

Coronal CT of both ankles demonstrates the middle facet with talocalcaneal coalition (*arrows*).

Answers

1. The lateral foot radiograph demonstrates the C shaped line (the C sign), which is formed by the medial outline of the dome of the talus and the postero-inferior outline of the sustentaculum tali.

2. Talocalcaneal coalition is most common in the middle facet.

3. Patients become symptomatic in early teenage years when the pre-existing cartilaginous coalition ossifies and reduces the joint mobility leading to repeated ankle sprains. Contraction and spasm of the peroneal muscles with forced inversion may occur. Mobility of the subtalar joint is reduced.

4. Talocalcaneal coalitions are characteristically seen on the medial side of subtalar joint.

5. Talar beak sign may be seen in cases of talocalcaneal coalition.

Pearls

- Tarsal coalition is an abnormal connection between tarsal bones that may be fibrous, cartilaginous, or osseous.
- Tarsal coalition is due to lack of segmentation during embryological development.
- Calcaneonavicular and talocalcaneal are two most common tarsal coalitions.

Suggested Readings

Crim JR, Kjeldsberg KM. Radiographic diagnosis of tarsal coalition. *AJR Am J Roentgenol.* 2004;182(2):323-328.

Taniguchi A, Tanaka Y, Kadono K, Takakura Y, Kurumatani N. C sign for diagnosis of talocalcaneal coalition. *Radiology.* 2003;228(2):501-505.

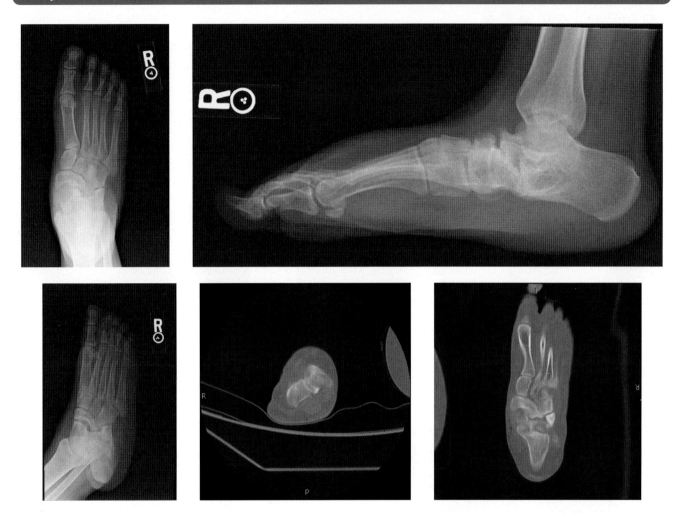

1. What are the findings?

2. At what period of life does this condition clinically present?

3. What is the etiology of this condition?

4. What percentage of this entity is bilateral?

5. What is the most common type of this entity?

Case ranking/difficulty:

Category: Lower extremities

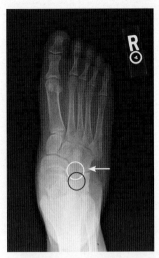

Frontal radiograph of the right foot reveals osseous fusion of the navicular and cuboid bones (*white circle*). There is close approximation of the adjacent calcaneocuboid (*arrow*) and calcaneonavicular articulations with sclerotic changes (*black circle*).

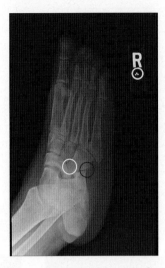

Oblique radiograph of the right foot reveals osseous fusion of the navicular and cuboid bones (*white circle*). There is close approximation of the adjacent calcaneocuboid (*black circle*).

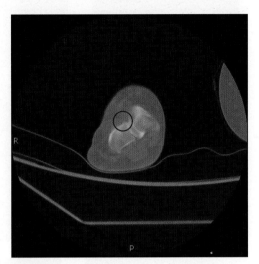

Axial CT of the right foot demonstrates bony fusion of the navicular and cuboid bone (*circle*).

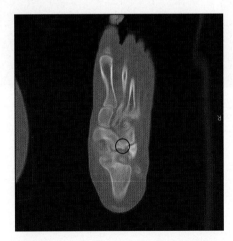

Coronal CT reveals osseous fusion and sclerosis of the navicular and cuboid bones (*circle*).

Answers

1. The findings are calcaneocuboid, navicular cuboid, and calcaneonavicular coalition. Pes planus is present.

2. The condition shown in the images usually presents during adolescence.

3. Coalition of the bones can be congenital; however, it can be acquired after a trauma.

4. Fifty to sixty percent of the cases are bilateral.

5. The most common types of tarsal coalitions in decreasing prevalence are calcaneonavicular, talocalcaneal, talonavicular, and calcaneocuboid.

Suggested Readings

Abrahams RB, Lewis, KN, Franco A. Tarsal Coalition. Unknown case #43. SPR web site January 4-22, 2011. <http://mirc.childrensmemorial.org/storage/ss12/docs/20101222133901390/MIRCdocument.xml>.

Taniguchi A, Tanaka Y, Kadono K, Takakura Y, Kurumatani N. C Sign for diagnosis of talocalcaneal coalition. *Radiology*. 2003;228(2):501-505.

Upasani VV, Chambers RC, Mubarak SJ. Analysis of calcaneonavicular coalitions using multi-planar three-dimensional computed tomography. *J Child Orthop*. 2008;2(4):301-307.

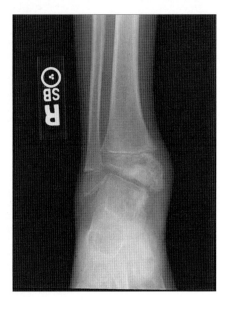 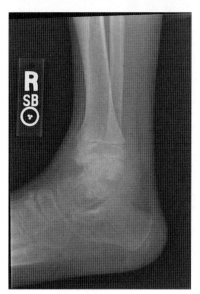

1. What are the findings?

2. Which tumor does this case resemble?

3. What is the frequency of this case?

4. In which part of the bone does this entity usually occur?

5. In which part of the body does this case most commonly occur?

Case ranking/difficulty:

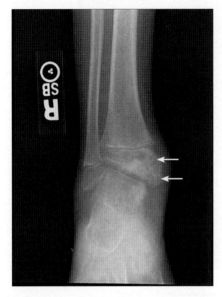

Frontal radiograph of the right ankle reveals a mass arising from the medial aspect of the distal tibial epiphysis (*arrows*). The mass is irregular and dense. The talus is tilted and soft tissue swelling noted.

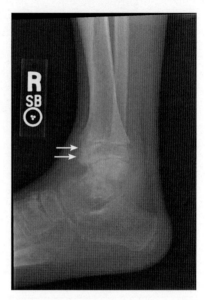

Lateral radiograph of the right ankle reveals a mass arising from the medial aspect of the distal tibial epiphysis (*arrows*). The mass is irregular and dense.

Answers

1. There is a bony mass arising from the medial aspect of the distal tibial epiphysis. Plain radiograph reveals that the periosteum of the tibial epiphysis is continuous and surrounds the mass.

2. Histologically Trevor's disease resembles osteochondroma.

3. The frequency of Trevor's disease is 1 per 1,000,000 population.

4. Trevor's disease usually involves only the lower extremities and on medial side of the epiphysis.

5. Trevor's disease involves most commonly the knees and the ankles. It has predilection to the medial side of the epiphysis. It is a benign lesion with no risk for malignant transformation.

Pearls

- Trevor's disease or dysplasia epiphysealis hemimelica (also known as Fairbank's disease) is a congenital bone developmental disorder.
- It always involves a single limb and the medial aspect of the epiphysis of a lower extremity.
- The condition consists of overgrowth of cartilage that resembles osteochondroma.
- Trevor's disease is a benign disorder, and no cases of malignant transformation have been reported.
- The classic radiographic appearance is of asymmetric epiphyseal growth with multiple ossific centers.

Suggested Readings

Keret D, Spatz DK, Caro PA, Mason DE. Dysplasia epiphysealis hemimelica: diagnosis and treatment. *J Pediatr Orthop*. 1992;12:365-372.

Kuo RS, Bellemore MC, Monsell FP, Frawley K, Kozlowski K. Dysplasia epiphysealis hemimelica: clinical features and management. *J Pediatr Orthop*. 1998;18(4):543-548.

Peduto AJ, Frawley KJ, Bellemore MC, Kuo RS, Foster SL, Onikul E. MR imaging of dysplasia epiphysealis hemimelica: bony and soft-tissue abnormalities. *AJR*. 1999;172:819-823.

11-year-old female with torticollis and restricted motion of the left shoulder

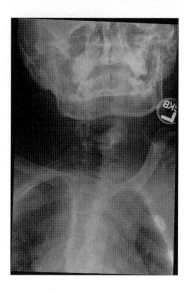 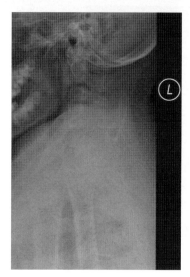

1. What are the findings?

2. Which associated anomalies of this case may be seen?

3. What is the process that was failed to achieve in utero that contributed to this anomaly?

4. What may be the clinical presentation?

5. What is the extent of the anatomical deformity of this case as classified by Cavendish grade IV?

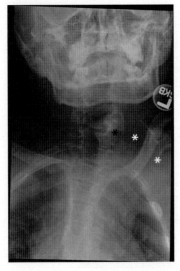

Frontal radiograph of the neck demonstrates elevation of the scapula (*white asterisks*). Omovertebral bone noted (*black asterisk*).

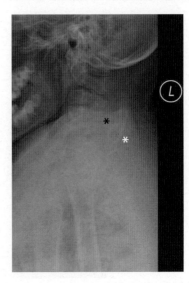

Lateral view of the neck demonstrates elevation of the scapula (*white asterisk*) and the omovertebral bone (*black asterisk*).

Answers

1. There is elevated left scapula and partial fusion of cervical vertebral bodies. There is omovertebral bone.

2. Associated anomalies with this entity may include scoliosis, Klippel-Feil syndrome, cervical rib, and cervical spina bifida.

3. This anomaly results from failure of the scapula to descend in utero.

4. Children with the shown entity usually present with torticollis, restricted forward flexion of the affected shoulder, and restricted abduction of the affected shoulder.

5. The extent of the anatomical deformity as classified by Cavendish grade IV is scapula elevated to the vicinity of the occiput.

Pearls

- Sprengel's deformity is the most common congenital malformation of the shoulder girdle.
- Sprengel's deformity, also termed congenital high scapula, is the result of failure of the scapula to descend in utero.
- Omovertebral bony connection between the superior pole of the scapula and the cervical spine may be seen.
- Management is guided by the patient's functional and cosmetic status, in addition to the extent of the anatomical deformity, classified by Cavendish grade.
- Definitive treatment involves surgical excision of omovertebral connections and re-positioning of the scapula.

Suggested Readings

Ahmad AA. Surgical correction of severe Sprengel Deformity to allow greater postoperative range of shoulder abduction. *J Pediatr Orthop*. 2010;30:575-581.

Chang MD, Franco A, Lewis KN. Left Sprengel Deformity and right radioulnar synostosis. <http://mirc.childrensmemorial.org/storage/ss12/docs/20100924123203640/MIRCdocument.xml>.

Hamner DL, Hall JE. Sprengel's Deformity associated with multidirectional shoulder instability. *J Pediatr Orthop*. 1995;15(5):641-643.

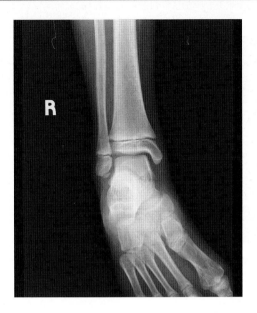
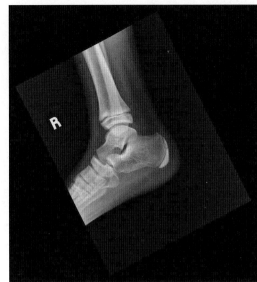

1. What is the structure that is adjacent to the tip of the lateral malleolus?

2. What is the etiology?

3. Why this condition may be symptomatic and cause pain?

4. What is the percentage of children having ossicles in the ankle and foot?

5. What are the treatment options?

Case ranking/difficulty: | **Category:** Lower extremities

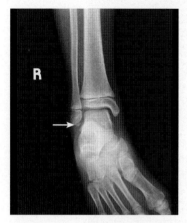

Oblique view radiograph of the right ankle demonstrates a separated ossicle at the tip of the lateral malleolus (*arrow*).

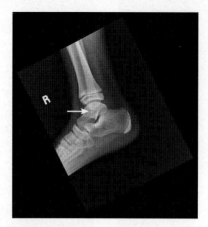

Lateral view radiograph of the right ankle demonstrates a separated ossicle at the tip of the lateral malleolus (*arrow*).

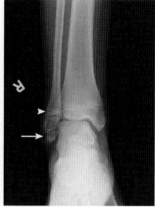

Frontal view of the right ankle of another 13-year-old male with asymptomatic os subfibulare (*arrow*). This patient was symptomatic due to a tiny non-displaced metaphyseal fracture (*arrowhead*).

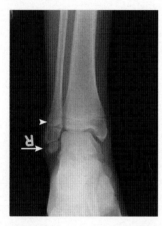

Oblique view of the right ankle of another 13-year-old male with asymptomatic os subfibulare (*arrow*). This patient was symptomatic due to a tiny non-displaced metaphyseal fracture (*arrowhead*).

Answers

1. The structure seen adjacent to the tip of the lateral malleolus is os subfibulare, which is a normal variant.

2. The etiology of os subfibulare is unclear. It can be due to unfused epiphyseal ossification center, supernumerary ossicle, or traumatic origin.

3. There are two theories regarding the origin of os subfibulare. One theory proposes that it is caused by an avulsion fracture attributable to pull of the anterior talofibular ligament, whereas the other theory proposes that it is the result of an accessory ossification center. Remote avulsion fracture and pull of the anterior talofibular ligament may cause pain. The ossicle noted in the image is well corticated and does not look like an acute fracture.

4. Twenty-two percent of normal children under the age of 16 have one or more accessory ossicles in the foot and ankle.

5. Excision of the ossicle and reattachment of the talofibular ligament provide symptomatic relief.

Pearls

- Ossification in lateral submalleolar area or in between lateral malleolus and talus has been reported to be a normal variant – os subfibulare.
- Perimalleolar ossifications can be found in three locations. Below the malleolar tip on medial side termed as os subtibiale, on the lateral side as os subfibulare, and along the lateral border of the lateral malleolus referred to as os retinaculi.
- The condition known as os subfibulare is sometimes a cause of ankle pain.
- Os subfibulare may or may not be associated with laxity of the anterior talofibular ligament.

Suggested Readings

Ferran J, Blanc T. Os subfibulare in children secondary to an osteochondral fracture. *J Radiol*. 2001;82(5):577-579.

Kono T, Ochi M, Takao M, Naito K, Uchio Y, Oae K. Symptomatic os subfibulare caused by accessory ossification: a case report. *Clin Orthop Relat Res*. 2002;399:197-200.

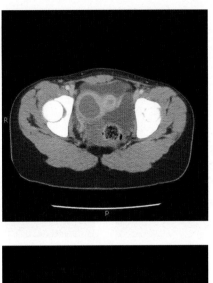
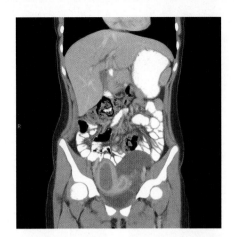
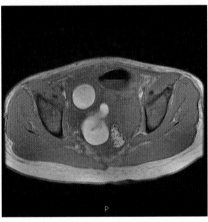
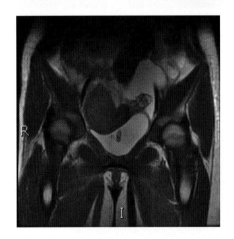

1. What is the differential diagnosis?

2. What type of anomaly is being shown?

3. Which of the body systems has high prevalence of associated anomalies with this case?

4. What is a complication of the shown entity?

5. The shown anomaly has a rudimentary horn. What is the long-term complication if the rudimentary horn is noncommunicating?

Case ranking/difficulty:

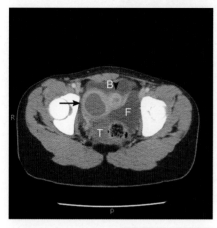

Axial CT of the pelvis reveals unicornuate uterus. There is a rudimentary non communicating horn dilated and filled with blood (*arrow*). The normal horn is shown (*arrowhead*). B, bladder; F, free fluid; T, hydrosalpinx.

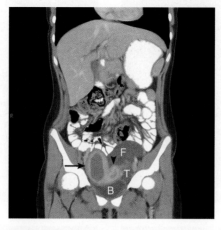

Coronal CT of the pelvis reveals unicornuate uterus. There is a rudimentary non communicating horn dilated and filled with blood (*arrow*). The normal horn is shown (*arrowhead*). B, bladder; F, free fluid; T, hydrosalpinx.

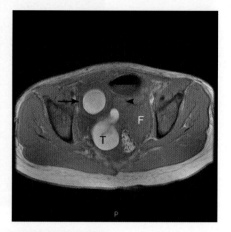

Axial MRI T1 of the pelvis reveals unicornuate uterus. There is high signal in a rudimentary non communicating horn that is dilated and filled with blood (*arrow*). The normal horn is shown (*arrowhead*). F, free fluid; T, hydrosalpinx.

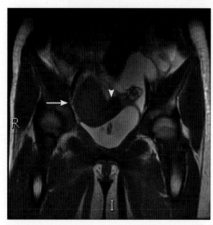

Coronal MRI T2 of the pelvis reveals unicornuate uterus. There is a rudimentary non communicating horn that is dilated and filled with blood (*arrow*). The normal horn is shown (*arrowhead*).

Answers

1. Differential diagnosis may include tubo-ovarian abscess, ruptured hemorrhagic ovarian follicle, bicornuate uterus with blood product retention in one of the uterine horn, pyosalpinx, and endometrioma.

2. The anomaly shown is Müllerian duct anomaly. One or both Müllerian ducts may not develop fully, resulting in abnormalities such as uterine agenesis or hypoplasia (bilateral) or unicornuate uterus (unilateral).

3. Renal tract anomalies are associated with Müllerian duct anomalies in up to 30% of cases because of the close embryologic relationship between the paramesonephric and mesonephric ducts.

4. Spontaneous abortion and premature labor may occur in pregnancies with a unicornuate uterus, and the poorest fetal survival among all uterine anomalies has been reported.

5. In patients that have a rudimentary horn on the contralateral side, when the rudimentary horn is noncommunicating, endometrial tissue expelled retrogradely through the fallopian tube during menstruation results in an increased frequency of endometriosis.

Pearls

- On MRI unicornuate uterus appears curved and elongated, with the external uterine contour assuming a banana shape. Uterine volume is reduced, and the configuration of the uterus is asymmetric. Normal myometrial zonal anatomy is maintained.

Suggested Readings

Imaoka I, Wada A, Matsuo M, Yoshida M, Kitagaki H, Sugimura K. MR imaging of disorders associated with female infertility: use in diagnosis, treatment, and management. *Radiographics.* 2010;23(6):1401-1421.

Junqueira BL, Allen LM, Spitzer RF, Lucco KL, Babyn PS, Doria AS. Müllerian duct anomalies and mimics in children and adolescents: correlative intraoperative assessment with clinical imaging. *Radiographics.* 2009;29(4):1085-1103.

Failure to pass meconium

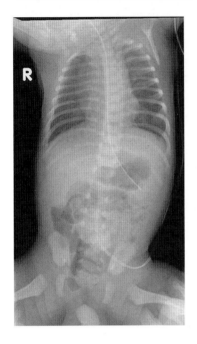 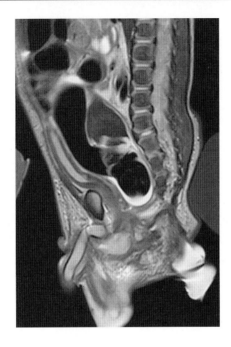 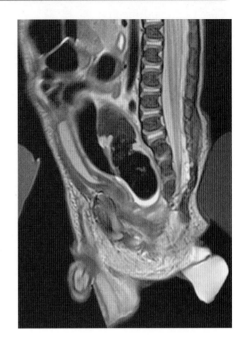

1. What are the findings?

2. What are the different types of anal atresia?

3. What is the normal height of the conus at birth?

4. What are possible complementary examinations?

5. Which examination is required before pelvic floor reconstruction?

Case ranking/difficulty: 🐸🐸🐸

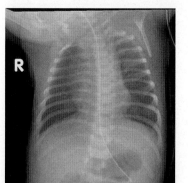

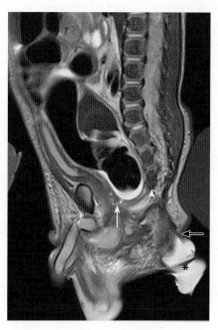

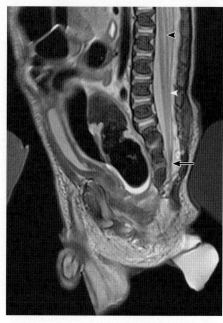

There is a segmentation anomaly of the S1-S2 sacral vertebra (*arrow*) and an absence of the distal sacrum/coccyx (*arrowhead*). Normal bowel gas distribution.

Dysgenesis of the sacrum with malformed and fused S2 and S3, absence of the distal sacral vertebrae and coccyx (*arrowhead*). There is a T2-hyperintense fluid collection on the posterior aspect of the anal cleft (*asterisk*) with a suggested canal pointing upwards to the distal end of the malformed thecal sac, representing an anterior myelomeningocele (*black outlined arrow*). There is a minute fistula ventral to the dilated rectal pouch showing contact to the preprostatic urethra (*arrow*).

There is a thickening of the distal cord with absence of the conus (*arrowhead*) and thickened filum terminale reaching the caudal open spinal canal (tethered cord, *black outlined arrow*). Within the medulla, a filiform T2-hyperintense syrinx can be seen (*black outlined arrowhead*).

Answers

1. The association between sacrococcygeal malformation, anorectal malformation, and presacral mass is characteristic for the Currarino triad.

2. According to the classification by Peña, there is no rectovaginal fistula, but the presence of a cloacal malformation (with an opening of the rectal fistula into the vaginal vestibulum) in girls. Perineal fistulas in both males and females are associated with so-called "low" anal atresia and mostly have normal pelvic floor musculature and sacrococcygeal bone.

3. Normal height of the conus at birth is L1/L2. If seen lower than L2/3, a tethered cord must be suspected.

4. A maximal distance of 1 cm between air limit and peritoneum in a cross table lateral X-ray allows primary repair without colostomy.

5. In the presence of a fistula, contrast is given into the distal rectal pouch through the enterostomy. Height and extension of the fistula are recorded in lateral projection.

Pearls

- Anorectal malformation (mostly anal atresia).
- Sacrum dysgenesis.
- Presacral mass.
- May be associated with tethered cord and renal anomalies.

Suggested Reading

Iyer RS, Khanna PC. Currarino syndrome. *Pediatr Radiol.* 2010;40(Suppl 1):S102.

Subject Index

Difficulty Level Index

Easy Cases

682, 641, 148, 93, 429, 1659, 661, 1008, 146, 636, 635, 633, 25, 421, 473, 373, 555, 426, 465, 358, 273, 219, 631, 402, 345, 368, 216, 73, 61, 91, 95, 386, 75, 640, 70, 128, 533, 424, 372, 16, 83, 129, 138, 667, 217, 68, 714, 67, 369, 92, 33, 29, 13, 59, 60, 242, 439, 84, 660, 349, 254, 126, 116, 113, 211, 654, 187, 112, 625, 215, 31, 2741, 2751, 77, 563, 624

Moderately Difficult Cases

1617, 630, 629, 452, 448, 408, 363, 210, 182, 115, 111, 76, 63, 51, 32, 430, 255, 669, 659, 658, 648, 198, 74, 2758, 647, 205, 197, 15, 417, 90, 350, 2743, 2744, 2748, 2750, 2749, 2759, 662, 638, 564, 370, 279, 253, 218, 712, 711, 644, 346, 1440, 133, 642, 556, 94, 334, 144, 82, 64, 106, 2037, 716, 708, 704, 671, 670, 666, 645, 486, 462, 458, 453, 432, 428, 425, 416, 411, 407, 403, 303, 269, 193, 188, 176, 125, 127, 120, 118, 88, 86, 85, 80, 55, 52, 532, 102, 707, 491, 376, 192, 233, 89, 2753

Most Difficult Cases

646, 706, 639, 427, 2745, 2762, 2742, 2746, 2763, 2754, 2752, 194, 213, 2747, 123, 422, 234, 100, 1624, 459, 443, 81, 149, 276, 415, 96, 56, 663, 643, 557, 559, 461, 460, 58, 2757, 525, 316, 304, 286, 124, 1003, 703, 665, 2765, 632, 598, 2760, 2756, 558, 543, 534, 445, 444, 121, 442, 65, 725, 2062, 2766

Author Index

Arie Franco

682, 641, 148, 93, 429, 1659, 661, 1008, 146, 636, 635, 633, 25, 421, 473, 373, 555, 426, 465, 358, 273, 219, 631, 402, 345, 368, 216, 73, 61, 91, 95, 386, 75, 640, 70, 128, 533, 424, 372, 16, 83, 129, 138, 667, 217, 68, 714, 67, 369, 92, 33, 29, 13, 59, 60, 242, 439, 84, 660, 349, 254, 126, 116, 113, 211, 654, 187, 112, 625, 215, 31, 77, 563, 624, 1617, 630, 629, 452, 448, 408, 363, 210, 182, 115, 111, 76, 63, 51, 32, 430, 255, 669, 659, 658, 648, 198, 74, 647, 205, 197, 15, 417, 90, 350, 662, 638, 564, 370, 279, 253, 218, 712, 711, 644, 346, 1440, 133, 642, 556, 94, 334, 144, 82, 64, 106, 2037, 716, 708, 704, 671, 670, 666, 645, 486, 462, 458, 453, 432, 428, 425, 416, 411, 407, 403, 303, 269, 193, 188, 176, 125, 127, 120, 118, 88, 86, 85, 80, 55, 52, 532, 102, 707, 491, 376, 192, 233, 89, 646, 706, 639, 427, 194, 213, 123, 422, 234, 100, 1624, 459, 443, 81, 149, 276, 415, 96, 56, 663, 643, 557, 559, 461, 460, 58, 525, 316, 304, 286, 124, 1003, 703, 665, 632, 598, 558, 543, 534, 445, 444, 121, 442, 65, 725, 2062

Jacques F. Schneider

2741, 2751, 2758, 2743, 2744, 2748, 2750, 2749, 2759, 2753, 2745, 2762, 2742, 2746, 2763, 2754, 2752, 2747, 2757, 2765, 2760, 2756, 2766

Acknowledgement Index

Chetan Shah
129, 219, 234, 29, 31, 32, 486, 56, 58, 61, 714, 716, 73, 74

Neil Borden
639, 646, 647, 648, 658, 659

Ramon Figueroa
194, 197, 198, 205, 215